ALLE ZEIT WACH

SJ

1842

# Glaucoma Update II

Glaucoma Society of the International
Congress of Ophthalmology
Carmel/California, October 22–27, 1982

Editors
G.K. Krieglstein and W. Leydhecker

With 83 Figures

Springer-Verlag Berlin Heidelberg
NewYork Tokyo 1983

Professor Dr. G.K. Krieglstein
Professor Dr. Dr. h.c. W. Leydhecker
Universitätsklinik und Poliklinik für Augenkranke
Kopfklinik
Josef-Schneider-Str. 11
8700 Würzburg

ISBN-13: 978-3-540-12422-1 e-ISBN-13: 978-3-642-69096-9
DOI: 10.1007/978-3-642-69096-9

**Library of Congress Cataloging in Publication Data**
International Congress of Ophthalmology (24th : 1982 : Carmel, Calif.)
Glaucoma update II.
Previous Glaucoma update published as: Glaucoma update / International Glaucoma Symposium, Nara, Japan, 1978, 1979. Bibliography: p. Includes index.
1. Glaucoma-Congresses. I. Krieglstein, G. K. (Günter K.), 1944–. II. Leydhecker, W. (Wolfgang), 1919–. III. International Glaucoma Symposium (1978: Nara-shi, Japan)
Glaucoma update. IV. Title. RE871.I5 1982 617.7'41 83-4716
ISBN 0-387-12422-5 (U.S.)



Typesetting: Fotosatz Service Weihrauch, Würzburg.
Printing and binding: Offsetdruck Beltz, Hemsbach
2122/3321-543210

# Glaucoma Society of the International Congress of Ophthalmology
Carmel/California, October 22–27, 1982

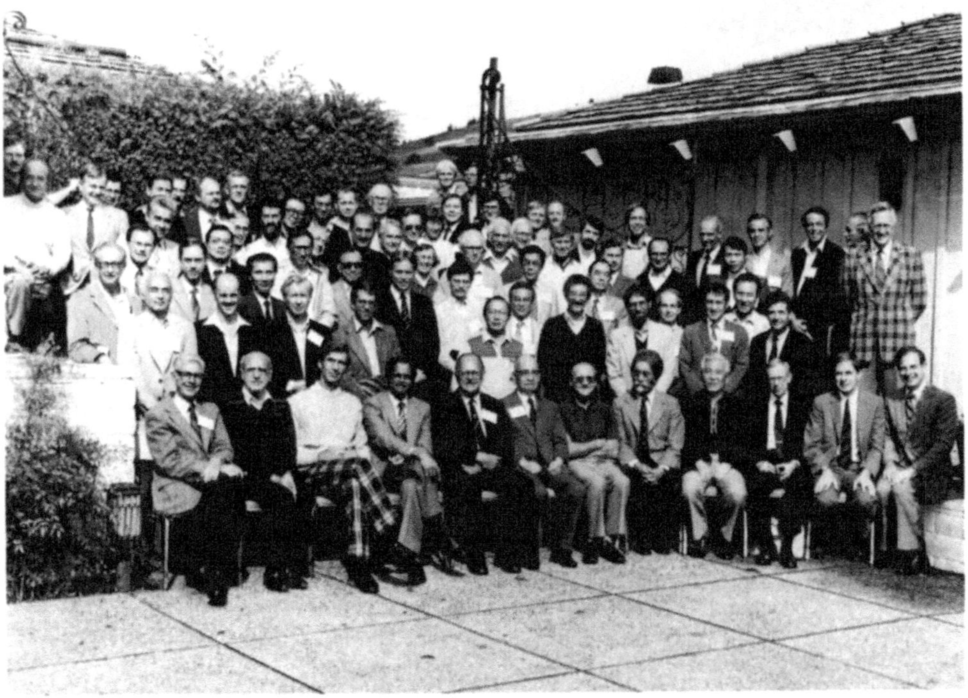

Participants of the committee meeting of the Glaucoma Society of the International Congress of Ophthalmology, Carmel/California, October 22–27, 1982

# Table of Contents

## Preface

The second Committee Meeting of the Glaucoma Society of the International Congress of Ophthalmology was held in Carmel Valley/California from October 22–27, 1982. Traditionally this meeting was closed and preceded the International Congress of Ophthalmology in San Francisco. A group of roughly 80 experts on glaucoma - active members of the committee and invited guests - exchanged latest scientific experiences on the progress in pathophysiology, diagnosis and treatment of the glaucomas. The aim of the meeting was to provide quite informal presentations grouped around main topics and ample, lively discussions.

The scientific and local organization was in the hands of Jack Hetherington Jr./San Francisco and Stephen M. Drance/Vancouver. It is the sincere wish of the society to express warmest thanks to Valerie Hetherington who took in a most charming and efficient way much of the burden of the local organization.

The idea of pre-circulation of all scientific presentations 2–3 months before the meeting to all participants and guests proved to be effective with respect to fruitful and stimulating discussions at the site of the meeting.

We thank all participants for their co-operation in sending their manuscripts in time.

The society is indebted to Chibret Int. Pharmaceutical Company for generous support of this publication.

Würzburg, 15. Febr. 1983

G.K. Krieglstein
W. Leydhecker

## List of Contributors

Anderson D.R., Bascom Palmer Eye Institute, University of Miami, School of Medicine, P.O. Box 016880, Miami, Florida 33101, USA

Akiba, Y., Institute of Medical Electronics, Faculty of Medicine, University of Tokyo, Tokyo, Japan

Araie, M., Department of Ophthalmology, Univ. of Tokyo, School of Medicine, 7-3-1, Hongo, Bunkyo-ku, Tokyo 113, Japan

Atkin, A., The Mount Sinai Medical Center, Dept. of Ophthalmology, One Gustave L. Levy Place, New York/NY 10029, USA

Azuma, I., Dept. of Ophthalmology, Osaka Medical College, 2-7 Daigakucho, Takatsuki/ Osaka, 569, Japan

Becker, B., Department of Ophthalmology, Washington Univ., School of Medicine, 660 South Euclid Avenue, St. Louis, Missouri 63110, USA

Berghoff, K., Institut für Physiologie und Chemie, Philipps-Universität, D-3550 Marburg/ Lahn, Federal Republic of Germany

Betinjane, A.J., Clinica Oftalmologica, Rua Prof. Artur Ramos, 96-8.0 And., Sao Paulo-01454, Brasil

Bill, A., Department of Physiology and Medical Biophysics, Box 573, S-751 23 Uppsala, Sweden

Bodis-Wollner, I., The Mount Sinai Medical Center, Dept. of Ophthalmology, One Gustave L. Levy Place, New York/NY 10029, USA

Brubaker, R.F., Mayo Clinic, 200 First Street S.W., Rochester, MN 55905, USA

Burke, J., Department of Ophthalmology, University of Arizona, School of Medicine, Tucson, Arizona

Calixto, N., Hospital Sao Geraldo, Faculdade de Medicina, Universidade de Minas Gerais, Belo-Horizonte, 30 000, Brasil

Carvalho, C.A., Clinica Oftalmologica, Rua Prof. Artur Ramos, 96-8.0 And., Sao Paulo-01454, Brasil

Coca-Prados, M., Dept. of Ophthalmology and Visual Science, Yale University, School of Medicine, 310 Cedar Street, P.O. Box 3333, New Haven, CT 06510, USA

Cronemberger Sobrinho, S., Hospital Sao Geraldo, Faculdade de Medicina, Universidade de Minas Gerais, Belo-Horizonte, 30 000, Brasil

Draeger, J., Universitäts-Augenklinik, Martinistraße 52, 2000 Hamburg 20, Federal Republic of Germany

Drance, S.M., Univ. of British Columbia and Vancouver General Hospital, Dept. of Ophthalmology, 2577 Willow Street, Vancouver, B.C. V5Z 3N9, Canada

Ernest, J.T., Department of Ophthalmology, University of Illinois at Chicago, Eye and Ear Infirmary, 1855 West Taylor Street, Chicago, Illinois 60612, USA

Go, F., Institut of Medical Electronics, Faculty of Medicine, University of Tokyo, Tokyo, Japan

Goldberg, Anna V., Glaucoma Service and Research Laboratories, Wills Eye Hospital, Thomas Jefferson University, Philadelphia, PA 19107, USA

Goldberg, William A., Glaucoma Service and Research Laboratories, Wills Eye Hospital, Thomas Jefferson University, Philadelphia, PA 19107, USA

Goldstick, T.K., Department of Chemical Engineering, Northwestern University, Evanston, Illinois 60201, USA

Gramer, E., Universitäts-Augenklinik Würzburg, Josef-Schneider-Straße 11, D-8700 Würzburg, Federal Republic of Germany

Hamanaka, T., Department of Ophthalmology, School of Medicine, Gunma University, Maebashi, Japan

Herschler, J., Department of Ophthalmology, University of Arizona, School of Medicine, Tucson, Arizona

Hoskins, H.D., Dept. of Ophthalmology, Glaucoma Clinic, Rm. A-775, San Francisco/ Cal. 94143, USA

Iwata, K., Dept. of Ophthalmology, Niigata Univ., 951 Niigata-City, Asahimachi 1, Japan

Kitazawa, Y., School of Medicine, Dept. of Ophthalmology, 7-3-1 Hongo, Bunkyo-ku, Tokyo 113, Japan

Kondo, K., Dept. of Ophthalmology and Visual Science, Yale University, School of Medicine, 310 Cedar Street, P.O. Box 3333, New Haven, CT 06510, USA

Krakau, C.E.T., University Eye Clinic, Dept. of exp. Ophthalmology, S-22 185 Lund, Sweden

Krieglstein, G.K., Universitäts-Augenklinik Würzburg, Josef-Schneider-Straße 11, D-8700 Würzburg, Federal Republic of Germany

Krupin, T., Department of Ophthalmology, Washington Univ., School of Medicine, 660 South Euclid Avenue, St. Louis, Missouri 63110, USA

Lakowski, R., Univ. of British Columbia and Vancouver General Hospital, Dept. of Ophthalmology, 2577 Willow Street, Vancouver, B.C. V5Z 3N9, Canada

Langham, M.E., The Wilmer Institute, Johns Hopkins University, Baltimore, Maryland 21205, USA

Laties, A.M., Department of Ophthalmology, University of Pennsylvania, Scheie Eye Institute, Philadelphia, PA 19104, USA

Leydhecker, W., Universitäts-Augenklinik Würzburg, Josef-Schneider-Straße 11, D-8700 Würzburg, Federal Republic of Germany

Lütjen-Drecoll, E., Anatomisches Institut der Universität Erlangen-Nürnberg, Krankenhausstraße 9, D-8520 Erlangen, Federal Republic of Germany

McGlinn, A., Department of Ophthalmology, University of Pennsylvania, Scheie Eye Institute, Philadelphia, PA 19104, USA

Mishima, S., Department of Ophthalmology, Univ. of Tokyo, School of Medicine, 7-3-1, Hongo, Bunkyo-ku, Tokyo 113, Japan

Moreno, F.J., Hospital Sao Geraldo, Faculdade de Medicina, Universidade de Minas Gerais, Belo-Horizonte, 30 000, Brasil

Motolko, M.A., Dept. of Ophthalmology, Univ. of Iowa, Iowa City/Iowa 52242, USA

Phelps, C.D., Dept. of Ophthalmology, Univ. of Iowa, Iowa City/Iowa 52242, USA

Podos, S.M., The Mount Sinai Medical Center, Dept. of Ophthalmology, One Gustave L. Levy Place, New York/NY 10029, USA

Poryzees, E.M., Glaucoma Service and Research Laboratories, Wills Eye Hospital, Thomas Jefferson University, Philadelphia, PA 19107, USA

Quigley, H.A., The Wilmer Institute, Johns Hopkins University, Ophthalmol. Research Unit., Baltimore/Maryland 21205, USA

Rohen, J.W., Anatomisches Institut der Universität Erlangen-Nürnberg, Krankenhausstraße 9, D-8520 Erlangen, Federal Republic of Germany

Rohrbach, M., Anatomisches Institut der Universität Erlangen-Nürnberg, Krankenhausstraße 9, D-8520 Erlangen, Federal Republic of Germany

Sampaolesi, R., Parana 1239.1., Buenos Aires, Argentina

Schachtschabel, D.O., Institut für Physiologie und Chemie, Philipps-Universität, D-3550 Marburg/Lahn, Federal Republic of Germany

Sears, M., Dept. of Ophthalmology and Visual Science, Yale University, School of Medicine, 310 Cedar Street, P.O. Box 3333, New Haven, CT 06510, USA

Shaffer, R.N., Univ. of California, Glaucoma Clinic A-775, San Francisco, Cal. 94143, USA

Shirato, S., Institute of Medical Electronics, Faculty of Medicine, University of Tokyo, Tokyo, Japan

Smith, R., Moorfields Eye Hospital, City Road, London EC1V2PD, England

Spaeth, G.L., Glaucoma Service and Research Laboratories, Wills Eye Hospital, Thomas Jefferson University, Philadelphia, PA 19107, USA

Stone, R.A., Department of Ophthalmology, University of Pennsylvania, Scheie Eye Institute, Philadelphia, PA 19104, USA

Svedbergh, B., Department of Physiology and Medical Biophysics, Box 573, S-751 23 Uppsala, Sweden

Takase, M., Department of Ophthalmology, Univ. of Tokyo, School of Medicine, 7-3-1, Hongo, Bunkyo-ku, Tokyo 113, Japan

Ujie, K., Department of Ophthalmology, School of Medicine, Gunma University, Maebashi, Japan

Winter, R., Universitäts-Augenklinik, Martinistraße 52, 2000 Hamburg 20, Federal Republic of Germany

Krieglstein G.K./Leydhecker W. (eds)
Glaucoma Update II


# Protein Phosphorylation in Cultured Human Ciliary Epithelia in Response to Activators of Adenylate Cyclase, Cyclic AMP and Analogues[1]

M. Coca-Prados, K. Kondo and M. Sears, New Haven

In many diverse cell systems intracellular production of cyclic AMP (cAMP) at an accelerated rate influences protein kinase activity so that the state of phosphorylation of specific substrate proteins is changed. It is accepted that study of the phosphorylation of endogenous proteins may increase our knowledge of how hormones, transmitters, and second messengers like cAMP regulate a biologic response, e.g. change in secretion, membrane permeability.

Isoproterenol is known to reduce intraocular pressure (IOP) (Weekers et al. 1955). Later it was reported that adrenergic activation of beta receptors or activation of adenylate cyclase by other agonists lowers IOP by reducing net flow (Eakins 1963; Gregory et al. 1981; Sears et al. 1981). The presence of adenylate cyclase activity and/or beta receptors (Waitzman and Woods 1971; Bromberg et al. 1980; Gregory et al. 1981) and $beta_2$ receptors (Nathanson 1981) in the ciliary epithelia and in tissues containing the ciliary epithelia (Neufeld and Sears 1974; Neufeld and Page 1977) have been documented. It was therefore desirable to search for evidence of cAMP induced phosphorylation of proteins from the cells involved in the production of aqueous humor, the ciliary epithelia. The purpose of this report, reflecting work in progress in our laboratory, is to present preliminary data that indicate that specific proteins from cultured ciliary epithelia are phosphorylated after stimuli by beta adrenergic agents and other activators of adenylate cyclase.

[1] This work was supported in part by U.S. Public Health Service grant EY-00237, EY-04328, EY-00785, Research to Prevent Blindness, Inc. and the Connecticut Lions Eye Research Foundation, Inc., and The New Haven Foundation

## Materials and Methods

*Drugs and isotopes:* (-) Isoproterenol HCl, (-) epinephrine bitartrate, (-) norepinephrine HCl, (-) phenylephrine HCl, (±) propranolol HCl, cholera toxin, dibutyryladenosine 3′:5′ cAMP, 8-bromoadenosine 3′:5′ cAMP, cyclic AMP and theophylline was obtained from Sigma Chemical Co., Timolol maleate a gift from Merck, Sharp & Dohme, Forskolin from Calbiochem, Phenoxybenzamine HCl a gift from Smith, Kline & French labs., Carrier-free $^{32}P$ as orthophosphate from Amersham. Molecular weight standards from Pharmacia. *Tissue source*: Human eyes were obtained from second-trimester fetuses from TAB's (Therapeutic Abortions) (Yale University), or post-morten through the courtesy of the Connecticut Eye Bank, Inc. *Cultures* were prepared from dissected ciliary processes (Coca-Prados, Kondo, Sears, in press). Cells grown in monolayer cultures with Dulbecco Modified Eagle Medium (DMEM) containing D-valine in place of L-valine and 5% DFCS, in an atmosphere of 5 to 10% $CO_2$ at 37 °C, were photographed under phase-contrast microscopy. Additional studies after thin-sectioning with an LKB ultratome were done under electron microscopy (Hitachi 600). Culture cells to a density of 1–2 $\times 10^5$ cells/dish were incubated at 37 °C in 1 ml phosphate-free minimum essential medium (MEM) (Gibco) with 2% DFCS, 500 µCi/ml of carrier-free $^{32}P$-orthophosphate and drugs. Subsequent operations were done using pre-cooled solutions (Coca-Prados and Sears, in press). SDS polyacrylamide gel electrophoresis (SDS-PAGE) was done in 5–18% gradient slab gels according to Laemmli (1970). Quantitation of $^{32}P$ in phosphorylated proteins was done by excising bands from the dried gels, adding 100 µl of water to each slice, incubating with 1 ml of Protosol (New England Nuclear) at 60 °C for

1 hour. Scintillation fluid (10 ml) was added and $^{32}P$ was determined in a Nuclear Chicago Mark II liquid scintillation counter and corrected for decay. Several autoradiographs were scanned using a Joyce-Loebl densitometer.

## Results

When epithelial cells cultured from human fetal ciliary processes (Fig. 1) were treated with beta adrenergic agonists or their analogues in the presence of $^{32}P$-orthophosphate, four major protein bands showed evidence of incorporation of larger amounts of $^{32}P$ relative to controls. Figure 2 describes the autoradiograph of the phosphorylated proteins resolved on SDS-PAGE from cultured human cells treated with equimolar amounts of drugs. Bands were identified in which major changes were reproducibly seen (repeated at least five times in SDS-PAGE slab gels) and are labeled in Fig. 2, 3, 4 as a, b, c and d. Molecular weights were assigned by markers: band a $\simeq$ 78K–79K; band b $\simeq$ 57K–58K; band c $\simeq$ 48K–49K; and band d $\simeq$ 36K–37K daltons. Bands a–d were identified as proteins by their resistance to RNase and DNase and digested by pronase. Regions between 94K and 34K of the autoradiographs (lanes 1–7) (Fig. 2) were scanned and the profiles compared (Fig. 4). Enhancement of phosphorylation of bands a–d by isoproterenol and epinephrine was qualitatively similar (Fig. 4; 2nd and 4th trace) but quantitatively was more effective (Coca-Prados and Sears, in press). Band b, of molecular weight 58 daltons, can be phosphorylated as high as twofold over control in the presence of $10^{-6}$M of isoproterenol, a greater effect obtained when compared with the other protein bands (a, c, d). The order of stimulated phosphorylation in bands a–d could be written: isoproterenol>epinephrine>norepinephrine>phenylephrine. The enhanced phosphorylation in the presence of beta-adrenergic agonists is saturable at $10^{-6}$M. When either timolol or propranolol, nonselective beta-adrenergic antagonists, at concentrations of $10^{-5}$M, were added together with a beta-adrenergic agonist to human CPE cells (Fig. 2; lanes 3, 5, 7) the pattern of phos-

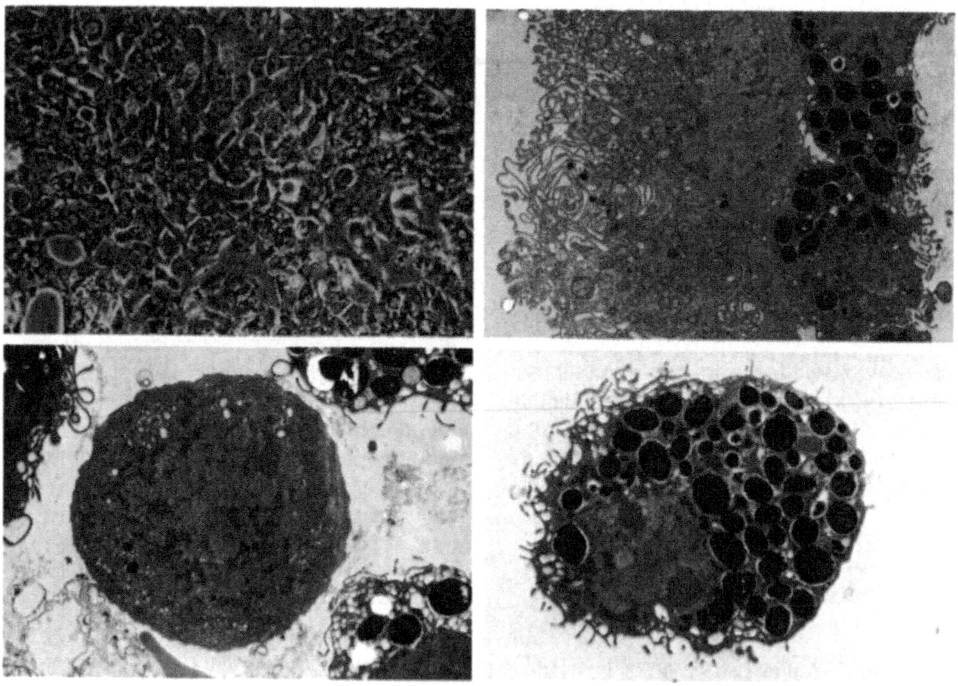

**Fig. 1.** *(Upper left)* low power (× 185) phase contrast micrograph of cultured human epithelia from fetal ciliary processes. *(Upper right)* Stage of progressive digestion of epithelia (× 2900). *(Lower left)* Nonpigmented epithelial cell (× 3350). *(Lower right)* Pigmented epithelial cell (× 3400)

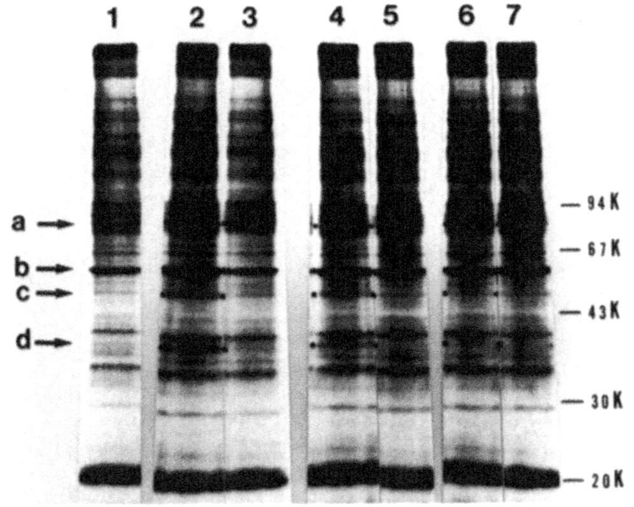


**Fig. 2.** Protein phosphorylation stimulated by equimolar amounts ($10^{-6}$M) of: isoproterenol (*lane 2*); epinephrine (*lane 4*); and norepinephrine (*lane 6*). Bands a–d correspond to proteins with increased $^{32}P$ incorporation in response to beta adrenergic agonists. Isoproterenol plus timolol ($10^{-5}$M) (*lane 3*); epinephrine plus timolol (*lane 5*); norepinephrine plus timolol (*lane 7*); control, no drugs added (*lane 1*). Molecular weights correspond to protein markers run on the same gel

phorylation is similar to controls (Fig. 2; lane 1). Densitometry confirmed these findings (see legend, Fig. 4).

Figure 3 shows that cholera toxin, forskolin, dibutyryl cAMP, 8-bromo cAMP or cAMP plus theophylline produced the same spectrum of phosphorylated proteins as did the beta-adrenergic agonists; 8-bromo cAMP caused the greatest stimulation of phosphorylation in band b, ≃ 2.5-fold versus the control.

## Discussion

This preliminary report is the first study of endogenous protein phosphorylation in

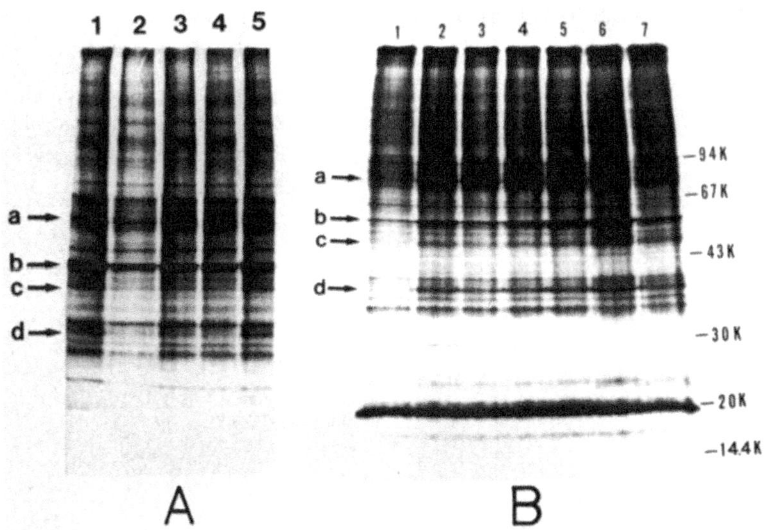


**Fig. 3 A, B.** Pattern of phosphorylated proteins in cultured human ciliary epithelial cells. **(A)** Isoproterenol ($10^{-6}$M), *lane 1;* phenylephrine ($10^{-6}$M), *lane 2;* phenylephrine ($10^{-6}$M) + phenoxybenzamine ($10^{-5}$M), *lane 3;* phenylephrine ($10^{-6}$M) + timolol ($10^{-5}$M), *lane 4;* forskolin ($10^{-6}$M), *lane 5.* **(B)** No drugs added, *lane 1;* isoproterenol ($10^{-6}$M), *lane 2;* dibutyryl cAMP (0.5 mM), *lane 3;* dibutyryl cAMP (1 mM), *lane 4;* cholera toxin (1 μg/ml), *lane 5;* 8-bromoadenosine cAMP (2 mM), *lane 6;* cAMP + theophylline, *lane 7*

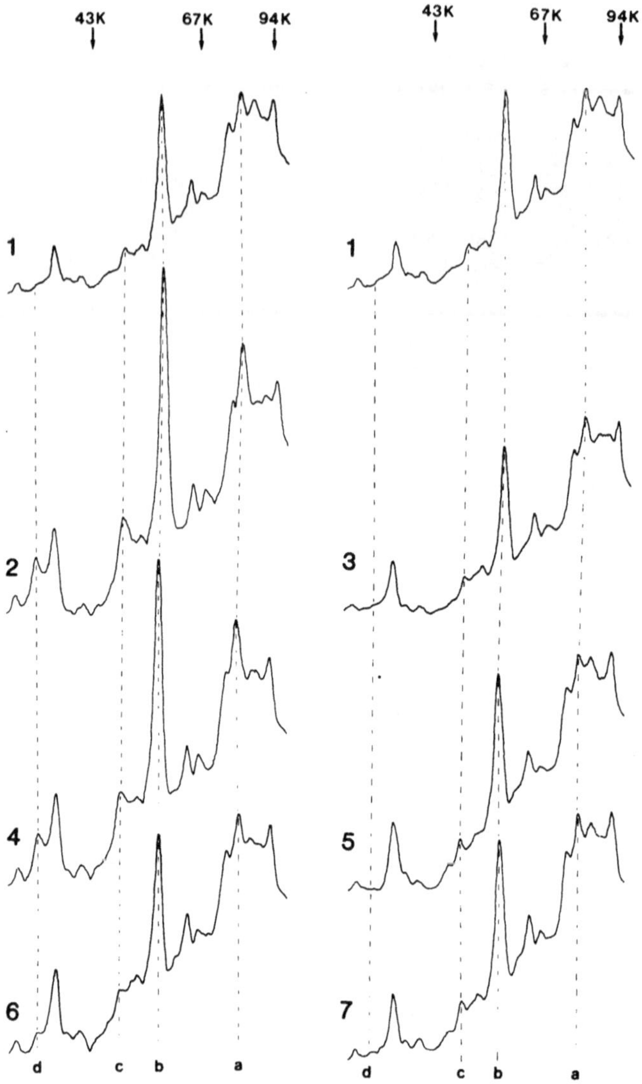


**Fig. 4.** Densitometer tracing $^{32}P$-orthophosphate labeled proteins from Fig. 2. *Arrows* indicate protein markers, *dash lines* positions of bands *a, b, c*, and *d* where changes in incorporation of $^{32}P$ occurred. For convenience only the 94K-34K region of the gel is displayed. *Upper trace:* control. *Second trace: left,* isoproterenol; *right,* timolol plus isoproterenol. *Third trace: left,* epinephrine; *right,* timolol + epinephrine. *Bottom trace: left,* norepinephrine, *right,* timolol plus norepinephrine

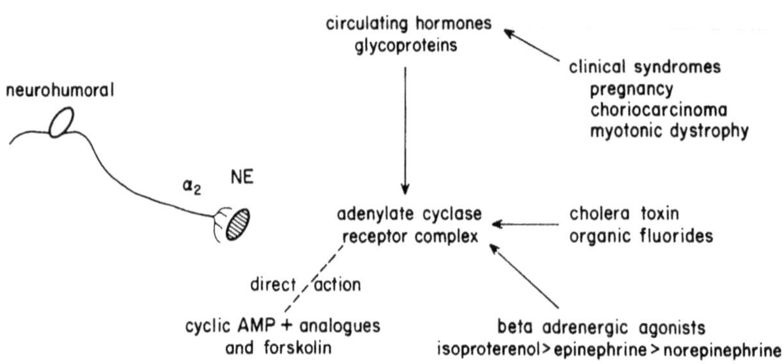


**Fig. 5.** Adenylate cyclase mediated reduction in aqueous net inflow

human cultured ciliary epithelial cells. A cell population comprising pigmented-like epithelial cells is shown in Figure 1. The observation that these cultured cells respond rapidly to hormones that elevate intracellular levels of cAMP supports the idea that the agonists exert their physiological effects in animal tissue by phosphorylating specific substrate proteins mediated by cAMP-dependent kinase(s), and indicates that the beta-adrenergic receptor adenylate cyclase system is coupled and functional. Such enhancement of $^{32}P$ incorporation into protein bands a–d with beta-agonists is specifically blocked by beta-antagonists such as timolol or propranolol but not by an alpha-antagonist such as phenoxybenzamine. The protein phosphorylation data (Fig. 2, 3, 4) demonstrated an order of potency for the catecholamines consistent with previous results obtained using homogenate preparations of human ciliary process epithelial cells (Nathanson, 1981) that a beta$_2$-adrenergic receptor is involved. The pattern of phosphorylated proteins induced by isoproterenol was mimicked by agents which raise cAMP levels (Fig. 3) such as cholera toxin or forskolin, as well as analogues of cAMP, dibutyryl cAMP, 8-bromoadenosine cAMP, or cAMP with theophylline. Finally, alpha-adrenergic agonists such as phenylephrine do not stimulate protein phosphorylation in bands a–d, as do beta-adrenergic agonists.

The identity of the four major phosphorylations (a–d) has yet to be determined. Band b, of about 57–58K dalton, is the more prominent of the proteins labeled in response to isoproterenol or epinephrine, up 2–3 fold over control. Study of this protein indicates that it is not tubulin. Other studies are in progress. In the meantime demonstration of pharmacologically induced phosphorylation of proteins derived from human ciliary epithelia substantiates another element of the adenylate cyclase complex in the ciliary epithelia by providing evidence for cAMP dependent kinases in these cells.

## References


Bromberg BB, Gregory DS, Sears ML (1980) Beta-adrenergic receptors in ciliary processes of the rabbit. Invest Ophthalmol Vis Sci 19:203–207

Eakins K (1963) The effect of intravitreous injections of norepinephrine, epinephrine and isoproterenol on the intraocular pressure and aqueous humor dynamics of rabbit eyes. J Pharmacol Exp Ther 140:79–84

Gregory DS, Bausher LP, Bromberg BB, Sears ML (1981) The beta-adrenergic receptor and adenyl cyclase of rabbit ciliary processes. In: Sears ML (ed) New Directions in Ophthalmic Research, New Haven, Yale University Press, p 127–145

Gregory DS, Sears ML, Bausher L, Mishima H, Mead A (1981) Intraocular pressure and aqueous flow are decreased by cholera toxin. Invest Ophthalmol Vis Sci 20:371–381

Laemmli UK (1970) Cleavage of structural proteins during the assembly of the head of bacteriophage $T_4$. Nature (London) 227:680–685

Nathanson JA (1981) Human ciliary process adrenergic receptor: pharmacological characterization. Invest Ophthalmol Vis Sci 21:798–804

Neufeld AH, Sears ML (1974) Cyclic AMP in the ocular tissues of the rabbit, monkey and human. Invest Ophthalmol Vis Sci 13:475–477

Neufeld AH, Page ED (1977) In vitro determination of the ability of drugs to bind to adrenergic receptors. Invest Ophthalmol Vis Sci 16: 1118–1124

Sears ML, Gregory D, Bausher L, Mishima H, Stjernschantz J (1981) A receptor for aqueous humor formation. In: Sears ML (ed) New Directions in Ophthalmic Research, New Haven, Yale University Press, pp 163–183

Waitzman MB, Woods WD (1971) Some characteristics of an adenyl cyclase preparation from rabbit ciliary process tissue. Exp Eye Res 12: 99–111

Weekers R, Delmarcelle Y, Gustin J (1955) Treatment of ocular hypotension by adrenalin and diverse sympathomimetic amines. Am J Ophthalmol 40:666–672


## Discussion

**Langham to Sears:** The discrepancies that have been noted on the effect of adrenergic drugs on aqueous humor formation and on the outflow resistance may find explanation in the complexity of the pre- and post-synaptic adrenoceptors. In this respect our traditional understanding of the adrenergic neuro-effector system has undergone significant change with the identification and characterization of adrenoceptors at pre-synaptic sites which regulate and modulate the release of the transmitter norepinephrine. Alpha ($\alpha_2$) presynaptic receptors have been found in ocular tissues. The ocular effector responses mediated by post-synaptic $\alpha$ and $\beta$ adrenoceptors will be modified by circulating levels of catecholamines as well as by the local level of adrenoceptor agonists and antagonists.

I would like to add a cautionary note when considering the use of inhibitors of the $Na_1K$ dependent ATPase to decrease intraocular pressure. Some years ago we reported that very small intravitreal injections of ouabain (1 pg) led to a prolonged but fully reversible decrease of intraocular pressure. However, it was evident that injected eye went blind within one hour. All one week the eyes appeared normal and intraocular pressure had recovered. In contrast histological and electromicroscopical studies revealed a complete loss of the neural retina. Biochemical studies showed that the normal retina had an extremely sensitive NaK dependent ATPase.

**Comment by Sears:** A reduction in aqueous humor formation mediated by the adenylate cyclase receptor complex in the ciliary epithelia is a concept that unifies all relevant clinical and experimental observations and several that we have been lucky enough to make both in our clinic and laboratory. Agents acting through adenylate cyclase receptor complex, like HCG (human chorionic gonadotropin), account for the low eye pressure seen in pregnancy and in choriocarcinoma. Patients with myotonic dystrophy also have been known for years to have hypotony. We have now pointed out that the hypotony is initiated by increased levels of gonadotropin-like substances that occur in these patients secondary to gonadal atrophy. Experimentally, we have shown that cholera toxin and organic fluorides lower intraocular pressure by reducing inflow and these are the classic stimulators of cyclase after interaction with the cyclase receptor complex. The drop in pressure with these agents or isoproterenol are too large to be accounted for by an increase in outflow. Furthermore, there are no receptors for these agents in the outflow channels. Finally, as we have shown in this paper, cyclic AMP and analogues act directly on a protein kinase, and, forskolin, an agent acting directly on the catalytic unit of adenylate cyclase, also activates a cyclic AMP dependent protein kinase and, indeed, forskolin lowers intraocular pressure in humans and rabbits (Caprioli, Sears et al., in press).

Blaming species differences for the inability of inadequate physiologic techniques to demonstrate clear cut changes in *net aqueous flow* is responsible for part of the confusion in the literature. NPE has its appex turned toward the blood side and adenylate cyclase stimulation will result in movement of fluid from the ocular chambers (and the base of lateral sides of the NPE, out their apex), into the ciliary channels between the NPE and PE, i.e. reducing *net* aqueous inflow. Improved physiologic technique will be necessary to demonstrate this effect.

Krieglstein G.K./Leydhecker W. (eds)
Glaucoma Update II


# Drug Effects on Fluorescein Kinetics

R.F. Brubaker, Rochester

## Drug Effects on Fluorescein Kinetics

A number of drugs are used clinically as topical medications or systemic medications to lower intraocular pressure, suppress inflammation, or to alter pupillary size. This paper will summarize a systematic study of the effect of some of these drugs on the rate of aqueous flow through the anterior chamber.

It would have been preferable to have measured the rate of aqueous humor formation in these eyes since some portion of the formed aqueous may not enter the anterior chamber. However, no technique has been described for measuring aqueous formation and no satisfactory method has occurred to us.

As a practical matter, the turnover of a fluorescent tracer in the anterior chamber can be measured in humans. This measurement can be made quite reliably and has been the basis of our studies. The fluorescent tracer can be applied as drops, by iontophoresis, intravenously, or orally. For a number of reasons, we chose to apply the dye by iontophoresis using the method described by Jones and Maurice (1966). This technique is disadvantageous since it does not permit individual measurement of $K_d$ and $K_f$, the loss coefficients due to diffusion and flow. Yet, it is advantageous for several reasons. One need not be concerned with plasma binding, systemic metabolism, posterior chamber dynamics, or the limbal depot effect. Major advantages of all fluorescent tracer techniques are that the eye need not be punctured and the intraocular pressure need not be disturbed.

It is known that the diffusional loss of fluorescein from the anterior chamber is quite small compared to its loss by flow (Goldmann 1951; Nagataki 1975; Araie et al. 1980; Pederson et al. 1978). In testing a drug, it is easy to establish that diffusional exchange between plasma and aqueous humor is not affected by the drug by doing a separate experiment in which the dye is given systemically and the initial rate of rise of fluorescence in the treated eye and the untreated eye are compared.

The specific details of how flow is derived from the initial dose of fluorescein in the corneal depot and from the time course of anterior chamber fluorescence need not be addressed in this discussion but must be considered very carefully by the investigator who applies such a technique to measure flow (Anselmi et al. 1968; Jones and Maurice 1966; Coakes and Brubaker 1979; Brubaker 1982). To understand the results of our drug studies, however, we must consider the accuracy and the reproducibility of the technique.

Accuracy can be addressed rather simply. The accuracy is unknown. There are no independent methods which are suitable to establish the exact rate of flow through the anterior chamber under the experimental conditions in which we have chosen to work, except for Holm's (1968) technique. Reproducibility, however, can be measured in two ways. First, one can compare the measured flow in one eye to that in the fellow eye in a group of normal, untreated subjects, or one can compare the flow in a single eye as measured on different occasions.

The variation of the differences of paired measurements can be expressed as a percent. With the least squares method of flow calculation (Nagataki and Brubaker 1982), the coefficient of variation is 16% when fellow eyes are compared and 15% when eyes are compared to themselves on separate occasions. The nomographic method (Coakes and Brubaker 1979), a simpler method, shows greater variability, 20% as expected. Some studies were done by this latter method, but most were done by the method of least squares.

The coefficient of variation can be used to estimate the magnitude of drug effect which can be detected reliably with a given sample size (Cochran and Cox 1957). For most drug studies, we have studied 20–25 subjects and have compared the flow in the drug-treated eye to that in the placebo-treated fellow eye. With the least squares method of data analysis this sample size can detect a 14% effect. Smaller drug effects may not be detected with this sample size. This point must be kept in mind as one interprets the results.

Some commonly used ocular drugs were tested, as shown in Table 1. In some instances, no drug effect was measurable. Included in this group were dexamethasone, phenylephrine, and thymoxamine. Two drugs produced a small increase in flow. Epinephrine produced a 15% increase and pilocarpine produced an 18% increase. In neither case was the increase large enough to be clinically significant. However, it is clear that neither drug could have lowered intraocular pressure in these test circumstances by reducing aqueous humor flow. Some other mechanism must have accounted for the lowering of pressure.

**Table 1a.** Drugs which did not produce measurable effect on flow

| | Flow, μL (mean ± SD) | |
|---|---|---|
| Drug | Untreated | Treated |
| Dexamethasone | 2.6 ± 0.5 | 2.6 ± 0.7 |
| Phenylephrine | 2.6 ± 0.7 | 2.6 ± 0.6 |
| Thymoxamine | 2.4 ± 0.6 | 2.5 ± 0.6 |

**b.** Drugs which increased aqueous humor flow

| | Flow, μL (mean ± SD) | |
|---|---|---|
| Drug | Untreated | Treated |
| Epinephrine | 2.5 ± 0.4 | 2.9 ± 0.7 |
| Pilocarpine | 2.4 ± 0.4 | 2.8 ± 0.6 |

**c.** Drugs which decreased aqueous humor flow

| | Flow, μL (mean ± SD) | |
|---|---|---|
| Drug | Untreated | Treated |
| Acetazolamide | 2.1 ± 0.5 | 1.5 ± 0.3 |
| Timolol | 2.3 ± 0.4 | 1.5 ± 0.3 |
| Combination | 2.1 ± 0.5 | 1.2 ± 0.2 |

Two drugs were found to lower the rate of aqueous humor flow. Acetazolamide reduced the flow by 27% and timolol reduced it by 34%. When these drugs were combined, a 41% reduction in flow was observed.

Two additional drug combinations were tested, timolol plus epinephrine and thymoxamine plus epinephrine. In the former case, the effect of timolol dominated; a 46% lowering of the rate of flow was observed. In the latter case, the effect of epinephrine dominated; a 17% increase in the rate of flow was observed.

None of the drugs tested had any appreciable effect on the rate of entry of fluorescein into the anterior chamber following systemic administration of the dye. Also, none of the drugs effected the permeability of the corneal endothelium to any measurable extent.

Acetazolamide and timolol were by far the most active and consistent drugs which affected the rate of fluorescein clearance from the anterior chamber. It is clear that their therapeutic effect is mediated via flow. It is probable that both drugs decrease the rate of aqueous humor formation. Their effects are partly additive, a fact which is of clinical significance since the dosages used in these experiments are those which are commonly used for the treatment of glaucoma.

With one drug, timolol, we carried out a long term experiment to determine if the chronically treated eye responded identically to the acutely treated eye. We found that the effect after one year's treatment was smaller than after one week's treatment, indicating that the eye partly but not completely adapts to the drug after chronic exposure.

Measurement of the clearance of fluorescein from the anterior chamber is a good method with which to study the effects of clinically useful drugs on aqueous humor flow. Although fluorescent tracer techniques have limitations, they are much more direct methods of measuring flow than are techniques which measure resistance or intraocular pressure. Most of the drug effects which we have observed confirm the work of others by the same technique or by different techniques, except in the case of epinephrine where the bulk of experimental evidence supports the idea that this drug either has no effect on flow or lowers it. The effect of epinephrine on flow remains a dilemma to us. Additional experiments with drugs which have more specific properties will probably be useful in establishing patterns of drug effects on aqueous flow. Such data should be useful to permit rational clinical use of these drugs either singly or in combination.

**References**

Anselmi P, Bron AJ, Maurice DM (1968) Action of drugs on the aqueous flow in man measured by fluorophotometry. Exp Eye Res 7:487–496

Araie M, Sawa M, Nagataki S, Mishima S (1980) Aqueous humor dynamics in man as studied by oral fluorescein. Jpn J Ophthalmol 24: 346–362

Brubaker RF (in press) The flow of aqueous humor in the human eye. Proc AOS

Brubaker RL, Nagataki S, Bourne WM (1982) Effect of chronically administered timolol on aqueous humor flow in patients with glaucoma. Ophthalmology (Rochester) 89:280–283

Coakes RL, Brubaker RF (1978) The mechanism of timolol in lowering intraocular pressure. Arch Ophthalmol 96:2045–2048

Coakes RL, Brubaker RF (1979) Method of measuring aqueous humor flow and corneal endothelial permeability using a fluorophotometry nomogram. Invest Ophthalmol Vis Sci 18:288–302

Cochran WG, Cox GM (1957) Experimental designs, 2nd ed, John Wiley & Sons, Inc., p 19

Dailey RA, Brubaker RF, Bourne WM (1982) The effects of timolol maleate and acetazolamide on the rate of aqueous formation in normal human subjects. Am J Ophthalmol 93:232–237

Goldmann H (1951) Abflußdruck, Minutenvolumen und Widerstand. Der Kammerwasserstromung des Menschen. Doc Ophthalmol 5–6:278–356

Higgins RG, Brubaker RF (1980) Acute effect of epinephrine on aqueous humor formation in the timolol-treated normal eye as measured by fluorophotometry. Invest Ophthalmol Vis Sci 19:420–423

Holm O (1968) A photogrammetric method for estimation of the pupillary aqueous flow in the living eye, I. Acta Ophthalmol 46:254–277

Jones RF, Maurice DM (1966) New methods of measuring the rate of aqueous flow in man with fluorescein. Exp Eye Res 5:208–220

Lee F (1958) The influence of epinephrine and phenylephrine on intraocular pressure. Arch Ophthalmol 60:863–867

Lee DA, Brubaker RF, Nagataki S (1981) Effect of thymoxamine on aqueous humor formation in the normal human eye as measured by fluorophotometry. Invest Ophthalmol Vis Sci 21: 805–811

Nagataki S (1975) Aqueous humor dynamics of human eyes as studied using fluorescein. Jpn J Ophthalmol 19:235–249

Nagataki S, Brubaker RF (1981) Early effect of epinephrine on aqueous formation in the normal human eye. Ophthalmology 88:278–282

Nagataki S, Brubaker RF (1982) Effect of pilocarpine on aqueous humor formation in human beings. Arch Ophthalmol 100:818–821

Pederson JE, Gaasterland DE, MacLellan HM (1978) Accuracy of aqueous humor flow determination by fluorophotometry. Invest Ophthalmol Vis Sci 17:190–195

Rice SW, Bourne WM, Brubaker RF (1983) The effect of topical dexamethasone on aqueous flow rate and endothelial permeability (in preparation)

Townsend DJ, Brubaker RF (1980) Immediate effect of epinephrine on aqueous formation in the normal human eye as measured by fluorophotometry. Invest Ophthalmol Vis Sci 19:256–266

## Discussion

**Yablonski to Brubaker:** Dr. A. Bill stated that perhaps isoproterenol failed to yield a detectable change in anterior chamber aqueous humor flow because in its resting state the secretory mechanism of the ciliary processes may be under maximal beta adrenergic stimulation. However, the effect on topical epinephrine on aqueous humor flow would not support this hypothesis. Brubaker and co-workers have reported an increase in aqueous humor flow of about 18% after one drop of epinephrine. Similarly, Schenker, H., Yablonski, M.E., Podos, S.M., and Leiner, L., Archives of Ophthalmology 99:1212–1216, 1981, reported an increase of 18% in aqueous humor flow after a week of topical epinephrine, 2%, twice daily.

Secondly, I would like to ask Dr. Brubaker if he measured anterior chamber volume after isoproterenol as well as before?

**Brubaker:** Measurements of anterior chamber volume were only made before drug administration.

**Yablonski:** I would like to offer a possible explanation for the failure of isoproterenol to cause an observable increase in aqueous humor flow in the study of Brubaker. If the drug for some reason caused an increase in anterior chamber volume this would mask of similar increase in aqueous humor flow measured fluorophotometrically unless taken into account.

**Spaeth to Brubaker:** What Brubaker has described is really "clearance" not "flow". Would it help to use the word "clearance" rather than the word "flow"?

Krieglstein G.K./Leydhecker W. (eds)
Glaucoma Update II


# Beta-Adrenergic Agonists and Antagonists: Clinical Pharmacokinetics

S. Mishima, M. Takase, M. Araie and Y. Kitazawa, Tokyo

Since introduction of β-adrenergic antagonists, there has been a burst of research works on the mechanism of their hypotensive effects, and the effectiveness of these drugs for the treatment of glaucoma is now well established. Not only the knowledge of the mechanism of their action, but also of pharmacokinetics is of value for designing logical therapeutic regimen. Therefore, the recent findings on the latter aspects of the β-adrenergic drugs are summarized in this paper.

## 1. Intraocular Penetration, Elimination and Pigment Binding in the Rabbit Eye

The mode of intraocular penetration of instilled drugs is similar between the human and rabbit eyes (Mishima 1981), and this makes the data of ocular pharmacokinetics compiled in the rabbit eye useful in considering pharmacokinetics in the human eye. The corneal epithelium is the main barrier for penetration of instilled drugs, and it is more permeable to lipophilic than to lipophobic drugs: the relative permeabilities of the rabbit corneal epithelium for various drugs are listed in Table 1. The permeability of the human epithelium was thought to be 50–70% of that of the rabbit epithelium.

After instillation of $^{14}$C-epinephrine in the albino rabbit, its content in the iris and ciliary body becomes much higher than in the aqueous humor. This is attributed largely to the active absorptive uptake of this drug by the varicose adrenergic nerves in these tissues (Mishima 1982).

Various drugs including epinephrine are bound to the uveal pigments, and this was thought responsible for a reduction of hypotensive effects of pilocarpine and epinephrine (Melikian et al. 1971). After instillation of timolol and befunolol in the pigmented rabbit, their content in the iris and cilary body becomes much higher than in the aqueous humor, and their elimination from the eye is greatly retarded in the pigmented than in the albino rabbit; these drugs are bound to the uveal pigments (Araie et al. 1982). It is possible that this binding accounts for a lower hypotensive effect of timolol in the dark than in the blue eyes (Katz et al. 1979).

**Table 1.** The relative permeabilities of the rabbit corneal epithelium to various drugs

| Drugs | Relative values of permeability |
|---|---|
| Epinephrine | 1[a] |
| Dipyvalyl-epinephrine | 53 |
| Timolol | 14 |
| Befunolol | 13 |
| Bupranolol | 9 |
| Pilocarpine | 10 |

[a] The value was estimated to be $1 \times 10^{-4}$ cm hr$^{-1}$, on the assumption that the initial tear concentration is equal to the drug concentration and the loss rate in the tears is 0.1 per minute (Mishima 1981)

## 2. The Hypotensive Effects of Drugs in the Human Eye

A linear correlation is found between the intraocular pressure (IOP) and its reduction after drug instillation (Fig. 1). An analysis on a large number of eyes revealed that the intercept of the relationship with the IOP axis averaged 9.0 ± 4.5 (S.D.) mmHg (n = 18), which agrees with the episcleral venous pressure, and that the slope of the regression line increases by increasing drug concentration. This indicates that the dose-response relationship of the hypotensive effect be studied using the reduction ratio of the outflow pressure (Mishima 1981); this permits a com-

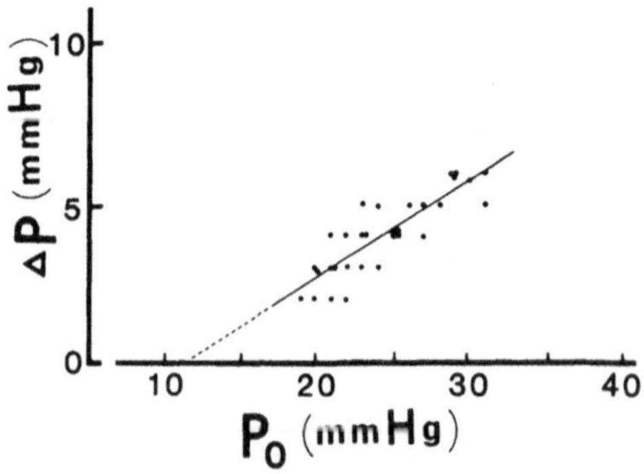


**Fig. 1.** Relationship between the reduction in the IOP ($\Delta P$) and the baseline IOP ($P_0$), 2 hours after instillation of 0.5% bupranolol solution. The correlation coefficient is 0.84. (Unpublished results of Takase et al.)

parison to be made between the results of IOP studies and those of other studies of clinical aqueous humor dynamics.

A transformation of Goldmann's equation on the aqueous outflow yields the following relationship applicable to small changes in the outflow pressure, outflow resistance ($R_r$) and the aqueous humor formation rate (F):

$$\frac{\Delta P_i}{P_i - P_e} = \frac{\Delta R_r}{R_r} + \frac{\Delta F}{F} \qquad (1)$$

where $P_i$ is the IOP and $P_e$ is the episcleral venous pressure which can be assumed to be 9 mmHg. The reciprocal of the tonographic outflow facility, the apparent outflow resistance, $R_{app}$, may be used for $R_r$ as an approximation, since the difference would be less than 20 percent. On this basis, the results of dose-response studies of the outflow pressure, the outflow facility or apparent outflow resistance and of the aqueous humor formation rate can be compared.

When Equation (1) is applied to the results of clinical aqueous humor dynamics in a large number of glaucoma patients, it is possible to estimate the relative contribution of the drug effects on the outflow resistance and aqueous formation rate to lower the IOP. Thus, the reduction ratios of the outflow pressure and the apparent outflow resistance were calculated from the published data, and their weighted averages computed. The fluorophotometry permits determinations of the aqueous humor formation rate in the human eye more accurately than by tonography, and the reduction ratios obtained by this method were also calculated (Table 2).

The reduction ratios of the outflow pressure and the apparent outflow resistance are similar with pilocarpine and epinephrine, but they differ significantly with acetazolamide and timolol. Furthermore, the reduction ratios of the outflow pressure and of the aqueous formation rate are similar with timolol. These results are consistent with the opinion that the hypotensive effects of pilocarpine and epinephrine are largely due to a reduction of the outflow resistance, and the effects of the latter two drugs are mainly due to a reduction in aqueous humor formation.

## 3. The Rate of Effect Disappearance

For a design of therapeutic regimen with a topical drug, the duration of its effect should be taken into consideration. The duration of the effect depends not only on the dose, but also on the rate at which the drug is eliminated from the eye and the least effec-

**Table 2.** The reduction ratios of the outflow pressure, the apparent outflow resistance and aqueous humor formation rate

| Drugs | $\Delta P_i/(P_i-P_e)$ | $\Delta R_{app}/R_{app}$ | $\Delta F/F$ | n |
|---|---|---|---|---|
| (1) Pilocarpin 4% | 0.48 | 0.49 | - | 12 |
| (2) Epinephrine 2% | 0.42 | 0.40 | - | 116 |
| (3) Acetazolamide (500 mg) | 0.19 | 0.07 | - | 17 |
| (4) Timolol | 0.41 | 0.13 | - | 109 |
| (5) | | | 0.39 | 67 |

(1) From Kronfeld 1971, (2) Weighted average from Mishima 1982, (3) From Becker and Constant 1955, (4), (5) Weighted averages from Mishima 1982

tive dose. Thus, the knowledge of these factors is of clinical value.

The least effective dose or concentration of the topical drug may be obtained by extrapolating the dose-response relationship. The least effective concentrations for the hypotensive effects were estimated to be 0.1–0.15% for pilocarpine and 0.1–0.2% for epinephrine ophthalmic solutions (Mishima 1981).

The rate of drug elimination from the eye may be calculated from the response changes for miotic or mydriatic drugs, since a simple relationship can be determined between the response and the drug concentration in the iris muscles. The elimination rate for pilocarpine was estimated to be 0.3–0.4 $hr^{-1}$. However, the IOP response is the final result of responses of various ocular tissues that are interrelated in a complex manner; a simple analysis of the IOP changes does not yield the rate of drug elimination. Consequently, the concept of the rate of effect disappearance was introduced.

Figure 2 illustrates a linear relationship between the logarithm of topical befunolol concentrations and the duration of its hypotensive effect which was defined as the time interval between the time of peak effect and the time of effect termination. The slope of the regression line gives the rate of effect disappearance and the intercept with the concentration axis gives the least effective concentration of the drug. Through this analysis, the rate of effect duration was estimated to be about 0.2 $hr^{-1}$ for bupranolol, 0.26 $hr^{-1}$ for befunolol and 0.06 $hr^{-1}$ for timolol. The least effective concentration was about 0.13–0.16% for bupranolol, 0.08% for befunolol and 0.045% for timolol.

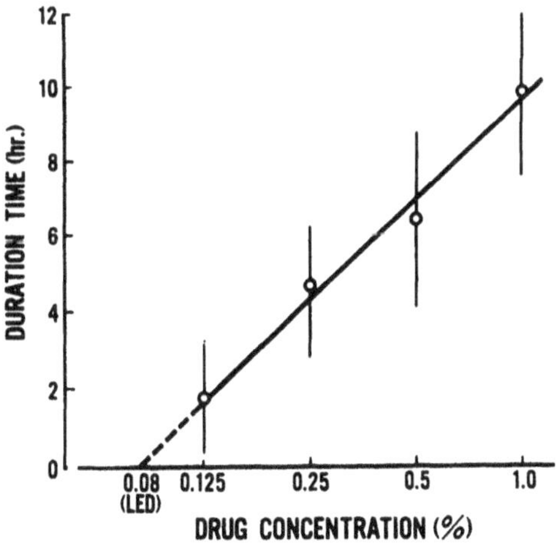


**Fig. 2.** Relationship between the average duration of the hypotensive effect and logarithm of befunolol concentration. *Vertical bars:* S.D. from the results of 8 normal volunteers. *LED:* least effective concentration. (From Mishima 1981)

The duration of the effect, T, of a topical drug with a concentration, C, may be computed from the rate of effect disappearance, k, and the least effective concentration, $C_{min}$, by the following equation:

$$T = 2.3 \text{ Log } (C/C_{min})/k \qquad (2)$$

The frequency of instillation may be determined on this basis so that the effect can be maintained over 24 hours. For example, we may propose instillation of 4 times a day with 1% pilocarpine, once or twice a day for 0.5% timolol.

## References


Araie M, Takase M, Sakai Y, Ishii Y, Yokoyama Y, Kitagawa M (1982) Beta-adrenergic blockers: ocular penetration and binding to the uveal pigments. Jpn J Ophthalmol 26 (in press)

Becker B, Constant MA (1955) Experimental tonography. The effect of carbonic anhydrase inhibitor acetazolamide on aqueous flow. Arch Ophthalmol 54:321–329

Katz IM, Berger ET (1979) Effects of iris pigmentation on response of ocular pressure to timolol. Surv Ophthalmol 23:395–398

Kronfeld PC (1967) The efficacy of combination of ocular hypotensive drugs. Arch Ophthalmol 78:140–146

Melikian HE, Lieberman TW, Leopold LH (1971) Ocular pigmentation and pressure and outflow response to pilocarpine and epinephrine. Am J Ophthalmol 72:70–73

Mishima S (1981) Clinical pharmacokinetics of the eye. Invest Ophthalmol Vis Sci 21:504–541

Mishima S (1982) Ocular effects of beta-adrenergic agents. Surv Ophthalmol 27 (in press)


## Discussion

**Comment by Mishima:** The effects of drugs, stimulation or inhibition depend on the original state of the tissue or organ. In this connection, I would like to cite the work of Dr. Bárány who showed that the effects of pilocarpine and of cholinolytic drugs on the outflow resistance depend on the original state of the outflow resistance. We can assume that at least under usual experimental conditions the state of the outflow resistance is in the middle range of its chargeable amplitude.

This also appears to be the case in aqueous humor formation. In the human eye timolol reduces the rate of aqueous formation and salbutamol increases it, and this would support the above consideration. However, the original state may undergo diurnal variation, and it is important to specify the time of the day when the experiment is carried out.

**Speath to Mishima:** Dr. Mishima's graphs relating pressure to change in pressure were described as linear. The three graphs he showed did not appear in actuality to be linear, rather to describe some other function, perhaps exponential. How was the lineality of these graphs calculated?

**Mishima to Spaeth:** The relationship between $\Delta P$ and $P_0$ is linear by regression analysis.

**Mishima to Simmons:** From published, data, we find that the reduction ratio of the outflow pressure, $\Delta P/(P_i-9)$ after argon laser trabeculoplasty (LTP) ranged from 0.38 to 0.55 and the reduction ratio of the apparent outflow resistance ranged from 0.4–0.5. In aphakic open angle glaucoma, $\Delta P/(P_i-9)$ was 0.2 from the date you published. We did not calculate this in pigmentary glaucoma.

**Mishima to Zimmermann:** Ocular pigments do bind various drugs and a great amount is required to saturate the binding sites. Even on repeated instillations the effects are less in the pigmented than in the lightly pigmented eyes. In addition, the clearance from the eye is very slow and the pigments act as a depot for the drugs.

Krieglstein G.K./Leydhecker W. (eds)
Glaucoma Update II


# Substance P-like Immunoreactive Nerves in the Anterior Segment of the Eye

R.A. Stone, A.M. Laties, and A. McGlinn, Philadelphia

The cholinergic and adrenergic components of the autonomic nervous system regulate important physiologic processes in the anterior segment of the eye. Not only do they control pupil size [1]; they also appear to influence blood flow [2], aqueous humor secretion [3] and aqueous humor outflow [4, 5].

Although significant species variation is acknowledged, there are general patterns of innervation by the two classical divisions of the autonomic nervous system [6]. In the cornea, the number of cholinergic and adrenergic fibers recognized is scant. In the filtration area, a modest adrenergic pattern is generally present along with a lesser and ill-defined cholinergic innervation. In contrast, for the ciliary process, there is a heavy subepithelial network of adrenergic fibers. The ciliary processes also receive modest cholinergic innervation. In asserting a lesser cholinergic innervation, there is a nagging concern that the methods for study may be of different sensitivity or that puzzling variations occur. This cholinergic innervation is histochemically more prominent in albino than pigmented animals. As would be expected, innervation to the smooth muscles of the anterior segment is markedly imbalanced. The ciliary muscle contains a dense network of cholinergic nerves accompanied by a minor but definite adrenergic innervation. The iris dilator receives a heavy adrenergic innervation but only a modest cholinergic innervation. In contrast to the dilator, the iris sphincter has a heavy cholinergic innervation but only a modest adrenergic innervation. Of immediate pertinence to the heterochromia of Horner's syndrome [7], anterior uveal melanocytes have a constant sympathetic innervation [8].

Paralleling these anatomical observations is the extensive use of autonomic agents in clinical ophthalmology for both diagnosis and therapy. Yet, our understanding of the autonomic control of anterior segment physiology is incomplete. Findings, such as the observation that both adrenergic agonists [5] and beta-adrenergic antagonists [9] lower intraocular pressure, underscore this limitation in our knowledge.

In recent years, a series of biologically active peptides have been found in both the central and peripheral nervous system that appear to act either as neurotransmitters or neuromodulators [10]. Because of the physiological studies and because prior histochemical studies of both cholinergic and adrenergic innervation have failed to demonstrate a nerve plexus pattern consistent with known innervation density, particularly in the cornea and filtration area, there is ample justification to search the anterior segment for the presence of additional neurotransmitters. Indeed, the existence of biologically active peptides, vasoactive intestinal peptide (VIP) and substance P have now been described for the eye.

VIP nerves are of limited distribution [11]. They are present in the ciliary processes, in the posterior portion of the ciliary muscle and around small to medium-sized choroidal blood vessels. They have not been seen in the iris. The pterygopalatine ganglion contains a large number of VIP-immunoreactive cell bodies, and destruction of this ganglion results in loss of the VIP nerves to the eye. The VIP network is similar to the facial parasympathetic innervation of the choroid [12, 13] and probably mediates vascular tone [13, 14].

Gathering but still incomplete evidence indicates that substance P plays an important role in ocular physiology. Intracameral injection of physiologic doses of substance P causes intense miosis [15, 16]. At higher concentrations, intracameral substance P causes protein leakage into the aqueous [17, 18] and an intraocular pressure elevation [16, 18]. Because prior iridectomy prevents this rise in intraocular pressure despite the protein release [16], the rise in intraocular pressure probably results from an angle closure glaucoma mechanism [16, 19]. Capsaicin, which depletes neuronal substance P, blocks the initial rise in intraocular pressure that follows application of nitrogen mustard [20]. In addition, the substance P antagonist (D-Pro [2], D-Trp [7, 9]) SP, reduces both the miotic response and the protein leakage caused by intraocular substance P injection or by infrared radiation [18]. Lastly, substance P is released into the aqueous humor after trigeminal nerve stimulation [17], and destruction of the trigeminal ganglion results in lowered tissue levels on the denervated side [21].

Histochemical localization of substance P depends on immunohistochemical technique. By this means substance P immunoreactivity has been discovered in retinal amacrine cells of an array of vertebrates extending from goldfish and frog to rat, rabbit and monkey [22–25] (unpublished observations). Of the studies published on the anterior segment [26–35], these are partially in conflict. For instance, substance P-like immunoreactive (S-PLI) innervation to the cornea has been reported in some studies [29–31, 33] while not in others [28, 34].

In the present studies [35], we used an established immunocytochemical technique to study the localization of substance P in the anterior segment of the eye of animals frequently used in glaucoma research – the rabbit, the cat, and both Old and New World monkeys.

## Experimental Procedures

### *Antisera*

Polyclonal rabbit anti-substance P antiserum was purchased from ImmunoNuclear Corp., Stillwater, Minnesota, while a monoclonal anti-substance P antiserum, raised in rats, was obtained from Pel-Freeze Biologicals, Rogers, Arkansas.

### *Tissue Preparation*

Two to three kilogram albino and Dutch-belted pigmented rabbits were killed by intravenous injection of sodium pentobarbital, and the eyes were removed immediately. Eyes were enucleated from adult cats under deep pentobarbital anaesthesia (immediately prior to death). Four adult squirrel monkeys *(Saimiri sciurea)* and one adult crab-eating monkey *(Macaca fascicularis)* were anesthetized with intramuscular pentobarbital. The eyes from selected monkeys were removed directly; other monkeys were perfused through the left ventricle with fixative (2% paraformaldehyde, 0.1 M lysine HCl and 0.01 M Na periodate in 0.5 M phosphate buffer) [36] prior to enucleation. Immediately after enucleation all eyes were immersed in fixative for 2–4 hours at 4 °C and washed overnight at 4 °C in 30% sucrose and 0.1 M phosphate buffer. 20 µ cryostat tissue sections were thaw-mounted on gelatin-coated slides. The sections were dried at room temperature and stored at −20 °C until stained by an indirect immunofluoresce technique.

### *Immunohistochemical Procedures*

For rabbit tissues, we used the anti-substance P antiserum derived from rats. For cat and monkey tissues, we used both rat and rabbit antisera.

Tissue sections, after a ten-minute wash in 0.1 M phosphate buffer at room temperature, were incubated for one hour at 37 °C in anti-substance P antiserum diluted at 1 : 250 in buffer containing 0.3% Triton X-100. The tissue sections then received two fifteen-minute washes in 0.1 M phosphate buffer and were then incubated at room temperature for thirty minutes with goat anti-rabbit IgG (Miles Biologicals, Elkart, Indiana), or goat anti-rat IgG (Cappel Laboratories, Cochranville, Pennsylvania), conjugated to fluorescein isothiocyanate at a dilution of 1 : 50 and containing 0.3% Triton X-100. All tissue sections finally were washed in 0.1 M phosphate buffer, cover-slipped in a Tris-glycerin mixture or in a 0.1 M phosphate buffer-glycerin mixture and examined under an epi-illumination fluorescence system.

To assess immune reaction specificity, the primary antisera were absorbed with 50 µM synthetic substance P (Peninsula Laboratories, Inc., San Carlos, California). The absorbed antisera then was substituted for the primary antisera in the immunohistochemical procedures. As another control, we incubated unreacted tissue sections with fluorescein isothiocyanate labelled IgG alone.

## Results and Discussion

SPLI nerves are present in a wide variety of anterior segment structures in the eye of the rabbit, cat, and monkey. In all instances, these nerve fibers have the typical meandering appearance of terminal autonomic nerves, with a fishnet distribution and characteristic varicosities. In our hands, immersion fixation brings out the SPLI nerves in the anterior segment of monkey eyes better than does perfusion fixation. We used immersion fixation exclusively for the anterior segment of the rabbit and cat eyes. Neither pre-absorbed antisera nor FITC alone react with ocular nerves. We find no difference between albino and Dutch-belted rabbit eyes. Nor is there a difference between the two different families of monkeys.

Immunohistochemical techniques are subject to an important limitation of all immunologic methods, a potential for cross-reactivity exists among related antigens [37]. As one of the tachykinin family of neuropeptides, there is justified caution in interpreting findings obtained with an antiserum raised against substance P as absolute proof of its identity in tissue section. Certain proof requires isolation and direct biochemical characterization of the neuropeptide. It is for these reasons that we and others use the term "substance P-like immunoreactive" in describing the nerves we visualized.

Yet, several lines of evidence strongly suggest that the nerve fibers identified in these studies do indeed contain substance P. For instance, we noted identical staining with two different antisera. One of these is monoclonal and is known to have very low cross-reactivity to a closely related tachykinin, eleidosin [38]. Further, radioimmune assay, which also depends on antibody recognition, has also indicated the presence of substance P in the anterior segment of the eye [21]. Lastly, and of great significance, physiological studies have indicated an extreme sensitivity of the iris to substance P [39].

In general, although occasional SPLI nerves are seen within the choroid of all three animals, the chief findings outside the neurosensory retina are in the anterior segment.

### *Cornea and Sclera*

In agreement with previous findings in the rat [29, 30], rabbit [31], and squirrel [33], we find SPLI nerve fibers in the cornea of all three animals studied, although only a small number of fibers can be visualized in each. SPLI nerves are present in distinct locations. Most often, they occur at the limbus and in peripheral cornea. More rarely, short segments of fine nerve fibers are seen just beneath the corneal epithelium (Fig. 1). The deep limbus just above the outflow apparatus also contains some SPLI reactive nerves in all three animals studied. In addition, occasional nerve fibers are seen in the anterior sclera surrounding intrascleral vessels.

Could substance P be the sensory transmitter of the trigeminal nerve supply to the cornea? Considerable evidence exists that substance P acts as a sensory neurotransmitter elsewhere in the body. The location of these SPLI nerve fibers in the cornea and the observation by Tervo et al. [31], that the trigeminal ganglion contains two distinct SPLI cell types both point in this direction. Their additional observation [31] that section of the first and second division of the fifth nerve leads to the disappearance of SPLI nerves to the cornea would further support such a hypothesis. Yet the evidence is incomplete, for a demonstration by immunohistochemistry of

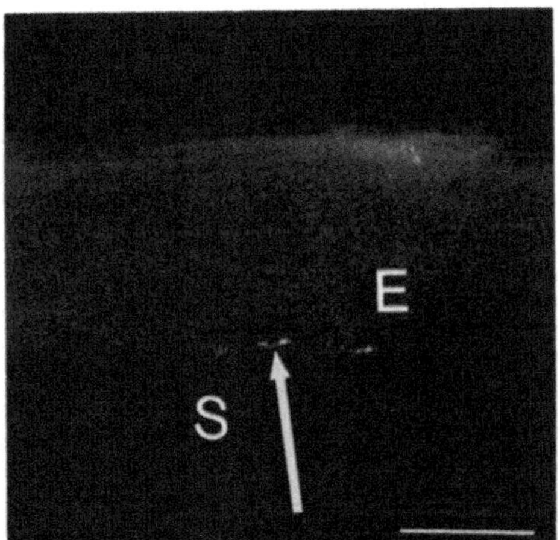


**Fig. 1.** Corneal innervation in the rabbit. A rare SPLI nerve is seen underneath the corneal epithelium *(E)*. *S*, corneal stroma. (Fluorescent micrograph; *bar*, 20 μ)

a SPLI nerve density comparable to the known richness of the corneal innervation is lacking. Instead Tervo [29, 31], Shimizu [33], and we [35] have been unable to demonstrate anything near in density to the plentiful corneal nerve plexus known to exist. Such a failure testifies either to a deficiency of method and/or to the presence of a different and still unrecognized neurohumor in the majority of corneal nerves. Certainly the method is delicate. For instance, even modest glutaraldehyde fixation profoundly reduces SPLI staining [28, 29]. Evidence compatible with but not proof of the presence of an unrecognized neurohumor in corneal nerves is provided by the results of application to the cornea of the substance P antagonist (D-Pro [2], D-Trp [7, 9]) SP. This antagonist blocks a response by the iris sphincter to exogenous substance P but fails to reduce corneal sensitivity [18]. Thus, substance P may very well not be a major sensory transmitter for corneal nerves.

Although most descriptions of corneal innervation emphasize the nerve supply to the epithelium and superficial cornea, there are several candidate structures to be served by a deep SPLI limbal innervation. To date, an innervation to the corneal endothelium has been described only for the rabbit [40] and frog [41]; SPLI nerves could supply this cell layer as well. These nerves could supply Schwalbe-line's cells, a recently recognized discontinuous cord of secretory cells located at the anterior end of the trabecular meshwork [42]. Moreover, the deep limbal region of the cat in particular has a dense population of melanocytes which again could claim an innervation. Questions of degree and balance among these possibilities await further study.

*Outflow Apparatus*

Of immediate pertinence to the topic of this symposium, the aqueous outflow apparatus of all three animals studied contain SPLI nerves. In the rabbit, such nerves are seen regularly in the pectinate ligament (Fig. 2a); the tissues of the ciliary cleft itself receive a sparse innervation. In the cat things are different: here SPLI nerves are only occasionally visualized within the pectinate ligament, while the deeper structures within the ciliary cleft receive a definite SPLI innervation. Among the animals we studied, SPLI nerves to the outflow apparatus are most prominent in the monkey [32]. They are found in the trabecular (Fig. 2b) and juxtacanalicular tissues as well as to either side of Schlemm's canal. They may extend the length of the trabecular meshwork to the edge of Descemet's membrane. Less frequently, they spill over beyond the meshwork into deep peripheral cornea.

Whether this SPLI innervation to the outflow is an afferent, an efferent, or for that matter a mixed pathway is unknown at present. Certainly, there is ample precedent for the existence of substance P in specialized sensory receptors; it has been localized immu-

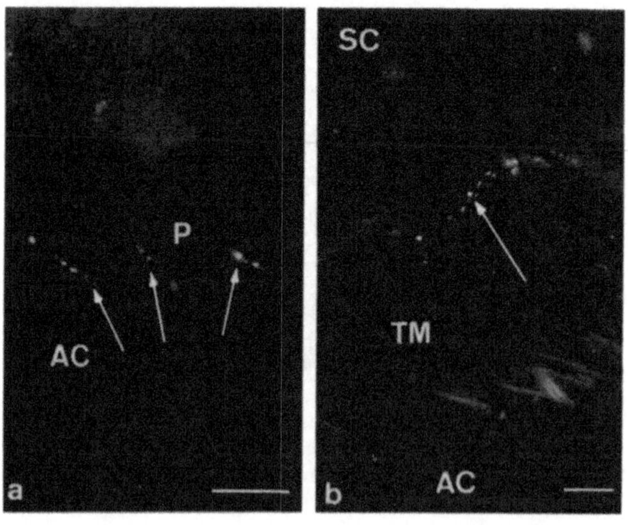


**Fig. 2.** Innervation to outflow pathways. **(a)** Three SPLI fibers *(arrows)* are seen in the pectinate ligament *(P)* of the rabbit eye. **(b)** An SPLI nerve *(arrow)* lies in the trabecular meshwork *(TM)*. *SC,* Schlemm's Canal; *AC,* Anterior Chamber; (Fluorescent micrographs; *bar,* 20 μ)

nologically in such structures as the carotid body [43] and taste bud [44]. There is also precedent for a role in autonomic regulation, as substance P is thought to be the transmitter at the first synapse of the systemic baroreceptor reflex [45, 46]. As a stimulus of further experiment, it seems permissible to speculate that SPLI nerves in the outflow could constitute part of a chemoreceptor or baroreceptor reflex arc in the anterior segment. Substantiation of such a hypothesis, however, requires a physiological demonstration of specific function.

*Ciliary Process and Ciliary Body*

A rich SPLI nerve network is seen in the ciliary and iridic processes of the rabbit. Nerve fibers course along the entire length of a process (Fig. 3a). They lie in close relationship to the blood vessels and frequently ramify just beneath the basement membrane of the pigmented epithelium at the tip of a process. These nerves, however, have not been seen to cross the basement membrane. The ciliary process of both the cat and monkey contain SPLI nerves in similar pattern but of lesser number. A distinct SPLI innervation to an individual ciliary process is also what occurs for the adrenergic innervation.

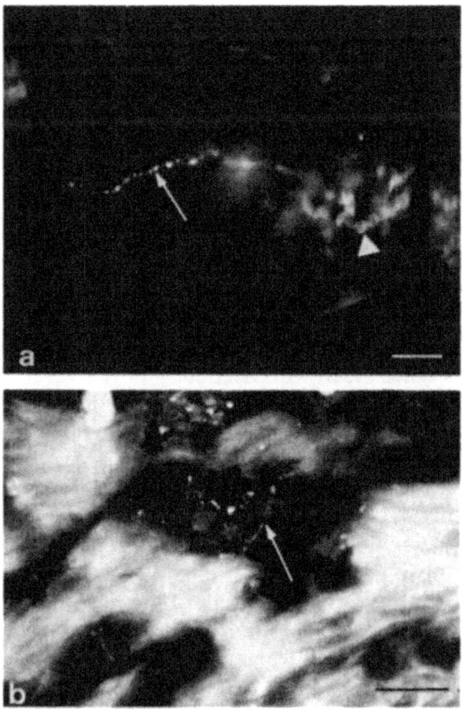



**Fig. 3.** Innervation to the ciliary body. **(a)** An SPLI nerve *(arrow)* extends along the core of a ciliary process in the rabbit eye. Blood elements autofluoresce *(arrowhead)*. **(b)** An SPLI nerve *(arrow)* is seen in association with a ciliary body melanocyte of the squirrel monkey eye. (Fluorescent micrographs; *bar*, 20 μ)

Unfortunately, just as is true for the adrenergic innervation, the histologic technique does not provide a tissue assignment sufficient to determine whether a nerve fiber serves the blood vessel, the epithelium or both. Yet favorable preparations reveal nerve fibers right at the basement membrane of the apical epithelium making neuropeptide diffusion to epithelial cells clearly possible. In this connection, substance P in the kidney exerts potent effects on salt and water excretion [47]. The search for a role for substance P in the ciliary process requires studies in this line.

Elsewhere in the ciliary body, SPLI innervation of melanocytes in a remarkable feature (Fig. 3b). Adrenergic neurons also innervate ciliary body and iris melanocytes [8]. Since the adrenergic innervation moderates iris pigment synthesis [7], it would be of interest to know whether substance P does likewise.

SPLI nerves are often present in the suprachoroid lamina. Blood vessels, particularly in the posterior ciliary body, also receive some SPLI nerves. Yet no nerves directly supplying the ciliary muscle are seen. Because of the proximity of muscle cells to melanocytes and blood vessels, however, the possibility of a minor SPLI innervation to ciliary muscle cannot be completely excluded at present.

*Iris*

The iris of all three animals contains a SPLI innervation, the nerve supply being richest in the rabbit. The rabbit peripheral iris has large nerve trunks, in which a fraction of the fibers stain for substance P (Fig. 4a). From these large trunks, SPLI nerve fibers issue to the layers of the iris.

SPLI nerves are present in the iris sphincter of all three animals. These nerves are seen with moderately high density in the rabbit (Fig. 4b). There is a slight but definite

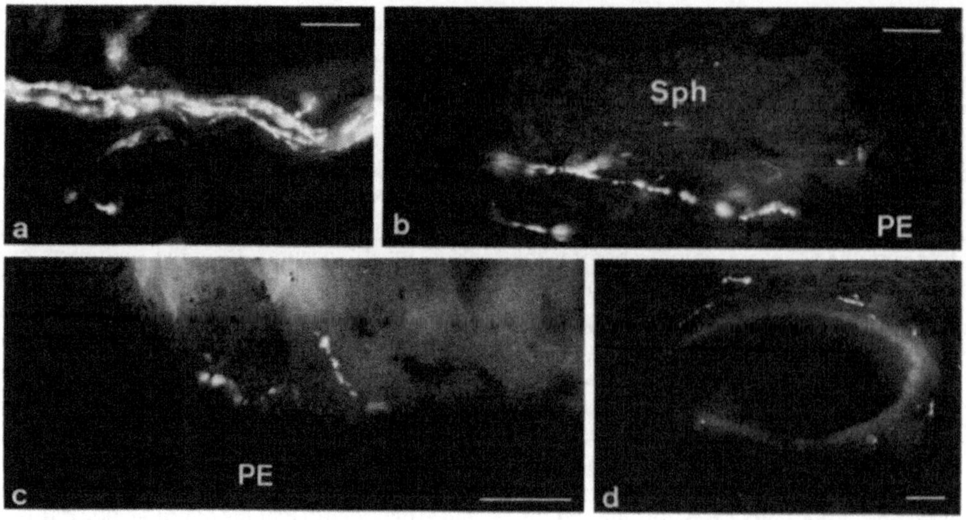


**Fig. 4.** Iris Nerves. **(a)** A nerve trunk in the rabbit iris contains SPLI nerves. Only a fraction of the fibers in such nerve trunks show immunoreactivity. **(b)** An SPLI nerve is seen in the iris sphincter muscle of the rabbit. **(c)** SPLI nerves run within the dilator muscle of the cat iris. **(d)** SPLI nerve fibers are seen frequently around large iris vessels, as illustrated here in the rabbit eye. *PE*, pigment epithelium; *Sph*, sphincter muscle; (Fluorescent micrographs; *bar*, 20 μ)

innervation in the cat; only a few fibers are seen in the monkey.

Even though the SPLI nerve density in the iris sphincter muscle is much less than the cholinergic nerve density, the iris sphincter's exquisite sensitivity to exogenous substance P [39] raises the question of whether or not the iris sphincter has still another visceral efferent supply. The known cholinergic muscarinic sphincter innervation mediates reflex pupillary constriction [48]. Anatomical and physiological evidence indicates that the lesser adrenergic innervation to the iris sphincter also participates in reflex dilatation [49]. In special circumstances, however the iris sphincter constricts by a mechanism that is neither cholinergic nor adrenergic. For instance, direct stimulation of the first division of the fifth cranial nerve induces pupillary constriction [50–53]. The topical application of noxious chemicals such as formaldehyde similarly induce miosis [54]. However, in contrast to cholinergic stimulation, atropine fails to block the pupillary response that follows either fifth nerve stimulation [51, 52] or the application of noxious chemicals [54]. Several experiments indicate that substance P may mediate these special pupillary responses [15–18, 39], and the demonstration of an SPLI innervation to the iris sphincter certainly provides additional evidence regarding a possible role for substance P in this phenomenon. Yet, presently available physiologic and anatomical studies still do not answer the question of whether or not there exists a third visceral efferent nerve supply to the iris sphincter. Clearly, whatever its role, the nature of the SPLI innervation to the iris sphincter differs from the previously described cholinergic and adrenergic innervation. Further studies clearly are needed.

SPLI nerves also are seen closely associated with the posterior iris epithelial layers and probably provide a modest innervation to the iris dilator (Fig. 4c). As in other iris structures, this innervation is most prominent in the rabbit. No physiological counterpart to this innervation is currently known.

The iris blood vessels of the rabbit have a prominent SPLI innervation; the larger vessels have the greatest nerve density (Fig. 4d). In the cat, the large vessels of the major arterial circle have a modest innervation. This innervation to iris may in some way be related to the breakdown in the blood-ocular barrier that occurs after intracameral injection of relatively large doses of substance P [17, 18].

In all three animals, SPLI nerves innervate iris stromal melanocytes, especially the melanocyte clusters at the anterior iris surface. Again, this innervation is most proment in the rabbit. The implication of iris melanocyte innervation is analogous to the ciliary melanocyte innervation just discussed. In the cat, an SPLI nerve fiber is occasionally seen among the deeper iris chromatophores but not among those more superficial. In contrast to melanocytes, SPLI nerves do not appear to innervate these cells.

## Overview

In general, the SPLI innervation to the cornea and sclera is less dense than the uveal innervation. Significantly, despite quantitative differences, such as a greater density of uveal innervation in the rabbit than in the cat and monkey, remarkable similarity is present among the three animals. Only in the aqueous outflow region, where the rabbit's innervation is largely confined to the pectinate ligament while that in the cat and monkey is more broadly distributed, does quantitative difference in innervation portend a possible functional difference. At present the meaning of the difference in the pattern innervation of the outflow pathways or of the quantitative differences among animals depends on physiological studies as yet undone.

With the large number of biologically active peptides already known, the present findings undoubtedly do not describe in full the peptidergic innervation of the anterior segment of the rabbit, cat, and primate eye. Yet, they do expand prior limits in knowledge indicating several potential roles for substance P while at the same time turning attention to the whole question of neuropeptides in the workings of the anterior segment of the eye.

Acknowledgments. Cheryl Wilson provided valuable technical assistance. This research was supported by a grant from the Pennsylvania Lions Sight Conservation and Eye Research Foundation, Inc., NEI grants 02942, 03444, and 04075, and the Gretel and Eugene Ormandy Teaching and Research Fund.

## References

1. Thompson HS (1981) Chap 12 The Pupil. In: Moses RA (ed) Adler's physiology of the eye. *7th edition. The CV Mosby Company,* St. Louis, pp 326–356
2. Alm A, Bill A (1973) The effect of stimulation of the sympathetic chain on retinal oxygen tension and uveal, retinal and cerebral blood flow in cats. Acta Physiol Scand 88:84–94
3. Uusitalo R, Palkama A (1971) Evidence for the nervous control of secretion in the ciliary processes. Prog Brain Res 34:513–521
4. Armaly MF (1959) Studies on intraocular effects of the orbital parasympathetic pathway III. Effect on steady-state dynamics. Arch Ophthalmol 62:817–829
5. Sears ML (1978) Perspectives in glaucoma research. Invest Ophthalmol Vis Sci 17:6–20
6. Laties AM, Jacobowitz D (1966) A comparative study of the autonomic innervation of the eye of the monkey, cat, and rabbit. Anat Rec 156:383–396
7. Laties AM (1974) Ocular melanin and the adrenergic innervation of the eye. Trans Am Ophthalmol Soc 72:560–605
8. Ehinger B, Falck B (1970) Innervation of iridic melanophores. Z Mikrosk Anat Forsch 105: 538–542
9. Phillips CI, Horwitt G, Rowlands DJ (1967) Propranolol as ocular hypotensive agent. Br J Ophthalmol 51:222–226
10. Hökfelt T, Johansson O, Ljungdahl Å, Lundberg JM, Schultzberg M (1980) Peptidergic neurons. Nature 284:515–521
11. Uddman R, Alumets J, Ehinger B, Håkanson R, Lorén I, Sundler F (1980) Vasoactive intestinal peptide nerves in ocular and orbital structures of the cat. Invest Ophthalmol Vis Sci 19:878–885
12. Ruskell GL (1970) An ocular parasympathetic nerve pathway of nerve origin and its influence on intraocular pressure. Exp Eye Res 10:319–330
13. Ruskell GL (1971) Facial parasympathetic innervation of the choroidal blood vessels in monkeys. Exp Eye Res 12:166–172
14. Stjernschantz J, Bill A (1980) Vasomotor effects of facial nerve stimulation: noncholinergic vasodilation in the eye. Acta Physiol Scand 109:45–50
15. Mandahl A, Bill A (1981) Ocular responses to antidromic trigeminal nerve stimulation, intracameral prostaglandin $E_1$ and $E_2$, capsaicin and substance P. Acta Physiol Scand 112:331–338
16. Stjernschantz J, Sears M, Stjernschantz L (1981) Intraocular effects of substance P in the rabbit. Invest Ophthalmol Vis Sci 20:53–60
17. Bill A, Stjernschantz J, Mandahl A, Brodin E, Nilsson G (1979) Substance P: release on trigeminal nerve stimulation, effects in the eye. Acta Physiol Scand 106:371–373
18. Holmdahl G, Håkanson R, Leander S, Rosell S, Folkers K, Sundler F (1981) A substance P antagonist, [D-Pro$^2$, D-Trp$^{7,9}$]SP, inhibits in-

flammatory responses in the rabbit eye. Science 214:1029–1031
19. Butler JM, Hammond BR (1980) The effects of sensory denervation on the responses of the rabbit eye to prostaglandin $E_1$, bradykinin and substance P. Br J Pharmac 69:495–502
20. Camras CB, Bito LZ (1980) The pathophysiological effects of nitrogen mustard on the rabbit eye. II. The inhibition of the initial hypertensive phase by capsaicin and the apparent role of substance P. Invest Ophthalmol Vis Sci 19:423–428
21. Butler JM, Powell D, Unger WG (1980) Substance P levels in normal and sensorily denervated rabbit eyes. Exp Eye Res 30:311–313
22. Brecha N, Karten HJ (1980) Localization of enkephalin, substance P, neurotensin and somatostatin immunoreactivity within amacrine cells of the retina. Anat Rec 196:225
23. Karten HJ, Brecha N (1980) Localization of substance P immunoreactivity in amacrine cells of the retina. Nature 283:87–88
24. Brecha N, Scharma SC, Karten HJ (1981) Localization of substance P-like immunoreactivity in the adult and developing goldfish retina. Neuroscience 6:2737–2746
25. Eskay RL, Furness JF, Long RT (1981) Substance P activity in bullfrog retina: localization and identification in several vetebrate species. Science 212:1049–1051
26. Hökfelt T, Johansson O, Kellerth J-O, Ljungdahl Å, Nilsson G, Nygårds A, Pernow B (1977) Immunohistochemical distribution of substance P. In: Euler US, Pernow B (eds) Substance P. Raven Press, New York, pp 117–145
27. Schultzberg M, Hökfelt T, Olson L, Ålund M, Nilsson G, Terenius L, Elde R, Goldstein M, Said S (1980) Substance P, VIP, enkephalin and somatostatin immunoreactive neurons in intestinal tissue transplanted to the anterior eye chamber. J Auton Nerv Syst 1:291–303
28. Neuhuber W, Groh V, Gottschall J, Celio MR (1981) The cornea is not innervated by substance P-containing primary afferent neurons. Neuroscience Letters 22:5–9
29. Tervo K, Tervo T, Eränkö L, Eränkö O (1981) Substance P immunoreactive nerves in the rodent cornea. Neuroscience Letters 25:95–97
30. Miller A, Costa M, Furness JB, Chubb IW (1981) Substance P-like immunoreactive sensory nerves supply the rat iris and cornea. Neuroscience Letters 23:243–249
31. Tervo K, Tervo T, Eränkö L, Eränkö O, Cuello AC (1981) Immunoreactivity for substance P in the Gasserian ganglion, ophthalmic nerve and anterior segment of the rabbit eye. Histochem J 13:435–443
32. Laties AM, Stone RA, Brecha NC (1981) Substance P-like immunoreactive nerve fibers in the trabecular meshwork. Invest Ophthalmol Vis Sci 21:484–486
33. Shimizu Y, Kuwayama Y, Fukuda M, Ishimoto I, Shiosaka S, Inagaki S, Takagi H, Sakanaka M, Senba E, Kawai Y, Takatsuki K, Tohyama T (1982) Localization of substance P-like immunoreactivity in the anterior eye segment of squirrels: an immunohistochemical analysis. Invest Ophthalmol Vis Sci 22:259–263
34. Tornqvist K, Mandahl A, Leander S, Lorén I, Håkanson R, Sundler F (1982) Substance P-immunoreactive nerve fibers in the anterior segment of rabbit eye. Cell Tissue Res 222: 467–477
35. Stone RA, Laties AM, Brecha N (1982) Substance P-like immunoreactive nerves in the anterior segment of the rabbit, cat and monkey eye. Neuroscience 7:2459–2468
36. McLean IW, Nakane PK (1974) Periodate-lysine-paraformaldehyde fixative: a new fixative for immunoelectron microscopy. J Histochem Cytochem 22:1077–1083
37. Hökfelt T, Lundberg JM, Schultzberg M, Johansson O, Skirboll L, Änggård A, Fredholm B, Hamberger B, Pernow B, Rehfeld J, Goldstein M (1980) Cellular localization of peptides in neural structures. Proc R Soc Lond [Biol] 210:63–76
38. Cuello AC, Galfre G, Milstein C (1979) Detection of substance P in the central nervous system by a monoclonal antibody. Proc Nat Acad Sci USA 76:3532–3536
39. Soloway MR, Stjernschantz J, Sears M (1981) The miotic effect of substance P on the isolated rabbit iris. Invest Ophthalmol Vis Sci 20:47–52
40. Wolter JR (1957) Innervation of the corneal endothelium of the eye of rabbit. Arch Ophthalmol 58:246–250
41. Léon-Felíu E, Gómez-Ramos P, Rodríguez-Echandía (1978) Endothelial nerve fibers in the cornea of the frog *Rana ridibunda.* Experientia 34:1352–1353
42. Raviola G (1982) Schwalbe line's cells. A new cell type in the trabecular meshwork of *Macaca mulatta.* Invest Ophthalmol Vis Sci 22:45–56
43. Lundberg JM, Hökfelt T, Fahrenkrug J, Nilsson G, Terenius L (1979) Peptides in the cat carotid body (glomus caroticum): VIP-, enkephalin-, and substance P-like immunoreactivity. Acta Physiol Scand 107:279–281
44. Lundberg JM, Hökfelt T, Ånggard A, Pernow B, Emson P (1979) Immunohistochemical evidence for substance P immunoreactive nerve fibers in taste buds of the cat. Acta Physiol Scand 107:389–391

45. Gillis RA, Helke CJ, Hamilton BL, Norman WP, Jacobowitz DM (1980) Evidence that substance P is a neurotransmitter of baro- and chemoreceptor afferents in nucleus tractus solitarius. Brain Res 181:476–481
46. Haeusler G, Osterwalder R (1980) Is substance P the transmitter at the first synapse of the baroreceptor reflex in rats and cats? Clinical Science 59:295s-297s
47. Gullner HG, Campbell WB, Pettinger WA (1979) Role of substance P in water hemeostasis. Life Sciences 24:2351-2360
48. Loewenfeld IE (1958) Mechanisms of reflex dilatation of the pupil. Doc Ophthalmol 12:185–448
49. Schaeppi U, Koella WP (1964) Adrenergic innervation of the cat iris sphincter. Am J Physiol 207:273-278
50. Magendie F (1824) De l'influence de la cinquieme paire de nerfs sur la nutrition et les fonctions de l'oeil. J Physiol Exp Pathol 4:176-182
51. Bernard C (1858) Lecons sur la Physiologie et la Pathologie du Système Nerveux. Vol 2. Baillière, Paris, pp 205
52. Perkins ES (1957) Influence of the fifth cranial nerve on the intraocular pressure of the rabbit eye. Br J Ophthalmol 41:257-300
53. Stjernschantz J, Geijer C, Bill A (1979) Electrical stimulation of the fifth cranial nerve in rabbits: effects on ocular blood flow, extravascular albumen content and intraocular pressure. Exp Eye Res 28:229-238
54. Butler JM, Unger WG, Hammond BR (1979) Sensory mediation of the ocular response to neutral formaldehyde. Exp Eye Res 28:577-589
55. Hökfelt T, Kellerth JO, Nilsson G, Pernow B (1975) Substance P: localization in the central nervous system and in some primary seneory neurons. Science 109:889-890

## Discussion

**Mishima to Stone:** Substance P may be involved in the manifestation of the irritative responses after autidromic stimulation of the nerves of application of chemical irritants. Is it possible to show changes in the substance P nerves by your technologies, after application of the irritants or nerve stimulation?

**Stone to Mishima:** Yes, at least in one special instance. If either manipulation severely depleted the neuronal content of substance P, then we would not get a reaction product and the slides would be blank. However, our technique is not quantitative, and a more modest change of concentration likely would be missed. We have not performed these experiments at present.

Krieglstein G.K./Leydhecker W. (eds)
Glaucoma Update II


# Ocular Effects of Vanadate[1]

T. Krupin, St. Louis, S.M. Podos, New York, and B. Becker, St. Louis

Sodium-potassium-activated adenosine triphosphatase ($Na^+$, $K^+$), ATPase, was first described in the crab nerve by Skou in 1957 [1]. The role of the enzyme in the formation of aqueous humor has been investigated in various laboratory animals and man. ($Na^+$, $K^+$) ATPase has been shown to be active in the re-establishment of membrane potentials after depolarization and in the formation of certain secreted fluids, including aqueous humor.

A ouabain-sensitive ($Na^+$, $K^+$) ATPase has been demonstrated in the ciliary epithelium [2, 3]. Cytochemical localization of the enzyme in the nonpigmented ciliary epithelium has been demonstrated by routine histochemistry [4] and by electron microscopy [5]. These studies used lead as the trapping ion. Lead not only inhibited the enzyme but also induced nonenzymatic hydrolysis of ATP. Using Ernst nitrophenylphosphate as the substrate with strontium as the capture ion, Ritch et al. demonstrated reaction products on the basal infoldings of both the inner nonpigmented as well as the outer pigmented ciliary epithelium [6]. Treatment of the specimens with ouabain or vanadate reduced the accumulation of reaction products.

Potent inhibitors of ($Na^+$, $K^+$) ATPase such as ouabain, lowered the rate of aqueous humor formation in rabbits [7], cats [3] and humans [3]. Lowering intraocular pressure (IOP) required systemic administration. The cardiac glycosides proved ineffective following topical administration. However, intravitreal injection of ouabain in rabbits produced a unilateral decrease in IOP [7]. Vanadate, a potent inhibitor of ($Na^+$, $K^+$) ATPase [8, 9], reduced IOP following topical administration to the eyes of rabbits and monkeys [10, 11]. This paper reviews our experience with the effects of vanadate on aqueous humor dynamics and on ciliary epithelium biochemical mechanisms.

## Vanadate

Vanadate has been demonstrated as an ubiquitous element found in the earth's crust, air, seawater, soil and the tissues of man and animals [12]. On usual diets, humans consumed 1 to 4 mg of vanadium per day. In human experiments no toxicity was noted after oral doses of 22 mg/day for five months except for the occurrence of a "green tongue" [13]. Vanadate has been reported to be a panacea for numerous medical conditions [14, 15].

Recent interest in vanadate originated with its identification as a contaminant in a commercial preparation of adenosine triphosphate derived from rabbit or equine muscle [8]. Vanadate has been shown to have a wide range of biochemical and pharmacological activities. It inhibited several ATPases [16, 17], acid and alkaline phosphatases [18, 19], and adenylate kinase [20]. Most significantly, vanadate proved to be a reversible inhibitor of membrane ($Na^+$, $K^+$) ATPase. It appeared to bind to the cytoplasmic surface of the membrane in contrast to ouabain which adhered to the extracellular membrane surface. In addition, vanadate decreased phosphofructokinase activity [21] and cholesterol synthesis [22], stimulated adenylate cyclase [23], and affected glucose metabolism of many tissues [24].

### *In vivo Studies*

Vanadate administered topically as sodium metavanadate ($NaVO_3$) or sodium ortho-

[1] This study was support in part by Research grants EY 00004, EY 03651, EY 01867, and a Research Career Development Award EY 00082 (Dr. Krupin) from the National Institute of Health, Bethesda, Maryland

vanadate ($Na_3VO_4$) lowered IOP in rabbits [10]. The mean IOP in unanesthetized rabbits was significantly lower 60 minutes following unilateral administration of $NaVO_3$ (1% or 2%) or $Na_3VO_4$ (0.3%, 0.5%, 1.0% or 2.0%), and the reductions persisted for at least 240 minutes. The mean baseline IOP in eight rabbits receiving 0.5% $Na_3VO_4$ was $17.0 \pm 0.9$ mmHg ($\pm$ SEM). IOP was significantly ($p < 0.01$) reduced at 60 minutes, $12.2 \pm 0.7$ mmHg, 120 minutes, $12.3 \pm 0.7$ mmHg, and 240 minutes, $13.5 \pm 0.7$ mmHg. IOP in the contralateral diluent treated control eyes was not altered during the testing interval.

Topically administered vanadate did not alter tonographic outflow facility. Episcleral venous pressure, as measured with a 3 mm applanating head attached to a force-displacement transducer and mounted on a Haag-Streit biomicroscope, was not altered two hours after topically administered 1% vanadate. Using the equation $F = (P_o - P_v)\,C$, aqueous humor flow averaged 1.9 µl/min in control eyes and 1.3 µl/min in vanadate-treated eyes. This represented a mean decrease two hours after topical 1% vanadate of approximately 30%.

After topically applied vanadate posterior chamber aqueous humor ascorbate concentration increased, compatible with a decreased entry of water into the posterior chamber. Two hours after unilateral topical $Na_3VO_4$ 0.5% anterior chamber ascorbate was similar in treated, $25.5 \pm 2.0$ mg/dl, and control, $25.0 \pm 1.9$ mg/dl, eyes. However, posterior chamber aqueous humor ascorbate was significantly ($p < 0.01$) higher in the treated, $41.1 \pm 2.3$ mg/dl, than in the control, $34.0 \pm 3.0$ mg/dl, eyes. Since the new anterior chamber steady-state value for ascorbate might not have been reached at two hours; the reduction in $k_{fa}/k_{dpa}$ could only be approximated at about 40%.

Vanadate has been noted to stimulate adenylate cyclase activity in isolated membrane preparations [23]. However, anterior chamber cyclic AMP was not different comparing treated and control eyes of nine rabbits that had received unilateral 0.5% $Na_3VO_4$. Cyclic AMP or its analogs have been reported to increase outflow facility [25]. The absence of increased outflow facility or elevation of aqueous humor cyclic AMP following topical administration of $Na_3VO_4$ implied that in rabbits the ocular effect of vanadate was not related to adenylate cyclase stimulation. In amphibian epithelia vanadate blocked cyclic AMP-induced stimulation of water and sodium transported [26]. This suggested a site of action beyond cyclic AMP generation which might be a mechanism by which vanadate could reduce the production of aqueous humor.

Vanadate has been reported to have vasoconstrictor action [27]. Ocular blood flow was measured in six rabbits three hours following unilateral delivery of 0.5% $Na_3VO_4$. The method used was that described by Alm and Bill [28] using radioactive microspheres injected directly into the left ventricle of artifically ventilated rabbits. Blood flow was similar in the iris-ciliary body, retina, choroid and optic nerve of the treated and control eyes.

An interaction between vanadate and catecholamines has been described due to a complexation and direct chemical reduction of vanadate to vanadyl by the catecholamine [29]. In rabbits topical epinephrine promptly reversed the IOP-lowering effects of vanadate. The measured increased secretion of aqueous humor following topical epinephrine administration to human eyes [30] might be related to reduced endogenous vanadate levels by the administered epinephrine with subsequent increased aqueous humor secretion.

The effects of vanadate on the sodium pump have been shown to be dependent on its state of oxidation [31]. Vanadate was reduced by ascorbate so that it no longer inhibited renal ($Na^+$, $K^+$) ATPase. Thus, in the eye, the high aqueous humor concentrations of ascorbate and its responsiveness to plasma levels might regulate the ciliary epithelial ($Na^+$, $K^+$) ATPase inhibition by vanadate. While subcutaneous or intravenous administration of isotonic ascorbate failed to alter IOP in rabbits, the similar injection of ascorbate prevented or partially reversed the lowering of IOP induced by topical vanadate [11].

### *In vitro Studies*

Ouabain-sensitive rubidium-86 ($^{86}Rb^+$) uptake by tissue slices has been used as an estimate of $Na^+ : K^+$ pump activity. ($Na^+$, $K^+$) ATPase, the enzymatic representation of the $Na^+$-pump, has been described as oriented within the plasma membrane of many ion-secreting and ion-transporting cell types as well as nervous tissue cells. The sodium activation site was at the cytoplasmic surface while the potassium activation site was at the extracellular surface. Uptake of $Rb^+$ was handled by the $Na^+ : K^+$ pump in the same manner as potassium. Ouabain was believed to prevent binding of potassium to the enzyme at the extracellular surface, whereas vanadate appeared to act at the intracellular site [32].

Rabbit iris-ciliary body (I-CB) preparations incubated in vitro for one hour in Tyrode's solution at 37 °C accumulated trace amounts of $^{86}Rb^+$ to a concentration averaging 20 times that of the incubation medium [11, 33]. This accumulation was time- and temperature-dependent, competively inhibited by potassium, and demonstrated saturation kinetics with nonlabeled rubidium. Ouabain $10^{-3}$ M inhibited 87% of the $^{86}Rb^+$ accumulation while ouabain $5 \times 10^{-7}$ M inhibited uptake by 50%. Higher concentrations of vanadate ($3 \times 10^{-3}$ M) were required to produce 50% inhibition of accumulation. The necessary higher vanadate concentration was probably related to the need for vanadate to be transported into the cell where it inhibited the cytoplasmic portion of the enzyme.

Membrane preparations from I-CBs were used to measure ATPase activity. Briefly, incubation of the tissue preparation was carried out with ATP and ATPase activity was measured by determining the liberated phosphate (Pi). Control determinations from 18 assays of rabbit I-CB membrane preparations showed $35.2 \pm 1.1$ of Pi liberated $hr^{-1}$ $mg^{-1}$ protein. Of the total ATPase activity ($Mg^+$ plus $Na^+, K^+$) $39.3 \pm 1.5\%$ was ouabain ($10^{-3}$ M) sensitive indicating the ($Na^+$, $K^+$) ATPase portion. The addition of vanadate to the assay mixture resulted in an inhibition greater than that observed with ouabain $10^{-3}$ M. In four preparations control activity (Pi liberated $hr^{-1}$ $mg^{-1}$ protein) was $32.2 \pm 1.7$. Ouabain $10^{-3}$ M reduced Pi liberation to $20.5 \pm 0.2$ ($35.8 \pm 5.8\%$). Vanadate $10^{-4}$ M reduced Pi liberation to $23.0 \pm 2.2$ while $10^{-3}$ M reduced Pi liberation to $16.4 \pm 0.8$. This greater reduction with vanadate $10^{-3}$ M than that observed with ouabain $10^{-3}$ M suggested a vanadate inhibition greater than just the ($Na^+$, $K^+$) ATPase fraction. $HCO_3^-$-ATPase was determined in the presence of ouabain $10^{-3}$ M to inhibit the ($Na^+$, $K^+$) ATPase component with the addition of sodium bicarbonate to the incubation mixture. Control $HCO_3^-$-ATPase (Pi liberated $hr^{-1}$ $mg^{-1}$ protein) in 18 rabbit I-CB membrane preparations was $3.3 \pm 0.4$. The addition of vanadate reduced $HCO_3^-$-ATPase activity at $10^{-5}$ M, $2.2 \pm 0.3$, and $10^{-4}$ M, $0.72 \pm 0.1$.

Topical vanadate did not elevate anterior aqueous humor cyclic AMP. However, since vanadate has been reported to stimulate adenylate cyclase, this was studied in vitro in rabbit iris-ciliary body homogenates [34]. In three experiments the basal adenylate cyclase activity was $220 \pm 50$ pmoles/mg/min. Vanadate $10^{-3}$ M increased this activity by 77 $\pm$ 5%. The significance of this observation on vanadate's effect on aqueous humor dynamics remained uncertain since this agent did not increase outflow facility, the effect observed following intracameral injection of cyclic AMP or its analogs [25].

Renal organic anion transport systems were linked in a direct manner to the function of ($Na^+$, $K^+$) ATPase [35]. In vitro accumulation of either $^3$H-PAH or $^{131}$I-hippuran by the rabbit I-CB also demonstrated a relationship between this enzyme activity and organic anion transport. Control $^3$H-PAH accumulation after one hour incubation in Tyrode's medium at 37 °C showed a tissue to medium ratio (T/M) of $12.6 \pm 1.1$. The addition of ouabain $2 \times 10^{-7}$ M or vanadate $10^{-4}$ M resulted in 50% inhibition of the T/M ratio. Control accumulation of $^{131}$I-hippuran under similar test conditions resulted in a T/M ratio of $10.0 \pm 1.2$. Inhibition was reduced 50% by ouabain $5 \times 10^{-6}$ M or vanadate $10^{-3}$ M. The higher concentrations required for vanadate probably related to vanadate's intracellular site of action on ($Na^+$, $K^+$) ATPase.

**Conclusion of Rabbit Data**

The mechanism by which topical vanadate lowers IOP in the rabbits, presumably by inhibition of aqueous humor secretion, remains unknown. Our data do not suggest a systemic effect since the reduction of IOP is unilateral. The in vitro studies demonstrate that vanadate is an inhibitor of ciliary body ($Na^+$, $K^+$) ATPase as measured with $^{86}Rb^+$ accumulation or direct ($Na^+$, $K^+$) ATPase measurement. However, in addition vanadate also inhibits $HCO_3^-$-ATPase and stimulates adeny-

**Table 1.** Topical vanadate and intraocular pressure in untreated ocular hypertensive patients

| Vanadate concentration | No. | Intraocular pressure (mean mmHg ± SEM) Baseline | Time after Vanadate 1 h | 4 h |
|---|---|---|---|---|
| 0.5% | 5 | 22.7 ± 1.4 | 21.4 ± 1.2 | 22.2 ± 1.0 |
| Diluent | | 23.4 ± 1.2 | 20.6 ± 1.3 | 22.2 ± 1.0 |
| 1.0% | 5 | 26.8 ± 1.8 | 26.0 ± 2.4 | 24.6 ± 3.1 |
| Diluent | | 25.1 ± 1.6 | 26.4 ± 1.8 | 25.4 ± 2.0 |
| 1.5% | 5 | 25.6 ± 3.9 | 23.4 ± 3.4 | 22.8 ± 3.0 |
| Diluent | | 23.6 ± 2.8 | 21.8 ± 2.8 | 22.8 ± 1.4 |

late cyclase activity. The relationship of the latter two observations to aqueous humor secretion is unknown. The effects of ($Na^+$, $K^+$) ATPase inhibitors and the I-CB in vitro organic anion transport system require in vivo studies to determine possible physiologic significance. Since traces of vanadate occur widely in animal tissues, it may constitute "a natural mechanism" for regulation of ($Na^+$, $K^+$) ATPase activity in vivo [8].

## Topical Vanadate in Patients with Ocular Hypertension

Topical vanadate 0.5%, 1.0% or 1.5% was studied in three groups of ocular hypertensive patients, five subjects per group. These patients were not receiving anti-glaucoma therapy. Vanadate was randomly delivered to one eye (Table 1). Vanadate 0.5% resulted in no reduction in IOP. The responses following 1.0% or 1.5% were minimal. The number of patients was too small for statistical analysis; however, vanadate's IOP effect in patients was markedly less than in rabbits.

A number of possible reasons for this included: a) Vanadate penetrated poorly in humans and thus insufficient drug entered the eye. b) Normal vanadate tissue levels were higher in humans so that additional topically applied vanadate was ineffective. c) Aqueous humor levels of ascorbate or epinephrine in humans inactivated the vanadate. d) Inhibitors of ($Na^+$, $K^+$) ATPase might not be effective agents for reducing aqueous humor production in humans.

## References


1. Skou JC (1957) The influence of some cations on an adenosine triphosphatase from peripheral nerves. Biochim Biophys Acta 23:394
2. Riley MV (1964) The sodium-potassium-stimulated adenosine triphosphatase of rabbit ciliary epithelium. Exp Eye Res 3:76
3. Simon KA, Bonting SL, Hawkins NM (1962) Studies on sodium-potassium-activated adenosine triphosphatase. II. Formation of aqueous humor. Exp Eye Res 1:253
4. Cole DF (1964) Location of ouabain-sensitive adenosine triphosphatase in ciliary epithelium. Exp Eye Res 3:72
5. Kaye GI, Pappas GD (1965) Studies on the ciliary epithelium and zonule. III. The fine structure of the rabbit ciliary epithelium in relation to the localization of ATPase activity. J Microscopie 4:497
6. Ritch R, Brodsky WA, Mermelstein J, Pokorny K, Shabto U, Podos SM (1980) Localization and vanadate inhibition of ciliary NaK-ATPase. Invest Ophthalmol Vis Sci, ARVO [Suppl] p 173
7. Becker B (1963) Ouabain and aqueous humor dynamics in the rabbit eye. Invest Ophthalmol 2:325
8. Cantley LC Jr, Josephson L, Warner R, Yanagisawa M, Lechene C, Guidotti G (1977) Vanadate is a potent (Na, K)-ATPase inhibitor found in ATP derived from muscle. J Biol Chem 252:7421
9. Bond GH, Hudgins PM (1979) Kinetics of inhibition of Na K-ATPase by $Mg^{2+}$, $K^+$, and vanadate. Am Chem Soc 18:325
10. Krupin T, Becker B, Podos SM (1980) Topical vanadate lowers intraocular pressure in rabbits. Invest Ophthalmol Vis Sci 19:1360
11. Becker B (1980) Vanadate and aqueous humor

dynamics: Proctor Lecture. Invest Ophthalmol Vis Sci 19:1156
12. Schroeder HA, Balassa JJ, Tipton IH (1963) Abnormal trace metals in man-vanadium. J Chronic Dis 16:1047
13. Somerville J, Davies B (1962) Effect of vanadium on serum cholesterol. Am Heart J 64:54
14. Berthail V (1899) Résultats Thérapeutiques de l'emploi des sels de vanadium. Thesis, Lyon
15. Proescher F, Seil HA, Stillians AW (1917) A contribution to the action of vanadium with particular reference to syphilis. Am J Syphilis 1:347
16. Goodno CC (1979) Inhibition of myosin ATPase by vanadate ion. Proc Natl Acad Sci USA 74:2620
17. Bond GH, Hudgins PA (1980) Inhibition of Red Cell $Ca^{2+}$-ATPase by vanadate. Biochim Biophys Acta 600:781
18. Etten RL van, Waymack PP, Rehkop DM (1974) Transition metal ion inhibition of enzyme-catalyzed phosphate ester displacement reactions. J Am Chem Soc 96:6782
19. Lopez V, Stevens T, Lindquist RN (1976) Vanadium ion inhibition of alkaline phosphatase-catalyzed phosphate ester hydrolysis. Arch Biochem Biophys 175:31
20. DeMaster EG, Mitchell RA (1973) A comparison of arsenate and vanadate as inhibitors of uncouplers of mitochondrial and glycolytic energy metabolism. Biochemistry 12:3616
21. Choate GL, Mansour TE (1978) Inhibition of sheep heart phosphofructokinase by ortho vanadate. Fed Proc 37:1433
22. Azarnoff DL, Brock FE, Curran GL (1961) A specific site of vanadium inhibition of cholesterol biosynthesis. Biochim Biophys Acta 51:397
23. Schwabe U, Puchstein C, Hannemann H, Sochtig E (1979) Activation of adenylate cyclase by vanadate. Nature 277:143
24. Tolman EL, Barris E, Burns M, Pansini A, Partridge R (1979) Effects of vanadium on glucose metabolism in vitro. Life Sci 25:1159
25. Neufeld AH (1978) Influences of cyclic nucleotides on outflow facility in the vervet monkey. Exp Eye Res 27:387
26. De Sousa RC, Grosso A (1979) Vanadate blocks cyclic AMP-induced stimulation of sodium and water transport in amphibian epithelia. Nature 279:803
27. Jackson DE (1911) The pharmacological action of vanadium. J Pharmacol 3:477
28. Alm A, Bill A (1972) The oxygen supply to the retina. II. Effects of high intraocular pressure and of increased arterial carbon dioxide tension on uveal and retinal blood flow in cats. Acta Physiol Scand 84:306
29. Cantley LC, Ferguson JH, Kustin K (1978) Norepinephrine complexes reduces vanadium (V) to reverse vanadate inhibition of the (Na, K)-ATPase. J Am Chem Soc 100:5210
30. Townsend DJ, Brubaker RF (1980) Immediate effects of epinephrine on aqueous formation in the normal human eye as measured by fluorophotometry. Invest Ophthalmol Vis Sci 19:256
31. Grantham JJ, Glynn IM (1979) Renal Na, K-ATPase: determinants of inhibition by vanadium. Am J Physiol 236:F530
32. Cantley LC Jr, Resh MD, Guidotti G (1978) Vanadate inhibits the red cell ($Na^+$, $K^+$) ATPase from the cytoplasmic side. Nature 272:552
33. Krupin T, Fritz CA, Becker B (submitted for publication) In vitro accumulation of rubidium-86 by the rabbit anterior uveal tissue
34. Mittag T (personal communication)
35. Sheikh MI, Maxild J, Møller JV (1981) Effect of vanadate on the renal accumulation of p-aminohippurate in the rabbit kidney tubules in vitro. Biochem Pharmacol 30:2141

## Discussion

**Kolker to Krupin:** Did patients with the "green tongue" toxicity syndrome have their IOP's measured while on vanadate?

**Krupin to Kolker:** No.

Krieglstein G.K./Leydhecker W. (eds)
Glaucoma Update II


# The Biology of the Aqueous Humor[1]

J. Herschler and J. Burke, Tucson

Classic thinking about the causes for increased intraocular pressure in patients with open angle glaucoma have been mechanical in orientation. Mechanistic analogies to the obstructions of drain pipes fit well with our current understanding of the pathophysiology of angle closure glaucoma.

However, "plumbing theory" as applied to the pathophysiology of open angle glaucoma, although attractive conceptually, has not been verified histopathologically in any convincing manner, no matter how great the magnification used. The trabecular meshwork of eyes from elderly patients with and without glaucoma have no significant morphological differences.

There is a paucity of information concerning the role that the fluid (aqueous humor) may play in the obstructive phenomena. Thus, if gross abnormalities such as cells or flare are not present, the clinician tends to assume all aqueous is the same. However, several laboratory studies suggest that aqueous humor is not an inert fluid. For example, biochemical analysis of aqueous humor has identified high molecular weight lens protein as a cause of elevated intraocular pressure in phacolytic glaucoma [1]. Further, ascorbic acid concentration has been reported to differ from normal in chronic open angle glaucoma, but this finding has not been repeatable [2].

Laboratory work has also shown that aqueous humor can effect the growth and maturation of various types of cells [3, 4, 5]. In 1980, we first reported that biological activity of aqueous varied from one glaucoma patient to another and between glaucomas and normals [6]. The study was undertaken to determine why filtration fistulas might remain open in some patients but not in others. In addition, we were looking for insight into why pressure regulation returns to normal following an operation in which a hole is made in the scleral coat of the globe.

Using a qualitative model to detect whether outgrowth occurred from an explant of Tenon's capsule in the presence of the patient's own aqueous humor, we were able to detect differences between glaucoma patients and cataract patients. Indeed, a difference was detected between glaucoma patients in whom filtration surgery was successful and those in whom the same surgical procedures failed. In successful glaucoma patients, explant outgrowth did not occur in aqueous humor, whereas explants from patients in whom failure of filtration occurred tended to show outgrowth.

In an experimental filtration operation in monkeys, we showed by sampling pre- and post-operative aqueous and Tenon's capsule that the aqueous humor was the dominant force, rather than the responding tissue, in determining whether growth of explants occurred [7].

For the past two years, we have been investigating growth effects of aqueous humor in a quantitative manner. Rather than employing explants of Tenon's capsule, monolayer fibroblast cultures derived from the explants were tested for responsiveness to varying concentrations of aqueous (0 to 100%). The cell cultures were incubated in aqueous-containing or aqueous-free media for 24 hours. Tritiated thymidine, which is incorporated into cells preparing for division, was present in the medium. Exposure to as little as 2% aqueous humor increased the number of proliferating cells over control cultures. Maximal stimulation occurred in 20% aqueous and the proliferation rate remained elevated through 100% aqueous.

[1] This study was supported by Public Health Service Research Grant EY 03655 from the National Eye Institute, National Institutes of Health, Bethesda, Maryland

How can the stimulatory activity we have found in our most recent work be reconciled with our previous reports of inhibitory activity? In part, the conflicting observations may be due to differences in the experimental procedures. In the previous studies, aqueous effects on long term cultures (14 days) of explanted tissue were examined. In the more recent experiments, short term monolayer fibroblast cultures (24 hours) were used. However, the observations may not be so conflicting as they initially appear. We have observed that exposure of fibroblast cell cultures to high concentrations of aqueous humor reduces cell survival. Cultures exposed to 50% aqueous, for example, have fewer cells surviving, but an elevated labeling rate in the surviving cells. In long term cultures of this type, the net effect may be no increase in cell number - an apparent inhibition of growth.

What does this mean? Our current feeling is that aqueous should be considered as a modulator of growth in which stimulatory agent(s) and cytotoxic factor(s) act in concert to affect changes in cell number, morphology and function. Understanding the nature of these modulators and their functions may provide the key to solving the problems of glaucoma filtration operations and perhaps glaucoma itself.

It is possible that derangement of the modulator system or other nutritional factors in the aqueous may be causative in decreasing outflow facility in chronic open angle glaucoma. One plausible hypothesis is that the composition of the aqueous humor is altered in some individuals leading to changes in the proliferative capacity, biosynthetic properties and ultimately the survival of cells of the trabecular meshwork resulting in an increased resistance to outflow.

## References


1. Epstein DL, Jedziniak JA, Grant WM (1978) Identification of heavy molecular weight soluble protein in aqueous humor in human phacolytic glaucoma. Invest Ophthalmol 17:398–402
2. Lam KW, Lee PF (1975) Analysis of ascorbate concentration in the aqueous humor by high pressure liquid chromatography. Invest Ophthalmol 14:947–950
3. Kornblueth W, Tenenbaum E (1956) The inhibitory effect of aqueous humor on growth of cells in tissue cultures. Am J Ophthalmol 42:70
4. Albrink WS, Wallace AC (1951) Aqueous humor as a tissue culture nutrient. Proc Soc Exp Biol Med 77:754
5. Benezra D, Sachs U (1974) Growth factors in aqueous humor of normal and inflamed eyes of rabbits. Invest Ophthalmol 13:868–870
6. Herschler J, Claflin AJ, Fiorentino G (1980) The effect of aqueous humor on the growth of subconjunctival fibroblasts in tissue culture and its implications for glaucoma surgery. Am J Ophthalmol 89:245–249
7. Radius RL, Herschler J, Claflin A, Fiorentino G (1980) Aqueous humor changes following experimental filtration surgery. Am J Ophthalmol 89:250–254


## Discussion

**Spaeth to Herschler:** Dr. Herschler is to congratulated on this important work. We have also been studying the effect of aqueous humor on cultured cells from episcleral tissue. In our studies we have noted that freezing the aqueous humor, or storing it for a prolonged period prior to utilizing it in the experimental technique appears to change its effect. Has Dr. Herschler noted that freezing aqueous alters its effect on tissue culture?

**Leydhecker to Herschler:** Did you investigate the influence of age? Clinically we see very often cicatrization in young patients after filtering surgery, much more often than in the elderly. In reoperations one sees that it is the subconjunctival tissue which forms the cicatrization, and not the conjunctiva. For this reason I excise the subconjunctival tissue as much as possible in patients with a tendency for cicatrization of filtering scars, for example in re-operations, or in patients below 40 years of age. However, in re-operations this excision does not prevent cicatrization, as one might have hoped, but I think that the cicatrization rate is lower than if I would not have excised the tissue.

Krieglstein G.K./Leydhecker W. (eds)
Glaucoma Update II


# Medical and Surgical Alterations in Outflow Facility[1]

A. Bill, B. Svedbergh, K. Ujie and T. Hamanaka, Uppsala, Maebashi

In high tension open angle glaucoma, as in most other glaucomas, there is a low facility of outflow resulting in a high IOP. Electron microscopy has indicated abnormalities in the drainage routes. It would be natural then to start therapy by attempts at increasing the facility and the ideal drug, of course, would be one that restituted facility to its normal level and the outflow routes to their normal appearance. The search for such an agent is very much hindered by the lack of understanding of the glaucomatous process in the chamber angle. At present we really do not know if the routes between the anterior chamber and the canal of Schlemm are reduced in number or size and if the critical region is in the juxtacanalicular, cribiform, part of the routes or within the uveal and corneoscleral meshwork.

The pathways from the anterior chamber into the canal of Schlemm are very complex. In a single section for light or electron microscopy one never finds a complete or nearly complete channel leading from the chamber into the canal. What can be seen is a large number of compartments. In serial sections it becomes clear that many of the compartments communicate and experiments with perfusion of the outflow routes with particles in gelatine have demonstrated that after 20 minutes almost all of the open spaces in the uveal and corneoscleral meshwork have been filled (Svedbergh and Bill, unpublished).

Recent experiments with filling of the outflow routes with a low viscosity plastic, subsequent dissolution of the tissue in KOH and scanning electron microscopy of the casts support the opinion (Bill and Svedbergh 1972) that the narrowest part is close to the canal of Schlemm, Fig. 1. The intertrabecular spaces communicated in such a way that they formed a system of flat pathways through the uveal and corneoscleral meshwork. In the uveal meshwork and the inner parts of the corneoscleral meshwork the intertrabecular channels confluenced at many places; the main direction was essentially parallel to that of the canal of Schlemm.

In the outer parts of the corneoscleral meshwork the intertrabecular channels were very flat and in the juxtacanalicular region there was irregular filling indicating very narrow passages. On casts of the canal of Schlemm one could see relatively few, 200–300, connections to the juxtacanalicular region. These connections probably represent the widest routes draining aqueous into the canal of Schlemm: wide invaginations into endothelial cells of the inner wall with 2–3 µm pores into the canal of Schlemm.

Agents which markedly increase the outflow facility are likely to do so by affecting the juxtacanalicular tissue either by increasing the conductance in the physiological routes or by creating new routes.

## Pilocarpine

During the last few years it has become quite clear that in primates the facility increasing effect of pilocarpine is due to its effect on the ciliary muscle and not to direct effects on the meshwork or the inner wall of Schlemm's canal. The basis for our understanding is the study by Kaufmann and Bárány (1976a, b) that demonstrated that after disinsertion of the ciliary muscle from the trabecular meshwork pilocarpine lost practically all of its effect.

It was suggested long ago (see Leydhekker, 1960) that the effect of pilocarpine on the outflow routes for aqueous humor were due

[1] Supported by US PHS Grant EY-00475 and a Grant B82-14X-00147 from the Swedish Medical Research Council

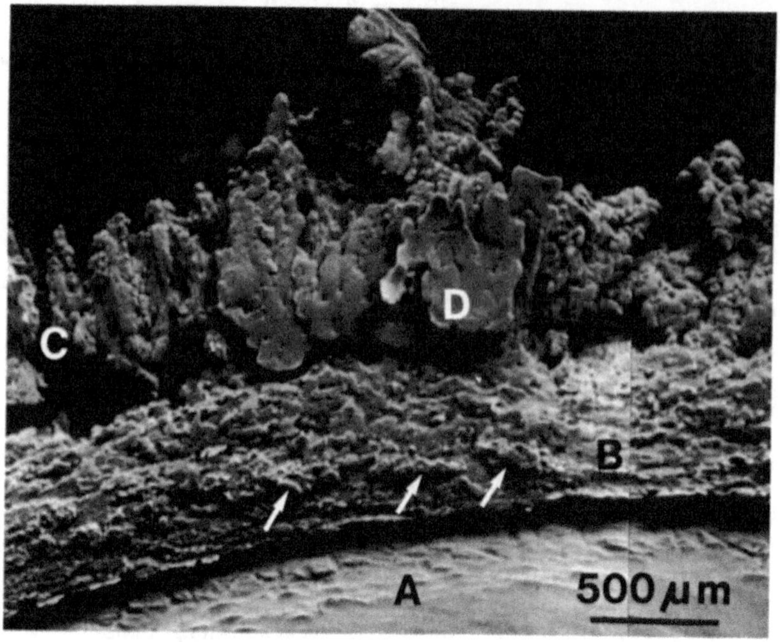


**Fig. 1.** Anterior view of the peripheral part of the plastic mass filling the anterior chamber. *A:* the anterior part of the anterior chamber. *B:* plastic present in the interspaces of the trabecular meshwork. Islands corresponding to the interspaces in the juxtacanalicular region at *arrows*. *C:* plastic filling the interspaces of the ciliary muscle. *D:* plastic filling the supraciliary space. Note furrow between *B* and *C–D* caused by the scleral spur. Nonfixed preparation perfused with Mercox-methylmethacrylate

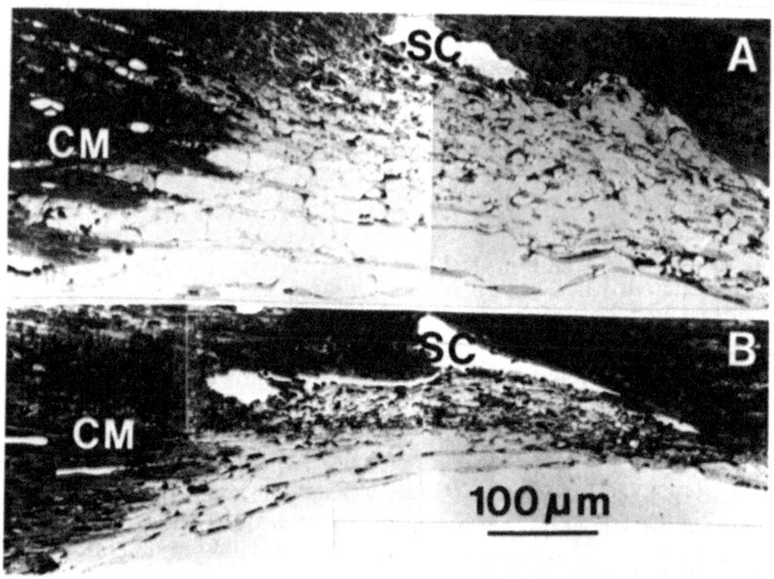


**Fig. 2A, B.** The tone of the ciliary muscle affects the trabecular meshwork markedly. **(A)** Eye treated with 20 µg pilocarpine i.c. **(B)** Eye treated with 0.75 µg atropine i.c. Contraction of the ciliary muscle caused unfolding of all parts of the trabecular meshwork. Vervet monkey. *CM:* Ciliary muscle. *SC:* Schlemm's canal

to contraction of the ciliary muscle which was considered to cause a widening of the spaces in the meshwork and the canal of Schlemm. This hypothesis has received a somewhat mixed support. Rohen, Lütjen and Bárány (1967) found indirect evidence indicating that pilocarpine acts by causing separation of trabecular lamelle and an increase in the filtering area of the canal of Schlemm. However, in the monkey Macaca arctoides, Lütjen-Drecoll (1973) found only a moderate increase in the area of the electron optically empty spaces close to the inner wall endothelium of Schlemm's canal. A dramatic distension of the juxtacanalicular meshwork was reported after pilocarpine treatment in human eyes (Grierson, Lee and Abraham 1978). In a subsequent study in baboons (Grierson, Lee and Abraham 1979) the effect was found to depend very much on the intraocular pressure. In experiments with prolonged stabilization of the intraocular pressure at 18 mmHg there was a marked distension. At the spontaneous intraocular pressure there was no striking effect.

In recent experiments in which great care was taken to avoid marked elevations in intraocular pressure and in which the outflow routes were perfused with latex particles in gelatine at the normal intraocular pressure (Svedbergh, Hamanaka and Bill, unpublished) it was found that pilocarpine-induced contraction of the ciliary muscle caused a marked widening of the outflow routes, Fig. 2. The results make it seem likely that the resistance to flow through all parts of the meshwork can be very much reduced by pilocarpine.

**Surgical and Laser Treatment**

Theoretically, holes made between the anterior chamber and the canal of Schlemm with trabeculectomy, electropuncture or by means of lasers can be expected to give a marked reduction in outflow resistance between the anterior chamber and the canal of Schlemm. The variable results of such procedures are probably due to at least two factors. One is that longitudinal flow in the canal of Schlemm normally may take place over only short distances and that the resistance to longitudinal flow in fact may be quite considerable (Moses 1979). The other problem is scar formation. In the trabeculoplasty procedure scar formation is probably a positive factor (Wise 1981). The laser is used to produce coagulation of the innermost part of the trabecular meshwork, which will cause some shrinkage and movement of the meshwork in the anterior chamber direction. Thus what is created with the laser is probably somewhat similar to the effect of pilocarpine treatment with respect to the movement of the outer parts of the meshwork.

**Wash-out**

It has been observed repeatedly that in experiments with prolonged perfusion of the anterior chamber in monkeys there is an increase in facility. In a study with prolonged perfusion at an elevated intraocular pressure Svedbergh (1974) could demonstrate that the increase in facility was quite marked. This effect seemed to be due to wash-out of material from the outflow routes especially the juxtacanalicular region. The effectiveness of wash-out procedures can be expected to depend to a large extent on the cell contact between the trabecular cells and also on that between the endothelial cells of the inner wall of Schlemm's canal. In the clinical situation it would seem to be a rather risky procedure to try and wash out material from the chamber angle if the wash-out required many hours of high intraocular pressure.

**Cytochalasins**

Cytochalasins are fungal metabolites that have very marked effects on many functions of cells. Many of these effects can be explained by the inhibitory effect of cytochalasins on the formation of microfilaments. When cytochalasin B was injected into monkey eyes it was observed that it caused a very marked increase in outflow facility within a short period of time and at microgram doses (Kaufman and Bárány 1977). The increase was reversible and could be repeated. Effects were obtained even after disinsertion of the ciliary muscle indicating that it was not due to a pilocarpine-like action. Studies on the ultrastructure of the monkey outflow routes after cytochalasin B (Svedbergh et al. 1978) demonstrated that there was marked separation and degeneration of trabecular cells, distension with separation of cells and loss of extracellular material in the juxtacanalicular region. In the inner wall of Schlemm's canal there was separation from the underlying tissue, abnormally large invaginations and even ruptures. It was observed in the experiments of Kaufman and Bárány that a rise in intraocular pressure above the normal level was important for the production of the increase in outflow facility. Cytochalasin thus seems to cause an enhanced wash-out effect.

## Chelating Agents

In cynomolgus monkeys the chelating agents EDTA and EGTA perfused through the anterior chamber in calcium free mock aqueous humor cause a very marked increase in outflow facility (Bill, Lütjen-Drecoll and Svedbergh 1980). The effect is rather rapid in onset and lasts for the period of perfusion with chelating agents but is then lost to a large extent if normal perfusate is used. Marked effects were seen at 4 mM EDTA but much lower concentrations are clearly effective, Fig. 3.

At high concentrations of EDTA or EGTA there were marked changes in the outflow routes in monkeys similar to those produced by cytochalasin B: in the trabecular meshwork there was cell separation due to splitting of cell junctions. There was also a distension of the juxtacanalicular meshwork and a wash-out of the extracellular material. In the inner wall of the Schlemm's canal there were frank ruptures. As with cytochalasins there were marked effects also on the corneal endothelium and in the ciliary muscle and sphincter pupillae muscle. It was suggested that EDTA or EGTA might be used as outlet cleaners in such cases of glaucoma in which the low facility can be attributed to pathological accumulation of some material in the outflow routes. Such materials could be erythrocytes, pigment or exfoliation material.

The observation that with EDTA or EGTA the increase in facility was shortlasting suggested that other treatments aiming at producing a prolonged disruption of cell junctions might be of interest. In cell biology a combination of EDTA and enzymes is sometimes used to produce efficient separation of cells. Since alphachymotrypsin has been used in ophthalmology without adverse effects if seemed of interest to study if this enzyme could produce a prolongation of the EDTA effect or if it might have an effect by itself (Bill 1980). Figure 3 shows an experiment in which a monkey eye was first perfused with EDTA and then with alphachymotrypsin. As soon as the EDTA perfusion was stopped there was a tendency to falling facility but after alphachymotrypsin the high facility was maintained for several hours.

Alphachymotrypsin alone is also quite effective in increasing the outflow facility, Fig. 4.

The results obtained with chelating agents and alphachymotrypsin suggest that these agents and other enzymes may be of interest in the treatment of glaucoma. For such treatment to be effective it will be of very great

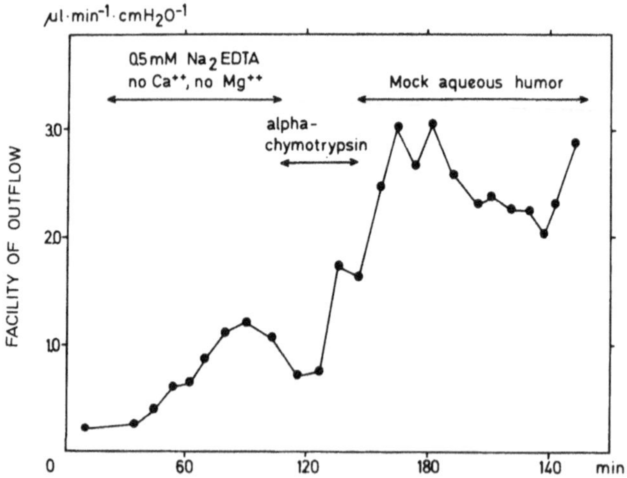


**Fig. 3.** The anterior chamber in a cynomolgus monkey was perfused with EDTA in calcium and magnesium free mock aqueous humor. There was a moderate increase in outflow facility. Subsequent perfusion with alphachymotrypsin caused a marked and prolonged increase in facility

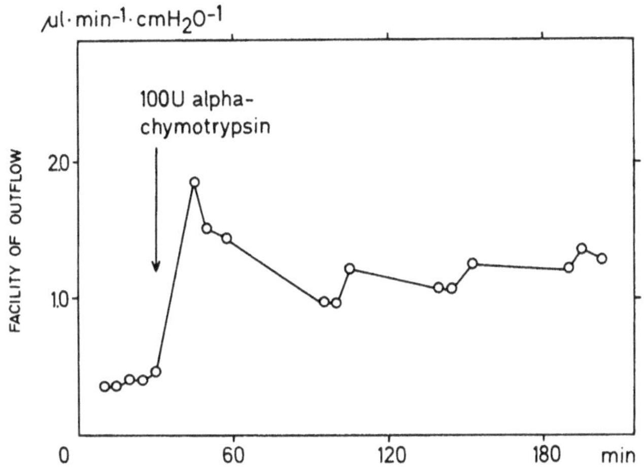


**Fig. 4.** 100 U alphachymotrypsin injected into the anterior chamber caused a prolonged increase in outflow facility

importance to analyze the juxtacanalicular tissue in glaucomatous eyes in order to ascertain the chemical nature of the material that tends to accumulate in the outflow routes. It may very well turn out that a specific enzyme, possibly in combination with chelating agents, can be used to dissolve and wash out clogging material from the outflow routes. The risk of damage to other parts of the anterior segment has to be kept in mind, however, and much work probably remains to be done before outlet cleaning with chemical agents can be used as a treatment in glaucoma.

## References

Bill A (1980) Effects of $Na_2EDTA$ and alphachymotrypsin on aqueous humor outflow conductance in monkey eyes. Ups J Med Sci 85:311-318

Bill A, Svedbergh B (1972) Scanning electron microscopic studies of the trabecular meshwork and the canal of Schlemm. An attempt to localize the main resistance to outflow of aqueous humor in man. Acta Ophthalmol 50:295-319

Bill A, Lütjen-Drecoll E, Svedbergh B (1980) Effects of intracameral $Na_2EDTA$ and EGTA on aqueous outflow routes in the monkey eye. Invest Ophthalmol Vis Sci 19:492-504

Grierson I, Lee WR, Abraham S (1978) Effects of pilocarpine on the morphology of the human outflow apparatus. Br J Ophthalmol 62:302-313

Grierson I, Lee WR, Abraham S (1979) The effects of topical pilocarpine on the morphology of the outflow apparatus of the baboon (Papio cynocephalus). Invest Ophthalmol Vis Sci 18:346-355

Kaufman PL, Bárány EH (1976) Loss of a acute pilocarpine effect on outflow facility following surgical disinsertion and retrodisplacement of the ciliary muscle from the scleral spur in the cynomolgus monkey. Invest Ophthalmol 15:793-807

Kaufman PL, Bárány EH (1977) Cytochalasin B reversibly increases outflow facility in the eye of the cynomolgus monkey. Invest Ophthalmol 116:47-53

Leydhecker W (1960) Glaukom. Springer, Berlin Heidelberg New York, p 402

Lütjen-Drecoll E (1973) Structural factors influencing outflow facility and its changeability under drugs. Invest Ophthalmol 12:280-294

Moses RA (1979) Circumferential flow in Schlemm's canal. Am J Ophthalmol 88: 585-591

Rohen JW, Lütjen-Drecoll E, Bárány E (1967) The relation between the ciliary muscle and the trabecular meshwork and its importance for the effect of miotics on aqueous outflow resistance. Albrecht von Graefes Arch Klin Exp Ophthalmol 172:23-47

Svedbergh B (1974) Effects of artificial intraocular pressure elevation on the outflow facility and the ultrastructure of the chamber angle in the vervet monkey (Cercopithecus ethiops). Acta Ophthalmol 52:829-846

Svedbergh B, Lütjen-Drecoll E, Ober M, Kaufman PL (1978) Cytochalasin B-induced structural changes in the anterior ocular segment of the cynomolgus monkey. Invest Ophthalmol Vis Sci 17:718-734

Wise JB (1981) Long-term control of adult open angle glaucoma by argon laser treatment. Ophthalmol 88:197-202

Krieglstein G.K./Leydhecker W. (eds)
Glaucoma Update II


# Morphological and Biochemical Studies on Cell and Tissue Cultures of Human Trabecular Meshwork

J.W. Rohen, Erlangen-Nürnberg, D.O. Schachtschabel, Marburg/Lahn, E. Lütjen-Drecoll, M. Rohrbach, Erlangen-Nürnberg and K. Berghoff, Marburg/Lahn

## Introduction

In the last few years, a number of investigations on monolayer cell cultures derived from isolated trabecular meshwork have been carried out (Rohen et al. 1976, 1978; Schachtschabel et al. 1977, 1982a, b; Grierson et al. 1980; Polansky et al. 1978, 1981; Alvarado et al. 1979). Since the explanted tissue pieces used for cell and tissue culture studies are composed of several cell types, the question arises as to whether those cells which later form the monolayer cultures are in fact derived from the cells covering the trabecular beams, or whether they grow out of other parts of the explanted tissue.

## Tissue Cultures of Human Trabecular Meshwork

To study the origin of these cells we started a series of experiments in which the entire chamber angle tissue comprising Schlemm's canal, the trabecular meshwork expanded between the scleral spur and the cornea and the adjacent corneosclera were explanted (so-called organ or tissue cultures). These explants were kept under tissue culture conditions for 2–10 days. The electron microscopic analysis of the explanted tissue showed great differences in behavior and morphological appearance between the various cell populations of the trabecular meshwork. During the first days after explantation, the endothelial lining of Schlemm's canal remained relatively unchanged. The endothelial cells form a complete layer of flat, elongated cells without any vacuoles or invaginations. Usually, after 5–7 days they degenerate and disappear (Rohen et al. 1982a).

In contrast, the subendothelial cells located in the cribriform or juxtacanalicular part of the meshwork gradually become activated. During the first 3 days they enlarge considerably and develop a conspicuous amount of rough surfaced endoplasmic reticulum, Golgi vesicles and ribosomes. Their nuclei become enlarged, thereby developing a great amount of nucleolar material. The mitochondria increase in number and size and show a highly electron dense intercristae matrix.

In contrast to these cribriform meshwork cells, the uveal and corneoscleral cells often degenerate and disappear within the first days after explantation. Although kept under the same tissue culture conditions they began to swell and disintegrate, losing their contact with the trabecular lamellae. After rupture of their plasmalemm, the cell organelles enter the intertrabecular spaces and finally degenerate (Fig. 1). Similar morphological changes were seen in both chamber angle explants of freshly enucleated monkey eyes and human autopsy eyes, enucleated within 6–8 h post mortem (Rohen et al. 1982a).

As a result of these experiments, it can be assumed that monolayer cell cultures of the isolated trabecular meshwork very likely derive from the cribriform meshwork cells rather than from cells of the uveal or corneoscleral portion of the trabecular meshwork. Why the uveal or corneoscleral trabecular cells appear to be less adaptable to the in-vitro environment than the cribriform cells is by no means clear.

To elucidate possible factors which may influence the survival and later activation of trabecular meshwork cells cultivated in organ cultures, we conducted a series of experiments in which either the composition of the medium or the composition of the explant (with or without the ciliary body) was changed (Fig. 2).

To quantify the effects on the survival and growth of the trabecular cells, the number of cells located in the 3 main portions of the trabecular meshwork were counted. The tissue

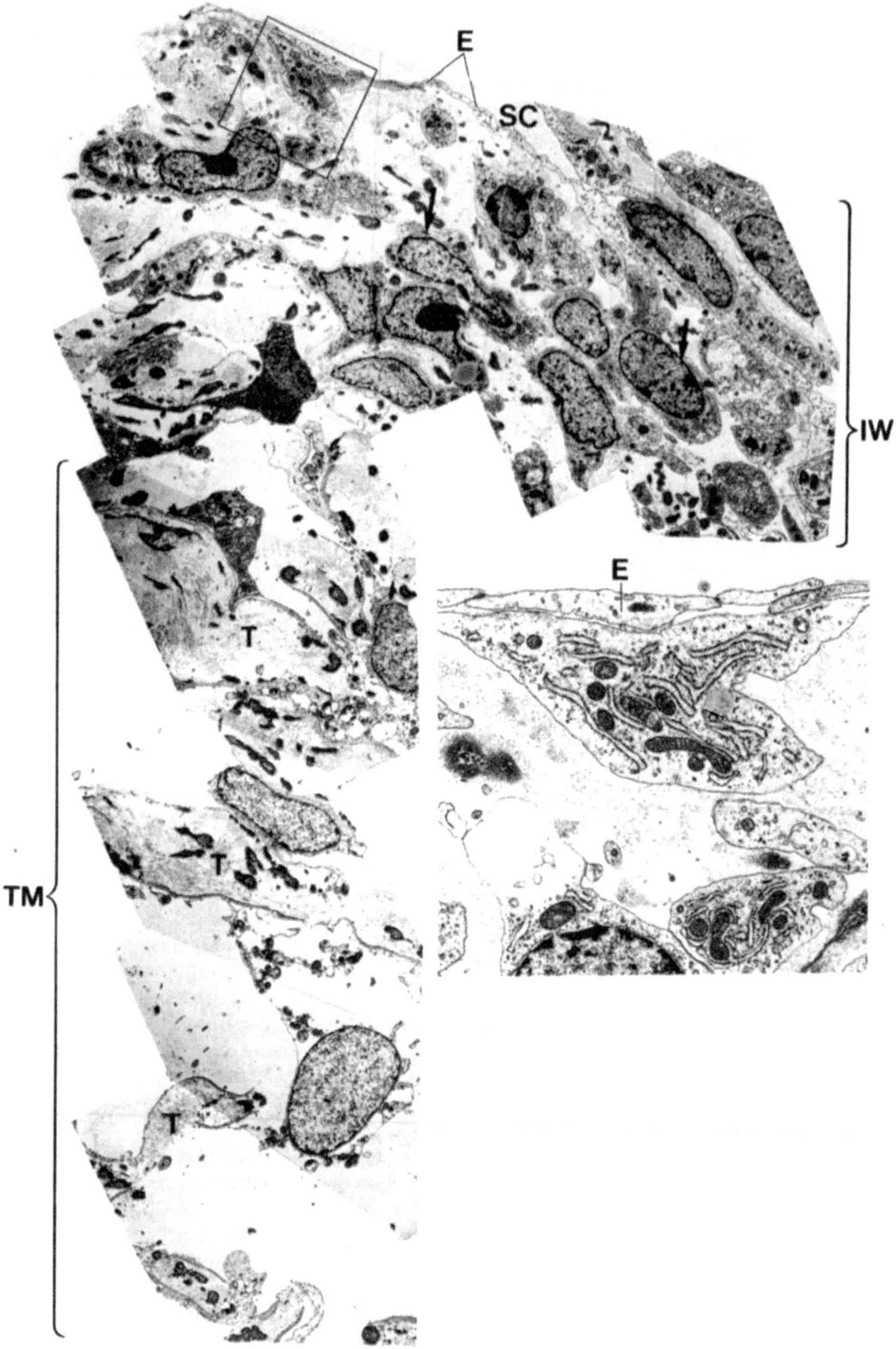


**Fig. 1.** Electron micrograph of the trabecular meshwork of a cynomolgus monkey 8 days after explantation (*survey picture*, 2735×; *inset* 9590×). Note the differences in the structure of the cribriform and corneoscleral uveal meshwork (after Rohen et al. 1982). *E:* Endothelial lining of Schlemm's canal; *IW:* Inner wall and cribriform layer; *SC:* Schlemm's canal; *T:* Trabecular beam; *TM:* Corneoscleral and uveal meshwork

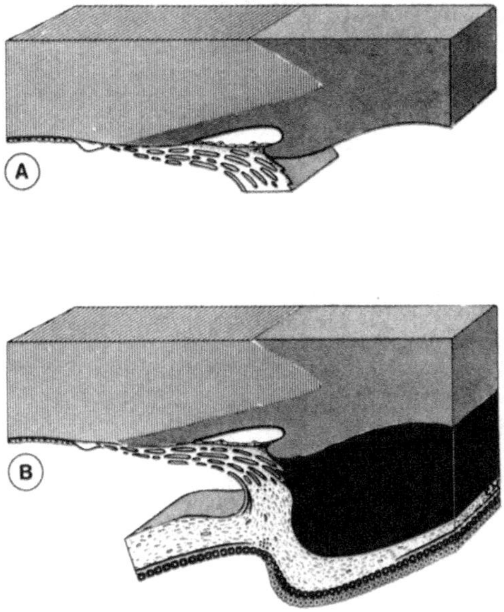


**Fig. 2A, B.** Schematic drawing of form and size of explants used in the experiments with "organ" cultures. **(A)** Trabecular meshwork without ciliary body. **(B)** Trabecular meshwork with ciliary body

cultures of the trabecular meshwork, which also contained the anterior part of the ciliary body with its epithelial lining were incubated for up to ten days. Following this period, an increase in the number of cells and cellular activation was observed, especially in the cribriform region of the trabecular meshwork, as compared with explants of the same eye containing only the trabecular meshwork and no ciliary body (Rohen et al., in press) (Fig. 3).

At present, no satisfactory explanation can be given for these stimulatory effects of the ciliary body on the trabecular meshwork.

## Histoautoradiographic Studies on Organ Cultures

Explants of human and monkey eyes containing trabecular meshwork and ciliary body were incubated with $^{14}$C-glucosamine or $^{35}$S-sulfate for several different time intervals. Histoautoradiographs revealed a particularly high amount of silver grains at the site of the non-pigmented ciliary epithelium, especially at the innermost part (crests) of the ciliary processes. In general, the labeling was weaker in the epithelium of the ciliary valleys.

The trabecular meshwork of these explants also showed some incorporation of the labeled precursors, though less than the ciliary processes. The greatest amount of silver grains was found in the cribriform layer, while less, if any, incorporation was seen in the uveal and corneoscleral part of the trabecular meshwork. This could either be due to an extensive deposition of labeled extracellular substances located in the cribriform meshwork or to an especially high activity in Glycosamino-glycan-(GAG)-synthesis of cribriform cells (to be published).

The capacity for GAG-synthesis of these cells was also studied following establishment of monolayer cultures derived from the trabecular meshwork of human autopsy eyes (Schachtschabel et al. 1982a, b).

## Studies on Monolayer Cultures

Incorporation of $^{14}$C-glucosamine or $^{35}$S-sulfate into GAGs was followed up to 74 h in activity proliferating monolayer cell cultures derived from the trabecular meshwork of human eyes. Incorporation of both precursors into cell-released GAGs occurred at a linear rate during the entire incubation period, while incorporation into cell-bound GAGs leveled off after about 30 h. The latter finding suggests that a cellular equilibrium between substrate uptake, GAG synthesis and possibly degradation product release and uptake was reached after this period.

Cell-bound and medium GAGs of these cultures have been characterized by enzymatic and electrophoretic methods. It was found that these cells produce hyaluronic acid, heparan sulfate, various kinds of chondroitin sulfates and dermatan sulfate.

Following $^{14}$C-glucosamine incorporation, 70–80% of the medium GAG-label was found in hyaluronic acid and 8–14% in heparan sulfate. About 30% of the cell-bound $^{14}$C-activity was associated with heparan sulfate and 60% with hyaluronic acid.

There was no significant change in this GAG synthesis pattern between primary cultures and phase II-cultures subcultured several times, as long as these cultures are in a proliferating state. Monolayer cultures of this kind, however, can enter a non-proliferating state with growth restriction and reduced metabolic activity, probably due to "senescence" and comparable to the phase III-

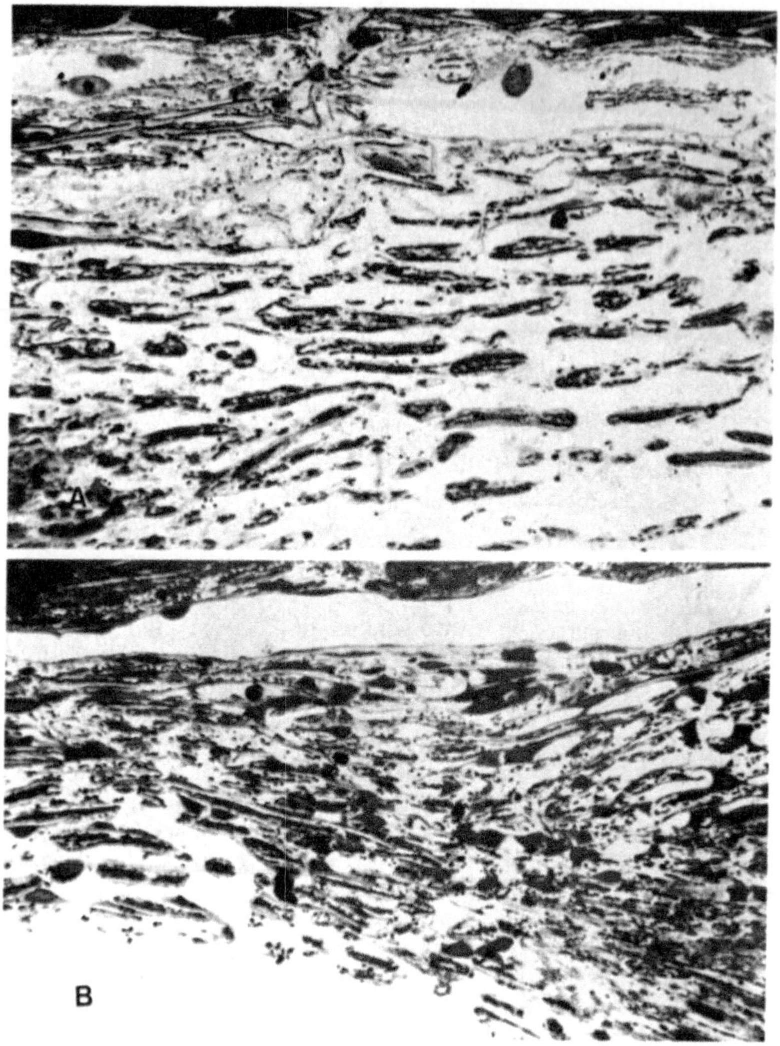


**Fig. 3.** Light micrographs of the human trabecular meshwork, kept under tissue culture conditions for 10 days (**A**) without and (**B**) with ciliary body (cf. Fig. 2); (× 480). Notice the cell loss in (**A**) and the increase in number and activity of the cells in (**B**)

phenomenon according to Hayflick and Moorhead (1961).

If such a culture was labeled several times (each time for 48 h following increasing culture periods) with $^{14}$C-glucosamine, a marked change in the GAG-pattern was observed. With increasing length of cultivation, such cultures reveal a progressively decreasing rate of GAG-synthesis. In trabecular meshwork cultures, consisting of "senescent" non-dividing cells, a characteristic change in the GAG-pattern was found when the observation time was prolonged up to 5 months.

The most striking finding of this study was the progressive decrease in the portion of hyaluronic acid and the concommitant increase of the heparan sulfate portion with increasing cultivation time. These findings could be relevant to the pathogenesis of glaucoma. If similar changes in the pattern of synthesized GAGs also occur during ageing in vivo, in particular a reduction in the synthesis and secretion rate of hyaluronic acid, it is conceivable that aqueous humor outflow resistance is affected by these alterations.

## References


Alvarado JA, Polansky JR (1979) Biologic activity of cultured human trabecular cells. Invest Ophthalmol, ARVO, Sarasota [Suppl] p 241

Grierson I, Robins E, Howes RC (1980) Preliminary observations on human trabecular meshwork cells in vitro. Albrecht von Graefes Arch Klin Exp Ophthalmol 212:173–186

Hayflick L, Moorhead PS (1961) The serial cultivation of human diploid cell strains. Exp Cell Res 25:585–621

Polansky JR, Gospodarowicz D, Weinreb R, Alvarado JA (1978) Human trabecular meshwork cell culture and glycosaminoglycan synthesis. Invest Ophthalmol Vis Sci, ARVO [Suppl] 17:207

Polansky JR, Weinreb R, Alvarado JA (1981) Studies on human trabecular cells propagated in vitro. Vision Res 21:155–160

Rohen JW, Schachtschabel DO, Figge H, Bigalke B (1976) Die Struktur der Kammerwasserabfluß-wege und ihre Veränderungen beim Glaukom: In vivo- und in vitro-Untersuchungen. Glaukom-Symposium Würzburg 1974, Enke, Stuttgart, pp 1–12

Rohen JW, Schachtschabel DO (1978) Morphological and biochemical studies of the human trabecular meshwork in tissue culture. Invest Ophthalmol, ARVO, Sarasota [Suppl] p 207

Rohen JW, Lütjen-Drecoll E, Rohrbach M (1983) Morphological studies on the trabecular meshwork in tissue culture. Albrecht von Graefes Arch Klin Exp Ophthalmol (in press)

Rohen JW, Lütjen-Drecoll E (1982) Biology of the trabecular meshwork. In: Lütjen-Drecoll E (ed) Basic aspects of glaucoma research. Schattauer, Stuttgart New York, pp 141–166

Rohen JW, Schachtschabel DO, Wehrmann R (1982c) Structural changes of human and monkey trabecular meshwork following in vitro cultivation. Albrecht von Graefes Arch Klin Exp Ophthalmol 218:225–232

Schachtschabel DO, Bigalke B, Rohen JW (1977) Production of glycosaminoglycans by cell cultures of the trabecular meshwork of the primate eye. Exp Eye Res 24:71–80

Schachtschabel DO, Rohen JW, Wever J, Sames K (1982a) Synthesis and composition of glycosaminoglycans by cultured human trabecular meshwork cells. Albrecht von Graefes Arch Klin Exp Ophthalmol 218:113–117

Schachtschabel DO, Wilke K, Wehrmann R (1982b) In vitro cultures of human and monkey trabecular meshwork. In: Lütjen-Drecoll E (ed) Basic aspects of glaucoma research. Schattauer, Stuttgart New York, pp 211–220

Krieglstein G.K./Leydhecker W. (eds)
Glaucoma Update II


# Timolol Maleate and Choroidal Blood Flow[1]

J.T. Ernest and T.K. Goldstick, Chicago, Evanston

**Abstract.** We have measured choroidal blood flow in cats by determining the rate of clearance of indocyanine green dye from the choroidal circulation. Measurements were made by rapidly (0.2 s) injecting indocyanine green dye (2.5 mg/ml), in 0.1 ml increments, into the common carotid artery and photoelectrically monitoring its concentration in the superior anterior ciliary vein. In the six normal cats studied, the choroidal blood flow during the control periods averaged 13.9 ± 2.7 ml/min/ml of choriocapillaris (mean ± S.E.) while in the five low flow cats it averaged 4.6 ± 0.6 ml/min/ml of choriocapillaris. Following a timolol maleate injection of 10 mg into the common carotid artery, the systemic blood pressure usually decreased and then returned essentially to control level within 5 to 20 minutes. The choroidal blood flow tended to parallel the systemic blood pressure but usually fell less. In the low flow cats, the blood flow increased briefly above control levels even when the blood pressure was below control. We conclude that timolol maleate does not constrict choroidal vessels in the cat.

## Introduction

Timolol maleate, a $\beta_1$ and $\beta_2$ adrenergic receptor blocking agent, has become a widely used anti-glaucoma drug [1-3]. The medication decreases aqueous humor formation without affecting outflow resistance [4], and it has been shown to have a similar effect in cats [5]. The mechanism of action is unknown but it appears to differ from that of carbonic anhydrase inhibitors [6]. In view of the extensive adrenergic innervation of the choroid in close approximation to the vasculature [7], we felt it important to investigate the possible effect of timolol on this circulation.

## Materials and Methods

Eleven cats weighing 3.5-5.5 kg were anaesthetized with 75 mg/kg of a 10% solution of α-chloralose in polyethylene glycol administered intravenously. A tracheostomy was carried out and the animals placed on a respirator (Model 607; Harvard Apparatus Company, Millis MA) and paralyzed with tubocurarine chloride (0.2 mg/kg) and gallamine triethiodide (0.5 mg/kg). The arterial blood pressure was monitored from a cannulated femoral artery with a pressure transducer (Model 1280C; Hewlett Packard, Waltham MA). The intraocular pressure was maintained at 15 mmHg by adjusting the height of an infusion bottle connected to an anterior chamber cannula through a second pressure transducer. The animal's temperature was measured with a rectal thermometer and maintained at 38.0 °C with a thermo-blanket. Arterial blood samples were analyzed throughout each experiment for pH, $PCO_2$, and $PO_2$ with a blood micro system (Models BMS 3 and PHM 72; The London Company, Radiometer A/S, Copenhagen, Denmark) at 38.0 °C. The animal's pH was maintained at approximately 7.40 by adjusting the respiratory rate and, with the tidal volumes used, this resulted in arterial $PCO_2$ levels of approximately 30 mmHg and $PO_2$ levels of approximately 95 mmHg.

The method of measuring the choroidal blood flow has been previously reported for monkeys [8] and cats [9]. Briefly, we used fiber optic bundles to pass near infrared light through the superior anterior ciliary vein and thereby obtained a continuous measurement of the dye concentration leaving the choriocapillaris. To reduce any motion artifact we

1 Supported in part by National Eye Institute Research Grant EY 04085 and a RPB Eye Research Professorship (J.T.E.); presented in part at the Spring Meeting of the Association of Research in *Vision and Ophthalmology*, Sarasota, Florida, May, 1979

occasionally, temporarily, disconnected the respirator but this made little difference. To measure choroidal blood flow, we injected a 0.1 ml bolus of a 2.5 mg/ml solution of indocyanine green dye, in 0.2 seconds, into the homolateral common carotid artery and continuously recorded the dye concentration in the superior anterior ciliary vein on a polygraph (Model 7758; Hewlett Packard) on which the arterial and intraocular pressures were recorded. The dye concentration was also recorded simultaneously on a separate, larger strip chart recorder (Model EU-20B; Heathkit, Benton Harbor, MI) the record from which was subsequently digitized by hand at 2 Hz. In addition, for most of the animals, the dye concentration was also digitized directly at 10 Hz and the data stored on a PDP 11/03. Later, the digitized dye concentration data were computer analyzed (CDC 6600) using a standard nonlinear regression, monoexponential fit routine to give the choroidal blood flow from the washout portion of the curve. This method has been shown to measure choroidal blood flow in cats [9].

To test the effect of timolol maleate, a bolus of 10 mg in 1 ml of 0.9 percent saline was injected into the homolateral common carotid artery in about 30 seconds. The timolol solution had been prepared just prior to its use. For the comparison of the results before and after timolol administration, we used as a control the average of up to three measurements taken within 20 minutes preceding the timolol injection. When repeated timolol injections were given to the same animal, the control average was taken from measurements made after we judged that the effect of the preceding timolol injection had dissipated, usually around 15 minutes.

## Results

Figure 1 shows typical indocyanine green dye clearance data (points) and the corresponding best fitting monoexponential (curve) for the washout region. The region of fit (between the last two vertical lines) was chosen as described elsewhere [9] such that the mean squared error was minimized and recirculation occurred at approximately the same time (fourth vertical line) in succeeding flow measurements on the same animal. The dye was injected at about -2 s but this value was not recorded because it was quite difficult to measure and was not used in the compu-

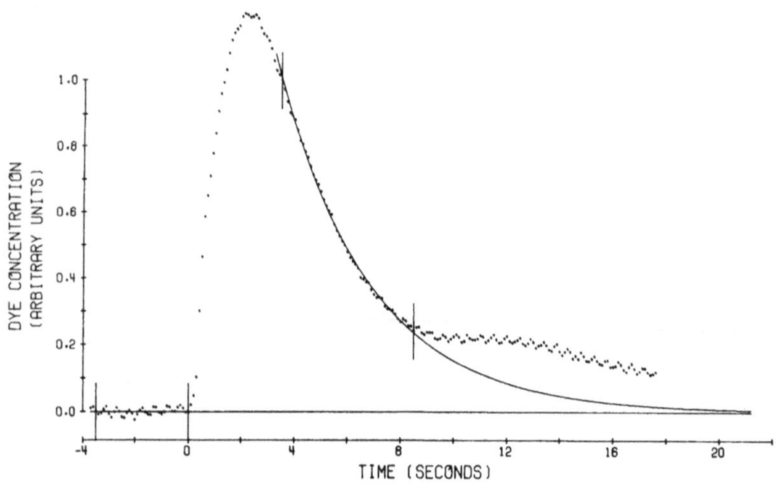


**Fig. 1.** Representative indocyanine green dye clearance curve for measurement of choroidal blood flow. These data were obtained during the control period from cat 6 when the perfusion pressure (mean systemic pressure minus intraocular pressure, always 15 mmHg) was 115 mmHg. The *points* are experimental, in this case directly digitized at 10 Hz. The *curve* is the best-fitting (nonlinear regression), computer-generated monoexponential. For these data, the blood flow rate (± S.E.) was 17.5 ± 0.1 ml/min/ml of choriocapillaris. The *vertical lines* delineate the boundaries of the baseline (35 *points* which were averaged) and the region of fit (51 *points*). *Zero* was arbitrarily taken as the end of the baseline

**Table 1.** Choroidal blood flow controls (ml/min/ml of choriocapillaris)

| | Cat 1 (5)[a] | Cat 2 (5) | Cat 3 (2) | Cat 4 (1) | Cat 5 (2) | Cat 6[b] (1) | Cat 7 (1) | Cat 8 (1) | Cat 9 (2) | Cat 10 (3) | Cat 11 (4) |
|---|---|---|---|---|---|---|---|---|---|---|---|
| | 3.6 | 6.0 | 4.2 | 3.3 | 6.6 | 17.5 | 9.5 | 23.3 | 8.2 | 11.3 | 7.9 |
| | 4.6 | 4.9 | 6.7 | 3.4 | 6.1 | 19.7 | 10.5 | 24.8 | 9.0 | 9.7 | 11.7 |
| | 4.1 | 3.9 | 6.3 | | 4.9 | 18.5 | 11.5 | 27.0 | 8.9 | 10.0 | 8.5 |
| | 3.6 | 3.3 | 7.4 | | 4.7 | | | | | 8.0 | 12.4 |
| | 3.8 | 3.4 | | | | | | | | 8.1 | 13.0 |
| | 4.0 | 2.8 | | | | | | | | 7.8 | 14.7 |
| | 3.9 | 3.1 | | | | | | | | 7.7 | 13.8 |
| | | 3.1 | | | | | | | | 7.2 | 12.2 |
| | | | | | | | | | | | 13.6 |
| Mean | 3.9 | 3.8 | 6.2 | 3.4 | 5.6 | 18.6 | 10.5 | 25.0 | 8.7 | 8.7 | 12.0 |
| S.E. | 0.1 | 0.4 | 0.7 | 0.1 | 0.5 | 0.6 | 0.6 | 1.1 | 0.3 | 0.5 | 0.8 |

Mean ± S.E. of all 11 cats is 9.7 ± 2.0, of the 5 cats with low flows (1–5), 4.6 ± 0.6, and of the 6 with normal flows (6–11), 13.9 ± 2.7 ml blood/min/ml of choriocapillaris; [a] Number in parentheses is number of timolol administrations given this animal; [b] For cat 6 a total of 19 flow measurements were actually made, one about every six minutes, during the two hours preceding the timolol injection. These values, in sequence, were: 18.8, 19.5, 19.3, 17.6, 19.0, 19.5, 18.1, 17.7, 16.8, 17.7, 19.4, 21.0, 17.4, 17.2, 19.6, 18.0, 17.5, 19.7, and 18.5 and their mean ± S.E. was 18.54 ± 0.25

tations. Although Fig. 1 was obtained with data digitized directly at 10 Hz, analysis of the same test using the clearance curve digitized by hand at 2 Hz gave virtually identical flow. The quality of the fit was the same before and after the timolol injection.

During the control periods the choroidal blood flow from the 11 cats studied varied considerably between animals with a mean (± S.E.) of 9.7 ± 2.0 ml/min/ml of choriocapillaris (Table 1). By contrast, the flow in a single animal was much more constant. For example, the mean of 19 measurements of blood flow obtained 6 minutes apart from one animal (cat 6) was 18.54 ± 0.25 ml/min/ml of choriocapillaris. For the six animals with normal choroidal blood flow the mean was 13.9 ± 2.7 ml/min/ml of choriocapillaris, while for the five with low control flows (less than 7 ml/min/ml of choriocapillaris) it was 4.6 ± 0.6 ml/min/ml of choriocapillaris. The normal value may be compared with our control values on 14 normal cats, measured in a different, later study [9], of 10.2 ± 0.6 ml/min/ml of choriocapillaris with a range of 8.5 to 14.0.

The effect of timolol maleate on the choroidal blood flow in a representative cat is shown in Fig. 2. The perfusion pressure (lower curve) is the mean systemic blood pressure measured in a femoral artery minus the intraocular pressure (maintained constant at 15 mmHg). The actual ocular perfusion pressure probably was somewhat lower than that we measured because the blood pressure in the ciliary arteries is lower than in the femoral arteries [10]. As shown in Fig. 2, there was often an initial, transient decrease in choroidal blood flow that paralleled the decrease in perfusion pressure immediately following the timolol injection. The blood flow, however, usually decreased less than the perfusion pressure. Often the flow then increased above control level. On the other hand, the perfusion pressure only slowly (5 to 20 min) returned toward control level and almost always remained slightly below control. There was no change in heart rate.

The data from all 11 of the cats (27 timolol administrations) are summarized in Table 2 where they are divided into a normal control flow (greater than 7 ml/min/ml of choriocapillaris) and a low control flow (less than 7 ml/min/ml of choriocapillaris) group. Although it might appear that the infusion of timolol had the opposite effect on the normal and low control flow cats, actually the results are quite comparable. The important point is the relationship between the change in perfusion pressure and flow, not the actual flow value. In the low flow group, the perfusion

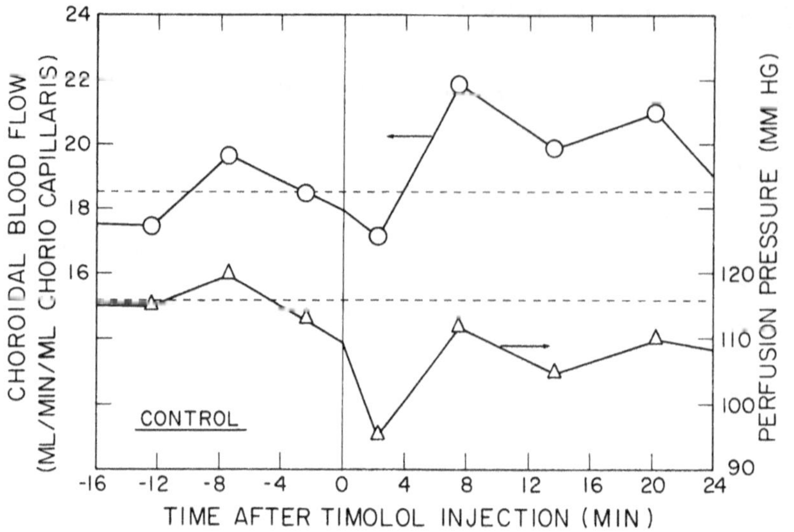


**Fig. 2.** *Top curve:* Cat choroidal blood flow before and following the common carotid artery injection of 10 mg of timolol maleate in cat 6. *Bottom curve:* Corresponding perfusion pressure. The *dashed lines* are the mean values during the control period. The times were taken from the beginning of the timolol injection to the mid-point of the region of fit (see Fig. 1)

pressure decreased less and the flow actually increased initially. In the normal flow group, timolol caused a greater reduction in perfusion pressure leading to a moderate reduction in flow. It is important to note that the timolol effect was over in 5 to 20 minutes. In four of the cats, measurements of choroidal blood flow were continued for from 40 to 90 minutes after the timolol injection but there appeared to be little effect of the timolol beyond 10 minutes.

The data from all 11 of the cats are pooled in Table 3. These data show that the perfusion pressure is significantly ($p < 0.001$) lowered in the first few minutes following the injection and that during the first 1 to 2 minutes the

**Table 2.** Choroidal blood flow and perfusion pressure following timolol

| Time After Timolol Injection (min) | Percent Change from Control Values (Mean ± S.E.) | | | | | |
|---|---|---|---|---|---|---|
| | LOW FLOW Control Less Than 7 ml/min/ml of Choriocapillaris | | | NORMAL FLOW Control Greater Than 7 ml/min/ml of Choriocapillaris | | |
| | No. of Measurements | Blood Flow | Perfusion Pressure | No. of Measurements | Blood Flow | Perfusion Pressure |
| 1–2 | 13 | 36.6 ± 10.1[a] | -8.8 ± 2.0[b] | 7 | -13.7 ± 4.6[a] | -21.6 ± 4.1[a] |
| 2–4 | 10 | -1.1 ± 7.5 | -7.3 ± 2.0[a] | 3 | -17.0 ± 5.3 | -16.3 ± 1.4[a] |
| 4–8 | 10 | 6.3 ± 8.1 | -3.1 ± 1.4 | 11 | 7.7 ± 5.5 | -4.6 ± 2.6 |
| 8–14 | 13 | -9.0 ± 4.5 | -2.8 ± 1.4 | 15 | 1.0 ± 3.7 | 1.1 ± 4.0 |
| 14–20 | 8 | -7.8 ± 7.8 | -3.2 ± 2.2 | 8 | 0.5 ± 4.2 | 3.2 ± 5.3 |

[a] Different from control values $p < 0.05$; [b] Different from control values $p < 0.001$

**Table 3.** Perfusion pressure, choroidal blood flow, and choroidal vascular resistance following timolol injection (pooled data)

| Time After Injection (min) | Percent Change from Control Values (Mean ± S.E.) | | | |
|---|---|---|---|---|
| | No. of Measurements | Perfusion Pressure | Flow | Resistance |
| 1- 2 | 20 | $-13.3 \pm 1.9^{b}$ | $19.0 \pm 6.7^{a}$ | $-22.3 \pm 3.5^{b}$ |
| 2- 4 | 13 | $-9.4 \pm 1.5^{b}$ | $-4.8 \pm 5.8$ | $-1.0 \pm 5.3$ |
| 4- 8 | 21 | $-3.9 \pm 1.5^{a}$ | $7.0 \pm 4.7$ | $-7.1 \pm 4.1$ |
| 8-14 | 28 | $-0.7 \pm 2.2$ | $-3.6 \pm 2.8$ | $4.8 \pm 3.0$ |
| 14-20 | 16 | $0.0 \pm 2.8$ | $-3.7 \pm 4.3$ | $7.1 \pm 5.9$ |

[a] Different from control values $p < 0.05$; [b] Different from control values $p < 0.001$

choroidal vascular resistance (defined as the perfusion pressure divided by the flow) is decreased.

## Discussion

The measurements obtained in this study agree well with those from other studies. For the cats with normal control flows, the mean choroidal blood flow was 13.9 ± 2.7 ml/min/ml of choriocapillaris with a range of 8.7 to 25.0 (Table 1), similar to the values we obtained on monkeys [8] and cats [9] with the same technique, 17.7 ± 1.8 and 10.2 ± 0.6 ml/min/ml of choriocapillaris, with ranges of 9.2 to 24.6 and 8.5 to 14.0 ml/min/ml of choriocapillaris. Also, the dye clearance curves obtained here from cats (Fig. 1) are remarkably similar to those obtained from monkeys [8], as has been discussed more extensively elsewhere [9]. This suggests that it is the washout rate of the choriocapillaris (i.e., blood flow in the units used here) which is the governing physiological parameter. As we also found [8, 9], the monoexponential fit of the dye clearance curve (Fig. 1) is extraordinarily good for a biological system.

The individual variability in choroidal blood flow between animals is quite large as has also been found by Bill [11] using a different technique. He attributed this to differences in choroidal vascular tone. We have previously shown [12] that the ocular vascular beds of the cat are responsive to sympathetic tone and while the intraocular pressure was controlled in the studies herein reported, the ocular nerves were intact. Moreover, the anesthetic we used, α-chloralose, does not suppress the nervous system [13]. There was usually rather less variability between measurements obtained from the same cat. This is evident from the extra data from cat 6 shown in Table 1 in which measurements were obtained every 6 minutes for two hours and the range of blood flow was only 16.8 to 21.0 ml/min/ml of choriocapillaris. This technique is thus ideally suited for the study of drug and perfusion pressure effects on the choroidal circulation where the animal can be used as its own control.

The infusion of a relatively large dose of timolol maleate into the carotid artery usually decreased perfusion pressure more than choroidal blood flow (Fig. 2, Table 2). The former reflects a decrease in the systemic blood pressure since the intraocular pressure was maintained at a constant level. It is significant that choroidal blood flow often increased above control values even though the perfusion pressure decreased and remained below control. The choroidal blood flow, however, responded to the fluctuations in the perfusion pressure, confirming previous observations [14].

We arbitrarily divided the results into low and normal blood flow groups (Table 2). Timolol had less effect on the perfusion pressure in the low flow group and actually increased choroidal blood flow. This may be of importance for its use in glaucoma where the perfusion pressure can be low due to elevation of the intraocular pressure.

The choroidal vascular resistance, defined as the perfusion pressure divided by the choroidal blood flow, decreased during the first 1 to 2 minutes following the injection of timolol (Table 3). This must be due to a vasodilatation of the choroidal vasculature. We do not know the mechanism by which timolol maleate caused choroidal vasodilatation. It apparently is not related to increased aqueous draining into the circle of Hovius and entering the superior anterior ciliary vein since timolol has no effect on aqueous outflow [5]. We have previously shown that hyperosmotic agents cause an increase in retinal oxygen tension, presumably secondary to increased blood flow [15]. However, there were no osmotic effects in the study herein reported since the timolol solution was isotonic with the blood.

The effects of timolol injections on the choroidal circulation do not appear to persist longer than 20 minutes even following repeated injections. In man timolol is usually applied topically once every twelve hours for months to years and separate studies are needed to see if there are any long term circulatory effects in human eyes. The most important conclusion to be drawn from our studies, however, is that timolol does not constrict the choroidal vessels. We were initially concerned that this might be part of the drug's intraocular pressure lowering effect but it is not.

*Acknowledgments.* We are grateful for the technical assistance of Debra Pate and Debbie Wing, for assistance in the computer analysis of data by Northwestern University students Kathryn Dirkes, Michael Fallert, Daniel Greenberg, Tracey Hudson, Rosalyn Jackson, Maurena Nacheff, John O'Riordan, Stuart Pulvirent, Andrew Seter and Alisa Stern, and for the manuscript preparation by Jackie Halik.

## References

1. Katz IM, Hubbard WA, Getson AJ, Gould AL (1976) Intraocular pressure decrease in normal volunteers following timolol ophthalmic solution. Invest Ophthalmol 15:489-492
2. Kaufman HE (1980) Timolol maleate. Ophthalmol 87:164-168
3. LeBlanc RP, Krip G (1981) Timolol. Canadian multicenter study. Ophthalmol 88:244-248
4. Coakes RL, Brubaker RF (1978) The mechanism of timolol in lowering intraocular pressure. In the normal eye. Arch Ophthalmol 96:2045-2048
5. Colasanti BK, Trotter RR (1981) Effects of selective $beta_1$- and $beta_2$ adrenoreceptor agonists and antagonists on intraocular pressure in the cat. Invest Ophthalmol Vis Sci 20:69-76
6. Liu HK, Chiou GCY, Garg LC (1980) Ocular hypotensive effects of timolol in cat eyes. Arch Ophthalmol 98:1467-1469
7. Laties AM, Jacobowitz D (1966) A comparative study of the autonomic innervation of the eye in monkey, cat, and rabbit. Anat Rec 156:383-396
8. Ernest JT, Goldstick TK (1979) Choroidal blood flow measurement in the monkey by clearance of indocyanine green dye. Exp Eye Res 29:7-14
9. Ernest JT, Goldstick TK (1983) Response of choroidal vascular resistance to hyperglycemia. Intl Ophthalmol 6:119-124
10. Bill A (1967) Uveal circulation, a review of methods and results. Glaucoma Symposium Tutzing Castle. Karger, New York, pp 52-72
11. Bill A (1962) A method for quantitative determination of the blood flow through the cat uvea. Arch Ophthalmol 67:62-68
12. Weiter JJ, Schachar RA, Ernest JT (1973) Control of intraocular blood flow. II. Effects of sympathetic tone. Invest Ophthalmol 12:332-334
13. Balis GU, Monroe RR (1964) The pharmacology of chloralose. A review. Psychopharmacologia 6:1-30
14. Alm A, Bill A (1970) Blood flow and oxygen extraction in the cat uvea at normal and high intraocular pressures. Acta Physiol Scand 80:19-28
15. Ernest JT, Stern WH, Trimble JL (1977) The effect of mannitol infusion on retinal function and oxygen tension. Invest Ophthalmol 16:670-673

## Discussion

**Yablonski to Ernest:** I would like to point out that contraction of the choroidal volume by itself would be expected to cause only a transient decrease in intraocular pressure the duration of which would conincide with the duration of the phase during which the choroid was actually contracting. Once the contraction phase is completed, despite the maintenance of a contracted choroidal volume, one would expect the intraocular pressure to quickly return to its pre-contraction level. Since the choroid could not undergo significant continued increasing contraction for a period of many hours, it is not reasonable to evoke this explanation for decreases of intraocular pressure which last many hours. Decreases of intraocular pressure of this duration would still be defined as an alteration in

the steady state level. Therefore, the change in I.O.P. could only occur if there were a change in one or more of four steady state parameters:
1. The rate of aqueous humor formation,
2. the outflow facility
3. the rate of uveoscleral flow, and
4. the level of episcleral venous pressure.

**Anderson to Ernest:** May I ask some questions about the methods used. If I understand the method correctly, it seems to me that not only must the front end of the bolus be a square wave, but also the back end of the bolus must be sharp. In addition, the length of the bolus must be small compared to the length of the exponential decay curve. Were these conditions met, or are they unimportant?

Secondly, the method depends on complete mixing in the capillary bed. Is this a reasonable assumption, or might the dye go through the capillary bed only partly mixed as a degraded bolus?

Thirdly, if there is a decreased volume of the bed along with an increased resistance and reduced volume of flow all as the result of vasoconstriction, might they not have balancing opposite effects on the decay curve so that it might seem unchanged when in fact the volume of flow had decreased?

**Leydhecker to Ernest:** The timolol effect has been compared one week after application with the effect after several months. I suggest to compare the effect on the first day with the later effect, since the lowering of the IOP is strongest on the first day. If you observed the same reduction in flow, would you then suggest that the better effect on the first day is due to a change of outflow facility? We have no indication that timolol changes the facility and I think we must conclude that on the first day the reduction of aqueous production is greater than on later days.

**Kolker to Ernest:** Have you performed studies of level blood flow with this method in animals treated with clonidine? Dr. Bill has shown his method that clonidine reduces uveal flow acutely.

**Ernest to Kolker:** I would like to thank Drs. Yablonski, Anderson, Leydhecker and Kolker for their discussions. I agree with Drs. Yablonski and Leydhecker and in response to Dr. Kolker, we have not studied clonidine. In answer to Dr. Anderson concerning the method, I would refer to our previous study published in INTERNATIONAL OPHTHALMOLOGY (ref. 9). In brief, first it is important to have a sharp bolus as you suggest. We have measured the half-time of the transient of our bolus in a ciliary artery and find it to be less than one second, compared to average choroidal washout half-times of over four seconds. Second, the increased dispersion of the dye caused by the choroidal vasculature indicates that there must be mixing. Based on all of our other studies, we feel the washout half-time is a good measure of choroidal blood flow. Third, if the volume of the vasculature in which mixing takes place decreases, our flow rate measurement would indeed appear to increase. However, we measured ocular volumes following timolol injections and they did not significantly change.

Krieglstein G.K./Leydhecker W. (eds)
Glaucoma Update II


# Relationship Between the Technique of Surgical Trabeculectomy and the Final Post-Operative Result

G.L. Spaeth and E.M. Poryzees, Philadelphia

Reports have suggested that varying the technique of trabeculectomy will alter the final result [1–12]. The present study was designed to test this hypothesis.

## Materials and Methods

The charts of 200 patients with primary open-angle glaucoma having trabeculectomy performed by the senior author were reviewed. Trabeculectomy was performed by modification of Watson's technique. A limbus-based flap was developed 8 mm posterior to the limbus and dissected to the corneoscleral sulcus. Wet-field cautery was applied where the sclera was to be incised; a one-third thickness scleral flap hinged at the corneoscleral sulcus was produced. A block of inner wall was then excised and sent for pathological examination. A peripheral iridectomy was performed. The scleral flap was closed. The conjuctival flap was closed in two layers with 8/0 chromic collagen. The anterior chamber was formed through a previously-placed paracentesis track. Atropine 1% was instilled throughout the procedure and continued post-operatively for two weeks. Phenylephrine 10% was given four times daily for two weeks post-operatively, as was dexamethasone 0.1% and a topical antibiotic four times daily, both for approximately one to two weeks.

Three aspects, and only three aspects, of the trabeculectomy technique were modified:

1. The size of the scleral flap and the block excised,

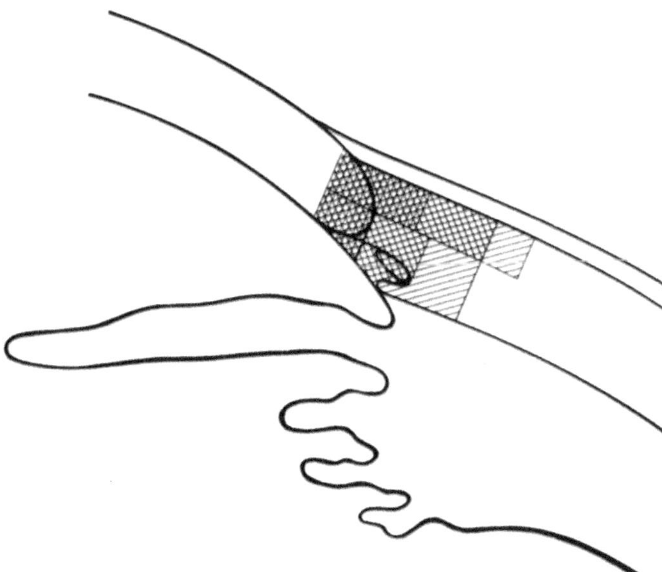

**Fig. 1.** *Cross-section* showing the three modifications of trabeculectomy utilized in this study. There are three different types of cross-hatching. The type of scleral flap corresponds with the similarly cross-hatched area of area of excised deeper tissue

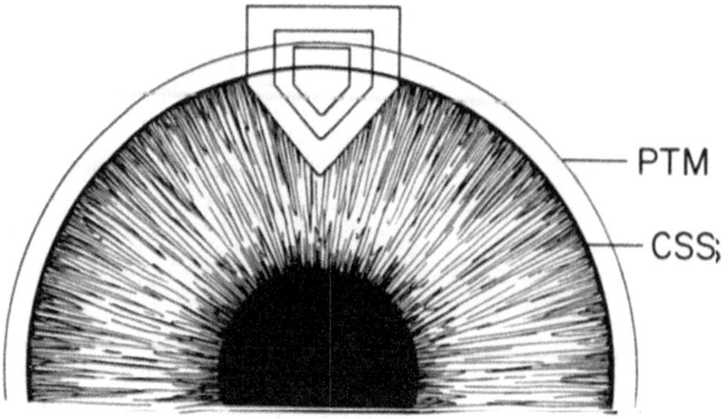


**Fig. 2.** Front view of the eye, showing the areas of the scleral flap and the excised block. Note that the *middle-sized block* just includes posterior trabecular meshwork *(PTM)*, and the *smallest-sized block* does not include posterior trabecular meshwork. The anterior extent is the same in all cases. *CSS*; corneascleral sulcus

2. The placement of the block excised with regard to its relationship to the scleral spur, and
3. The amount of leakage through the scleral flap at the conclusion of the procedure (Figs. 1 and 2).

In one group of cases, the scleral flap was made either large (5 mm × 4 mm × 5 mm), medium (4 mm × 4 mm × 4 mm), or small (3 mm × 3 mm × 3 mm). The anterior edge of the excised block was always incised just anterior to the corneoscleral sulcus. The posterior edge was incised either just anterior to the posterior trabecular meshwork (anterior), just anterior to the scleral spur and including the posterior trabecular meshwork (middle), or posterior to the scleral spur requiring disinsertion of the ciliary body from the scleral spur (posterior). The scleral flap was closed so that there was either no perceptible leakage through the cut edges even when the anterior chamber was filled with saline (no leakage), so there was a minimal ooze through one of the cut edges (oozing), or so there was a gross flow (leaking).

The indication for surgery was documented or anticipated deterioration of the optic nerve or visual field due to glaucoma despite maximum tolerated medical therapy, the deterioration occurring at a rate sufficiently rapid to interfere with the patient's lifestyle. The type of modification performed in each case was selected by a previously arranged plan based on the day of the week.

The post-operative care was similar in all our cases.

The charts were reviewed to collect data regarding the following: pre- and post-operative visual acuity; pre-operative intraocular pressure and post-operative intraocular pressure at one to three weeks, six months and one year; the nature of the bleb; and the incidence and type of complication.

The data were then analyzed to determine if there were any correlations between modifiation of technique and final result.

## Results

Results with regard to the effect of surgery on intraocular pressure are shown in Table 1.

The complications are shown in Tables 2 and 3.

Forty-eight cases (24%) of the 200 trabeculectomies required post-operative medication to help bring the pressure down towards the level felt necessary to correct the progressive optic nerve damage. The overwhelming majority of cases were treated with epinephrine. All of the various modification groups required medication with approximately equal frequency.

## Discussion

Several other studies have attempted to determine the effect of changing the technique of trabeculectomy on the final result [1–12].

This study showed a slight correlation between the final post-operative pressure and type of modification of trabeculectomy. However, the differences were not thoght to be of clinical consequence.

It appeared that the size of the block excised did not materially affect the final intraocular pressure. The group with the highest final intraocular pressure (those with small blocks excised), had higher intraocular pres-

**Table 1.** Relationship between modification of trabeculectomy and final intraocular pressure

| | | Percentage of 200 cases | Preoperative intraocular pressure[a] | Postoperative intraocular pressure[a] | Difference between pre- and post-operative intraocular pressure[a] |
|---|---|---|---|---|---|
| Size of flap and block | SMALL | 19 | 29.51 | 16.91 | 12.60 |
| | MEDIUM | 68 | 25.48 | 14.05 | 11.44 |
| | LARGE | 13 | 27.33 | 13.21 | 14.13 |
| Posterior edge of block in relation to scleral spur | ANTERIOR | 26 | 26.64 | 12.83 | 13.71 |
| | MIDDLE | 39 | 27.31 | 14.85 | 12.46 |
| | POSTERIOR | 35 | 26.47 | 14.74 | 11.73 |
| Amount of leakage through scleral flap | NO LEAKAGE | 14 | 26.20 | 13.85 | 12.35 |
| | OOZING | 58 | 28.23 | 13.46 | 14.77 |
| | LEAKING | 28 | 24.95 | 14.50 | 10.45 |

[a] Intraocular pressure in mmHg

sure to start with; the fact that the final intraocular pressure was also higher probably does not indicate less effect from the surgery. There was no significant difference statistically or clinically, for example, between cases with small or medium-sized blocks. A slightly lower pressure was obtained with a larger incision, but this was not a statistically significant difference, because the range of final pressures was large.

**Table 2.** Incidence of hyphema in 200 cases of trabeculectomy

| Size of Hyphema | | Small[c] %[b] | Medium[d] %[b] | Large[e] %[b] | Total % |
|---|---|---|---|---|---|
| Size of flap and block | SMALL | 17 | 0 | 0 | 17 |
| | MEDIUM | 18 | 5 | 1 | 24 |
| | LARGE | 25 | 0 | 0 | 25 |
| Posterior edge of block in relation to scleral spur | ANTERIOR | 13 | 4 | 0 | 17 |
| | MIDDLE | 23 | 3 | 3 | 29 |
| | POSTERIOR | 17 | 3 | 0 | 20 |
| Amount of leakage through scleral flap | NO LEAKAGE | 0 | 5 | 0 | 5 |
| | OOZING | 22 | 2 | 0 | 24 |
| | LEAKING | 16 | 4 | 4 | 24 |
| Percentage of 200 cases | | 19.5 | 3 | .5 | 23 |
| Total number of cases | | 39 cases | 6 cases | 1 case[a] | 46 cases |

[a] Note: One case had a medium, middle, leaking trabeculectomy; [b] Expressed as a percentage of the number of cases having the specific modification listed. Thus, one case with a medium, middle leaking trabeculectomy had a large hyphema, and that one case represents one percent of all trabeculectomies with a medium size flap, three percent of all trabeculectomies with a middle placement of the excised block, and four percent of all trabeculectomies with a leaking flap; [c] Small means hyphema less than 1 mm; [d] Medium means hyphema larger than 1 mm, but not thought to influence final operative result; [e] Large means hyphema may have affected final post-operative result

**Table 3.** Incidence of flat anterior chamber following 200 cases of trabeculectomy

| | | Slightly Shallow[a] | Moderately to Markedly Shallow[a] | Reformation Required[a] | Total[a] |
|---|---|---|---|---|---|
| Size of flap and block | SMALL | 12 | 12 | 3 | 27 |
| | MEDIUM | 5 | 3 | 1 | 9 |
| | LARGE | 13 | 13 | 4 | 30 |
| Posterior edge of block in relation to scleral spur | ANTERIOR | 8 | 4 | 0 | 12 |
| | MIDDLE | 9 | 5 | 4 | 18 |
| | POSTERIOR | 6 | 7 | 0 | 13 |
| Amount of leakage through scleral flap | NO LEAKAGE | 0 | 0 | 0 | 0 |
| | OOZING | 9 | 7 | 0 | 16 |
| | LEAKING | 9 | 2 | 2 | 13 |
| Percentage of cases | | 7.5 | 5.5 | 1.5 | 14.5 |
| Total number of cases | | 15 cases | 11 cases | 3 cases | 29 cases |

[a] in percentage

With regard to the position of the block excised, there was no statistically significant difference between any of the groups; there was a trend toward a greater effect from the more anteriorly placed incisions.

There was no difference in the final intraocular pressure between cases in whom the scleral flap was sutured so tightly that there was no leakage, and those in whom a purposeful leak of aqueous was developed. The smallest fall in intraocular pressure occurred in the group in which the aqueous leakage was most marked, but the difference was not clinically significant.

It appeared that none of the modifications employed in this study had a clinically significant effect on the final intraocular pressure.

Complications were slightly fewer in cases in which the scleral flap was sutured tightly. This was particularly apparent when considering the occurrence of post-operative flat anterior chambers. While only three cases of the 200 needed to have their anterior chamber re-formed following trabeculectomy, in no instance was this necessary where the flap was sutured tightly (Table 3). No cases required drainage of hyphema post-operatively, but the frequency with which hyphema occurred was lower in cases in which the scleral flap had been tightly closed.

Presumably, the less tissue that is disturbed and the more atraumatically surgery is performed, the less damage will be done to an eye receiving glaucoma surgery. Furthermore, if repeated surgery is required, there will be a greater untraumatized area in which to place the second procedure. Since small, anteriorly-placed, non-leaking trabeculectomies appear to work as well as larger, more posteriorly-placed, leaking trabeculectomies, it appears sensible to prefer the less traumatizing type of surgery. Furthermore, since the complication rate in trabeculectomies in which the scleral flap is tightly sutured is lower than in those cases where more leakage is permitted, it would also appear preferable to close the scleral flap securely.

**Abstract.** Two hundred cases of primary open-angle glaucoma were treated with modifications of Watson's trabeculectomy. Modifications of surgical technique included three different sizes of scleral flap, three different positions of the block excised, and three differences tightnesses of closure of the scleral flap. The final intraocular pressure was not significantly different in any of the groups; the modifications did not appear to affect the final intraocular pressure. The initial intraocular pressure for the entire group was 26.6 mmHg and the final intraocular pressure 14.7 mmHg. Twenty-four percent of all cases required medications post-operatively.

The incidence of post-operative shallow anterior chamber or post-operative hyphema was significantly lower in those cases where the scleral flap was closed tightly. Considering all cases, reformation of the anterior chamber was required in three cases (1.5%) and a significant hyphema occurred in seven cases (3.5%).

Since more extensive surgery (a large scleral flap, a larger, more posteriorly-placed block of excised tissue, and a greater amount of filtration immediately post-operatively) does not give a better result than less extensive surgery, it seems preferable to perform a trabeculectomy with a scleral flap no larger than 3 mm × 3 mm, a corneoscleral block excised totally anterior to the scleral spur, and a scleral flap which is tightly closed. Continued experience in the future may indicate that even less extensive surgery is equally satisfactory.

## References


1. David R, Sachs U (1981) Quantitative trabeculectomy. Br J Ophthalmol 65:457–459
2. D'Ermo F, Bonomi L, Doro D (1979) A critical analysis of the long-term results of trabeculectomy. Am J Ophthalmol 88:829–835
3. Duzanec Z, Krieglstein GK (1981) Die Beziehung zwischen Druckregulierung und anatomischer Lokalisation sowie Trepangrossebei der Goniotrepanation. Eine prospektive Studie. Klin Monatsbl Augenheilkd 178:431–435
4. Fronimopoulos J, Lambrou N (1980) The significance of the scleral flap for the surgery of glaucoma. Surv Ophthalmol 25:121–122
5. Joseph NH, Spaeth GL (1972) Modified trabeculectomy with iridectomy. Wills Eye Hospital Annual Clinical Conference Program (Abstract)
6. Krasnov MM (1969) Microsurgery techniques for glaucoma. Am J Ophthalmol 67:857–864
7. Luntz MH (1980) Trabeculectomy using a fornix-based conjunctival flap and tightly sutured scleral flap. Ophthalmol 87:985–989
8. Mascarell EV, Taboada J, Menezo JL (1979) Various techniques of trabeculectomy. Palestra Oftalmologica Panamericana 3:40–47
9. Parrish RK, Spaeth GL (1980) Why trabeculectomies fail. Poster, American Academy of Ophthalmology Program (Abstract)
10. Spaeth GL (1980) A prospective, controlled study to cmpare the Scheie procedure with Watson's trabeculectomy. Opththalmic Surg 11:688–694
11. Stewart RH, Kimbrough RL, Bachh H, et al. (1979) Trabeculectomy and modifications of trabeculectomy. Ophthalmic Surg 10:76–80
12. Taylor HR (1976) A histologic survey of trabeculectomy. Am J Ophthalmol 82:733–735


## Discussion

**Kitazawa to Spaeth:** I like to know about the protocol of your follow-up during the immediate post-operative study. Through our prospective, follow-up study of trabeculectomized patient that involved more than 140 operations we learned by examining them twice daily for 7 consecutive, post-operative days it is not uncommon that the shallowing of anterior chamber with or without choroidal detachment takes place anytime between the first and the seventh post-operative day and disappears within a matter of 6 to 8 hours spontaneously. Based on this observation I like to emphasize that the incidence of shallow anterior chamber and/or choroidal detachment could be estimated quite variably depending on the timing of observations.

**Leydhecker to Spaeth:** I could not see any difference of the result whether the new exit for aqueous is cut round (trephine), or square (trabeculectomy, goniectomy). Some patients get repeated scarring of the filtering site whatever you do, even with excision of the subconjunctival tissue or with Dexamethason treatment.

**Sampaolesi to Spaeth:** I want to make two remarks. 1. In the last years I performed 200 trabeculectomies. I controlled them with two diurnal pressure curves in a year and one spot check intraocular pressure each month.

When I controlled the results I obtained:

After 1 year 90% of good results
After 3 years 75% of good results and
After 6 years 70% of good results.

35% of the patients with not regulated IOP were controlled with medical therapy and 5% I had to reoperate.

2. Regarding the size of the piece of trabeculectomy I make it 4 mm to 3 mm in order to get a bigger piece for histology.

On this slide I show you that I cut the specimen at the posterior end of the scleral spur.

Krieglstein G.K./Leydhecker W. (eds)
Glaucoma Update II


# Laser Iridotomy

H.A. Quigley, Baltimore

## Introduction

While surgical peripheral iridectomy is a simple, uncomplicated and well-established procedure for the therapy of pupillary block glaucoma, the last ten years have seen the replacement of this procedure by use of lasers in many centers. The early reports of Khuri (1973), Abraham and Miller (1975), and Pollack and Patz (1976) represented studies of the early success at routine utilization of laser energy to produce iris holes. This report will not deal in any depth with the history of the development of this technique-obviously, as with any new modality, the most common finding is that a number of insightful investigators contributed. With the extensive experience we have now had with the procedure, this exposition can concentrate upon the relative indications for laser iridotomy, some brief aspects of the methods demonstrated to be most useful so far, results, complications, and future research needed.

## Indications

It should be pointed out immediately that it is the opinion of the author that the indications for producing an iris hole have not been changed by the introduction of laser methods. Clearly, those who have mastered the technique are impressed that: 1) no retrobulbar anesthesia is required; 2) there is no chance of endophthalmitis; 3) wound leaks cannot occur; 4) intraocular hemorrhage is now reported but rare; 5) visual recovery is nearly immediate (and hospitalization is not used); and the conjunctiva is not disturbed for future filtering surgery when needed. It is a rare patient who experiences either intra-operative or post-operative pain. However, damage to intraocular structures clearly occurs, though at an apparently acceptable level with present lengths of follow-up (see below). The inherent risk of the procedure must therefore be justified by serious risk of vision loss from pupillary block glaucoma or other forms of glaucoma that would be helped by an iris hole. The indiscriminate treatment of eyes with narrow chamber angles but no other direct or indirect evidence of pupillary block tendency should be avoided.

Laser iridotomy is therefore useful in the treatment of acute, intermittent and chronic angle closure glaucoma. We have used it in the middle of acute attacks, failing only where prolonged intraocular pressure elevation has caused significant corneal clouding. Treatment of the fellow eye of patients suffering acute angle closure may have become much easier than in the days when the patient perceived "surgery" on an (as yet) uninvolved eye as too frightening. Eyes with iris bombe, aphakic pupil block, and incomplete surgical iridectomies represent some other frequent uses of laser iridotomy in my practice.

## Methods

I use the continuous wave argon laser almost exclusively, though recently a krypton (red) laser has been used with similar success. The relatively uniform absorption of light throughout the visible spectrum by melanin probably makes the wavelength of minor importance. It is, of course, the melanin pigment of the iris that absorbs the laser light energy and is most important to the production of the hole. Pilocarpine drops are instilled pre-operatively to prevent iris motion - the iris musculature contracts on laser stimulation. Topical anesthesia is required and that only because of the placement of a contact lens. This lens is a standard fundus lens with plano surface onto which is glued a plano-convex lens (focal length = 15 mm). The lens prevents lid blinking during treatment, may absorb heat energy that would otherwise be delivered to the corneal epithelium, provides greater focusing of the incident beam (increasing power density and penetration), and allows treatment in the more peripheral iris by its prismatic effect.

The treatment is carried out at high magnification, usually on the superior-nasal iris, where the chamber is often deepest. Advantage is occasionally taken of apparently thinner spots in the iris stroma elsewhere when these are present. The delivery system should always be aimed away from the fovea, lest energy be able to reach the posterior retina by refraction by the crystalline lens. The 12 o'clock position is avoided since bubbles of gas form during treatment and float to this area; if the treatment is carried out at 12 o'clock, these soon obscure the view. The clearest possible view of iris detail and the most precise focus are vital to success. This means the arcus senilis must be avoided, and if cloudy spots in the cornea develop during treatment, the patient is directed to look upward or downward to allow further iris treatment through clearer media. Failure to do so results in no iris hole and unnecessary cornea damage.

I use initial laser settings of 0.2 second duration, 50 micron spot size and between 0.5 and 1.0 watt energy. While a number of "catchy" names of methods have been popularized (the hump method, chipping away, etc.), there is no reason in my opinion to do anything other than begin attempting to make a hole in one spot. When little or no reaction is obtained with the initial deliveries, the energy is increased to a maximum of 1.5 watt at the same site. In only the most difficult irises does this fail to produce an actual hole with 10–15 burns. Then, further energy is directed at the edges of the hole to enlarge it, optimally to about 0.5 mm in largest diameter, clearing all debris from the center with perfectly placed burns only on tissue (never straight through the hole).

When difficulty is experienced in making a hole at the first spot attempted, one should move immediately to a second location, frequently with immediate success. When about 75 deliveries have been made in one eye at one sitting and no hole is present, it is best to stop, bringing the patient back in 1–2 weeks for a second treatment after the cornea and media clear. This is particularly true for the first few cases of any surgeon.

Topical steroids are given four times daily for one week and preoperative glaucoma medications are continued until the new pressure level is determined. The eye is not patched and vision is blurred one or two Snellen lines for 24 hours. Both eyes are treated at one session where indicated. During the first post-operative week, detailed examination is carried out and the pupil dilated under observation to assure no pressure rise and to prevent posterior synechiae (this is done, of course, only when a definite hole is present).

The identification of laser holes can present minor difficulty initially. The most reliable criterion is direct visibility of lens capsule, zonule, or ciliary processes. In dark irides, bright transillumination of the hole is helpful, but in blue eyes there is frequently a large area of transillumination (removal of iris pigment epithelium) even in areas with iris stroma still intact.

## Results

The success of any procedure improves with the experience of the surgeon. I demonstrated this in this procedure by noting the number of successful permanent holes I made in one session rising from 50% in my first 100 eyes to 85% in my most recent 100. The data to be given is comprised of 260 eyes I have personally treated and observed, along with reference to another 750 additional eyes treated by Irvin Pollack, Arnall Patz, and Alan Robin of the Wilmer Institute. Hopefully, others can benefit from our mistakes and achieve successful iris holes after fewer cases and with less difficulty in their first attempts.

Iris color makes a true difference among eyes in ease of penetration. Light brown eyes are easiest, due to the combination of a moderate melanin content (to absorb energy) and relative thinness (not a long way to go through). Blue eyes are more difficult because they have little pigment and higher energy levels and more deliveries are often necessary. Dark brown eyes have a good pigment content, but are quite thick, hence also often requiring more energy and/or more treatment sessions.

As a rule, iris holes that are open at six weeks after treatment remain open indefinitely, often enlarging with passing years. There have been two exceptions, however. In some early cases, we were able to produce only a small hole, or a group of small holes (50 micron diameter). In two such eyes, an apparent regrowth of iris pigment epithelium or macrophages occurred, obscuring the opening. Since one cannot be certain that the iridotomy would then be functional, these two eyes were retreated (quite easily) and have remained open since. The second group of eyes in which reclosure has occurred is iris bombe associated with chronic uveitis or rubeosis iridis. While the laser provides an acceptable and immediate means for ending pupil block in these eyes, the largest possible holes should be produced compatible with safety, since the inflammatory or neovascular tissue can grow over the opening, requiring retreatment or wide surgical iridectomy.

Since laser holes are smaller than surgical iridectomies as a rule, it was initially questioned whether they would be big enough to prevent pupil block. First, it can be easily seen directly at the time of treatment in over two-thirds of eyes that the peripheral angle deepens markedly. Second, in a series of over 100 eyes with either pre-treatment angle closure attacks or positive provocative testing, mydriatic provocative tests were repeated post-treatment. In none was the test positive, despite some of the holes being only 200 microns in diameter.

Many eyes with chronic angle closure glaucoma appear to benefit from iridotomy, not only in the prevention of acute attacks and progressive angle closure, but even in the resting pressure level. In 46 such eyes, I compared the intraocular pressure control before and after iridotomy (one year follow-up). In 14 eyes, pressure was normal on therapy before treatment and remained so afterward on similar medication. In the 32 eyes with pressures above 21 mmHg preoperatively, 14 (44%) had an improvement in pressure of 5 mmHg or more on either the same or less medication. This may have resulted from eliminating a relative pupillary block. In 11 further eyes, pressure was above 21 mmHg on maximum tolerated medical therapy. In five of these eyes, pressure dropped below 21 and the field loss has been stable without filtering surgery, while in the other 6 trabeculectomy became necessary. In the past, this decision was a difficult one, that is, should a surgical iridectomy or filtering surgery be done. Iridectomy might be sufficient, but if not, a second intraocular procedure (and retrobulbar anesthetic) was necessary. On the other hand, the risk of filtering surgery was too great to carry it out on all such patients when some would do well with iridectomy alone. Laser iridotomy provides a means of determining the need for filtration surgery or not with only one actual surgical intervention. It is interesting that I could not have predicted which patients would have needed to go on to filtration surgery from the degree of peripheral anterior synechiae, the extent of field loss (all had some) or the duration of glaucoma.

Another similar circumstance in which laser iridotomy can be used as a diagnostic tool is the aphakic eye with shallow or flat chamber and high pressure. Here, the differentiation between aphakic pupil block and malignant glaucoma can be made by laser iris hole. If the chamber does not deepen, vitreous surgery is required.

## Complications

Our greatest concern is decrease in visual acuity from laser iridotomy. This could occur from direct laser injury to the retina or from indirect effects on the lens or cornea. I have not recognized a retinal lesion produced by treatment. In eyes followed for nearly two years in my practice (Quigley, 1981) and in a larger group followed for up to five years by Robin and Pollack (1982), somewhat less than 15% of eyes had lost more than two lines (Snellen) of vision in the years after treatment. Evaluation of this group showed them to be older than those who maintained stable vision and to more frequently exhibit pre-treatment cataract. Almost every case of decreasing vision, then, represented a predictable progression of cataract in this minority group. Comparison with similar cataract progression in surgical iridectomy series (see Robin and Pollack, 1982) does not show any major difference in this respect between laser and surgical methods, though comparisons are limited by differences in patient selection. Corneal damage was not detected in primate studies (Hirst et al. 1982) and specular microscopy of our patients has delineated no major cell loss, though our clinical studies of this question are not complete. No patient has had a permanent decrease in vision related to corneal decompensation.

There is a mild inflammatory response to treatment and in some eyes intraocular pressure rises in the first 24–48 hours after treatment. When such rises were seen to be mild and nearly always inconsequential, we discontinued use of oral carbonic anhydrase inhibitors or osmotic agents to cover this period.

### Future Investigation

While laser-produced iridotomies have replaced the surgical method in our practice, further improvements would still be welcome. There is the occasional eye that responds inadequately. And, it would be more esthetically pleasing to perform the procedure with one delivery instead of the multiple, painstaking ones we utilize now. To this end, Pollack, Gaasterland, and others have begun experimental work with other lasers, including the Q-switched ruby laser. This instrument was recently used to produce a "one-shot" iris hole in a human eye. It delivers large amounts of energy in nanoseconds, probably without even heating up the tissue. I look forward to a continued exciting new time for the careful testing of newer technological advances.

### References


Abraham RK, Miller GL (1975) Outpatient argon laser iridectomy for angle closure glaucoma: a two year study. Trans Am Ophthalmol Soc 79:529–538

Hirst LW, Robin AL, Sherman S, et al. (1982) Corneal endothelial changes after argon laser iridotomy and panretinal photocoagulation. Am J Ophthalmol 93:473–481

Khuri CH (1973) Argon laser iridectomies. Am J Ophthalmol 76:490–493

Pollack IP, Patz A (1976) Argon laser iridotomy: an experimental and clinical study. Ophthalmic Surg 7:22–30

Quigley HA (1981) Long-term follow-up of laser iridotomy. Ophthalmol 88:218–224

Robin AL, Pollack IP (1982) Argon laser peripheral iridotomies in the treatment of primary angle closure glaucoma. Arch Ophthalmol 100:919–923


## Discussion

**Schwartz to Quigley:** I wish to make two points in relation to laser iridotomies. We have observed in several cases the spontaneous enlargement of laser iridotomies over a period of several years. We have been able to document this enlargement photographically (Sachs und Schwartz 1982). When we compared patients who showed spontaneous enlargements of the iridotomy with those who did not, we were not able to determine any related factors, either ocular or systemic. We are unaware of any observations in the literature indicating that surgical iridectomies increase spontaneously and, therefore, wonder whether there is something unique about the laser technique in producing an iridotomy that may spontaneously become enlarged.

Secondly, we noted in several cases that, following a patent laser iridotomy, the whole angle, as observed by slit-lamp gonioscopy, was not entirely opened. Instead, it was opened only in the quadrant which contained the laser iridotomy. Assuming that perhaps posterior synechiae had developed around the laser iridotomy, we proceeded to perform a surgical iridectomy on these eyes. Subsequent to the surgical iridectomy the entire angle opened. Therefore, we wish to emphasize the importance of evaluating the effectiveness of the laser iridotomy by gonioscopy and not simply by control of ocular pressure. The iridotomy is only effective when pupillary block is removed, as evidenced by the opening of the angle.


Sachs S, Schwartz B (1982) Enlargement of laser iridotomies over time. Am J Ophthalmol (submitted for publication)


**Spaeth to Quigley:** There is a significant difference between the argon laser iridectomy and the iridectomy performed with an instrument which causes much shorter more powerful bursts, as would occur with the Q-switched laser. With a Q-switched laser the effect on tissue is mechanical, and the tissue is vaporized. This, then, eliminates one of the problems of argon laser iridectomy, which is a dispersion of the tissue throughout the rest of the anterior segment, with deposition of the tissue in the trabecular meshwork. Presumably it would be better for the eye with this tissue vaporized rather than were is redistributed.

Krieglstein G.K./Leydhecker W. (eds)
Glaucoma Update II


# Corneal Sensitivity and Intraocular Pressure

J. Draeger and R. Winter, Hamburg

Nutrition and metabolism of the eye is affected by rise in intraocular pressure.

This not only is valid for the optic disc, for choroid and retina, but also for more anteriorly situated tissue. Change in blood supply will affect many metabolic processes. But pressure rise in the surrounding tissue may also affect directly nervous function. Corneal sensitivity is a very sensitive indicator for such a nervous function. In principle already Kal'fa and Paramonov (1955) have discussed a correlation between sensitivity threshold and glaucoma. But so far - to our knowledge - there are no experimental or clinical investigations published dealing with this specific subjects. Probably methodological problems are the reason. This obviously is due to the fact, at the threshold of sensitivity especially in the center of the cornea is exceedingly low. This on the other hand means that pathological changes can be diagnosed early and very precisely. Although this has been recognized since von Frey published his original investigations, aesthesiometry is not yet widely used because of the difficulties of the technique. Because of the low threshold values the applied force also must be very small; furthermore the measurement has to be rapid and reproducible. Up to now the methods used have not met these requirements: fibre filaments have been used in modern instruments but these vary with age, and are affected by humidity and the temperature of the air. The 'speed and angle of the approach and the elasticity of the filament vary, not to mention the skill of the examiner, so that the unreliability of the measurement has long hampered its use both clinically and in research.

Now we are in the position to use a new electronic-optical aesthesiometer which is extremely precise and independent of external changes in temperature and humidity (Fig. 1).

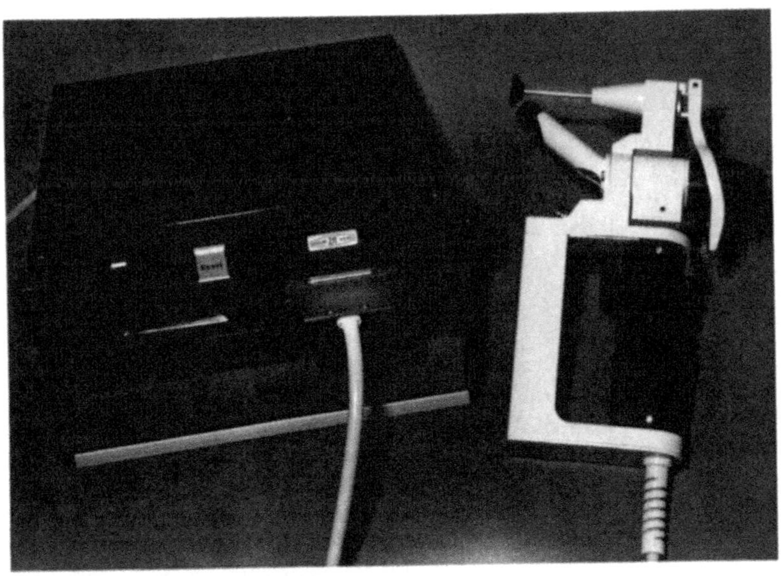

**Fig. 1.** Electronic-optical aesthesiometer, instrument and display

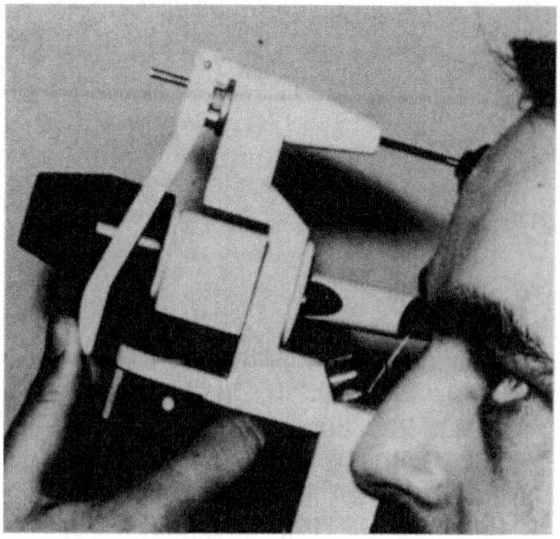

**Fig. 2.** Aesthesiometer applied to right eye

One hand holds the instrument. With the fingertip the motion of the contact pin is released and at the same time the force applied is diminished or increased. Optical control of the measurement is mandatory in order to determine the precise location of contact with the corneal epithelium (Fig. 2).

The contact pin touches the cornea rapidly at a predetermined speed which is automatically controlled.

The focus adjustment is facilitate by focusing cross lines. The illumination is part of the instrument. The threshold profile of corneal sensation is determined first. Before touching the corneal epithelium the forward motion is slowed down to avoid any ballistic effect.

A digital display continously indicates the force applied. This increase is faster the more the force increases. The upper limit is $1000 \times 10^{-5}$ N.

By division of the images in the eye-piece the corneal profile and the lateral location of the contact pin can be observed simultaneously (Fig. 3).

At the corneal centre very low values are found, i.e. between 0,8 and 2,5 units according to age – this corresponds to the value of $29 \times 10^{-5}$ N in the horizontal and $38 \times 10^{-5}$ near the limbus in the vertical meridian (Fig. 4).

The correlation between corneal sensitivity and age is determined next.

The mean value in the juvenile group at the 12 o'clock position near the limbus is 14,7; $31 \times 10^{-5}$ N is necessary to release the corneal reflex in the over-60 age group.

Investigating corneal sensitivity threshold of patients suffering from glaucoma different parameters had to be considered: as many eye diseases and especially eye surgery also affect the values only primary chronic glaucomas had to be selected.

Therefore two selected groups only are evaluated in our study: one group was on a 'medical therapy only, the other group was treated by a strictly standarized filtering procedure.

The sensitivity profile in patients with primary chronic open angle glaucoma compared to a group of normals shows a slight rise but only low statistical significance of the difference. Very much different is the result after fistulizing surgery: gonic-trephanation at 12 o'clock forming a bleb in the superior conjunctiva leads to a marked increase of the threshold all over the cornea, even in the lower circumference.

Cararact extraction, as earlier could be shown, results in a similar disease of sensitivity threshold.

As these values are measured within the first year after surgery, we are not yet able to estimate long term follow up. Possibly a similar recovery, as shown in our cataract cases, could be expected.

Significant correlation was proven between sensitivity and duration of the disease (Fig. 5). The longer the duration of the disease, the higher the threshold was.

Due to our limited number of cases we

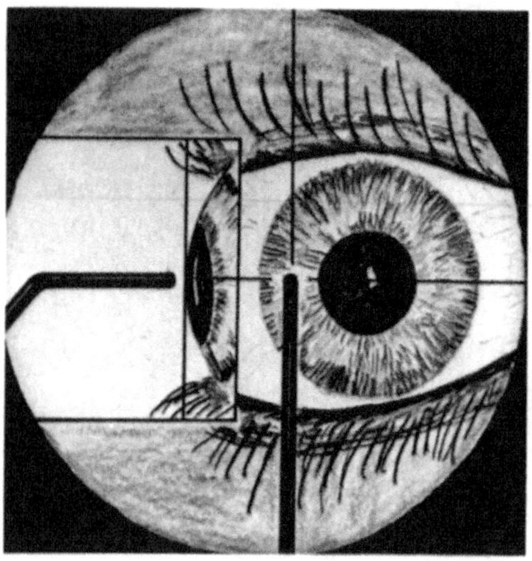

**Fig. 3.** Divided images in the eye-piece

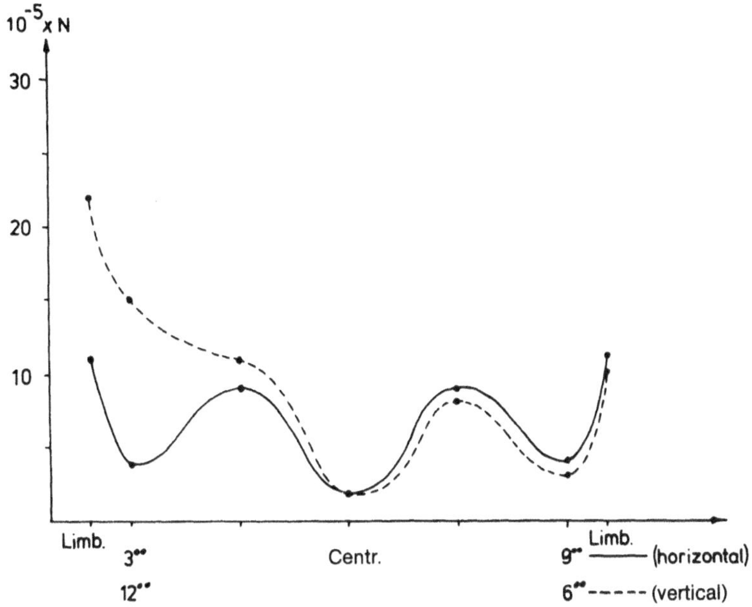


**Fig. 4.** Topography of corneal sensitivity. C = centre

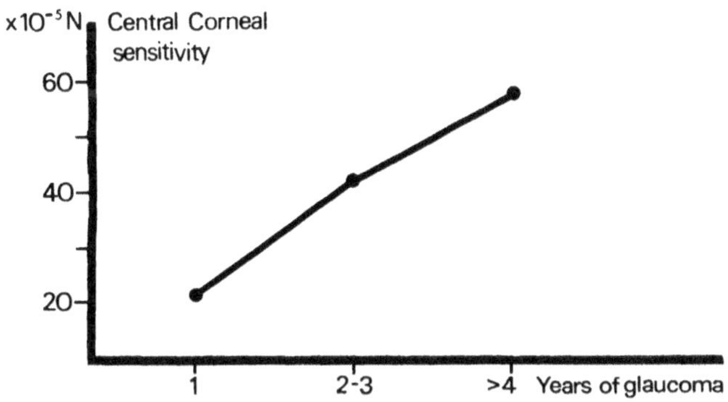


**Fig. 5.** Corneal sensitivity and duration of chronic glaucoma

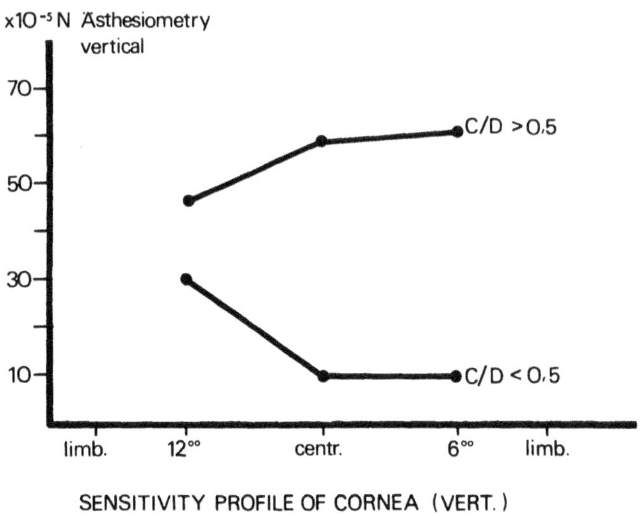


**Fig. 6.** Corneal sensitivity and c/d

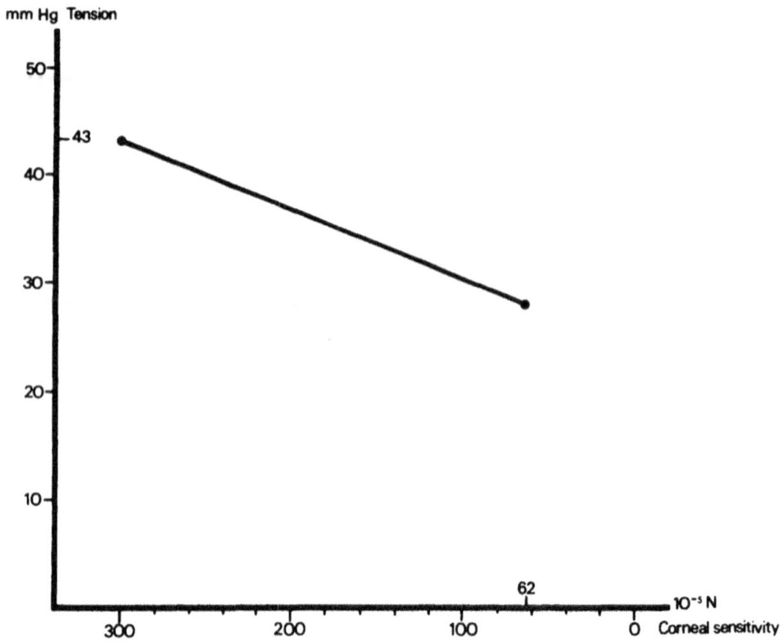


**Fig. 7.** Patient J.B. (28 years). Corneal sensitivity at 12 o'clock position, correlation with intraocular pressure

could not differentiate the individual case was regulated at the time of the examination or not.

Also significant was a result in cases where marked cutting and field loss were to be observed (Fig. 6). If the c/d ratio exceeded 0,5 a significant change of sensitivity threshold could be observed.

Furthermore corneal sensitivity also may be influenced by sudden rise in pressure (Fig. 7).

20 years old patient was admitted, intraocular pressure at this time 43 mmHg. The sensitivity threshold at the 12 o'clock position was significantly reduced. Only 90 minutes later, intraocular pressure now 28 mmHg, corneal sensitivity had improved from $300 \times 10^{-5}$ N to $62 \times 10^{-5}$ N. This result supports a direct correlation between nerve function and pressure in the surrounding tissue (Fig. 8).

In a lower pressure range this difference is less marked but still statistically significant.

This preliminary study proves a correlation between

1. - Duration of glaucoma disease and increase of sensitivity threshold, and
2. correlation between intraocular pressure and sensitivity threshold.

Looking at these figures one has to keep in

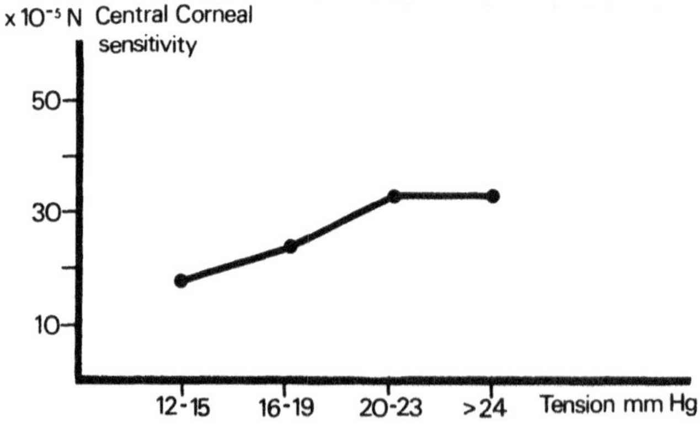


**Fig. 8.** Corneal sensitivity, center correlated with intraocular pressure

mind that not only the disease itself but also the medication influences corneal sensitivity: Already more than 10 years ago the unexpected local anaesthetic offect of beta-blocking-agents was detected. From our own experimental studies we know that most of the currently used beta-blocking-agents, besides their specific effect on intraocular hydrodynamics, may depress corneal sensitivity! To investigate this side effect 60 healthy patients of the age-group between 20 and 60 years were investigated. In detail the following procedure was adopted: Primarily we determined the sensitivity threshold at 6 h position. After that a drop of the candidate beta-receptor-blockers was instilled into the cul-de-sac and the measurements were taken for a quarter of an hour minutely. Thereby stimuli were recorded which just lead to contact sensation.

## Results

*1. Propanolol (Fig. 9)*

Far from the other drugs the Propanolol exhibits the strongest local anaesthetic potential. Its effect starts instantaneously and is comparable to that of the other local anaesthetic used in ophthalmology. The maximum-value amounted to $320 \times 10^{-5}$ N and was constant at this level for several minutes.

*2. Bupranolol (Fig. 10)*

Also with this drug the local anaesthesia manifests instantaneously although the maximum intensity is clearly much lower as determined for Propanolol. The main increase amounted to $10{,}9 \times 10^{-5}$ N. After 15 minutes the initial status was practically restored.

*3. Timolol (Fig. 11)*

Timolol as well shows a comparable local anaesthetic effect. However the initial sensitivity is restored within 8 minutes. Outstanding here was the fact that in the case of young people of 20–40 years practically no local anaesthesia was confirmed. This is in Contrast to the otherwise determined age dependent local anaesthetic effect of Propanolol and Bupranolol (Buhr-Unger et al. 1980).

*4. Metipranolol (Fig. 12)*

Application of 0,25% Metipranolol leads to an immediate local anaesthetic effect. The

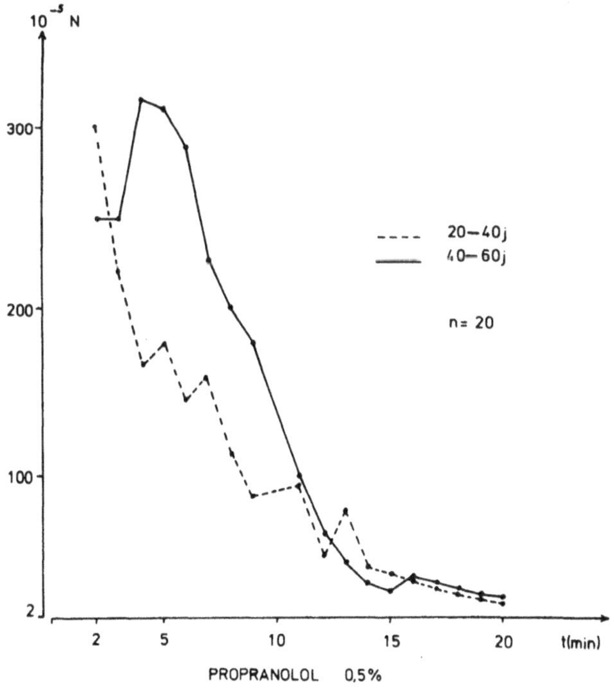


**Fig. 9.** Time dependent changes in the threshold-values in the 6 h position after Propanolol-eyedrops

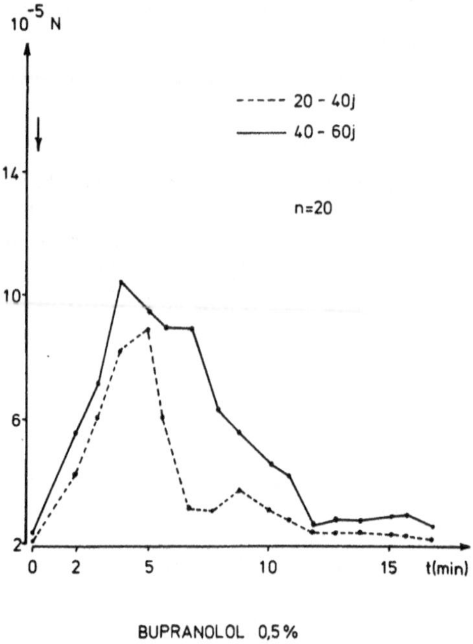


Fig. 10. Time dependent threshold profile at 6 h position as measured for Propanolol

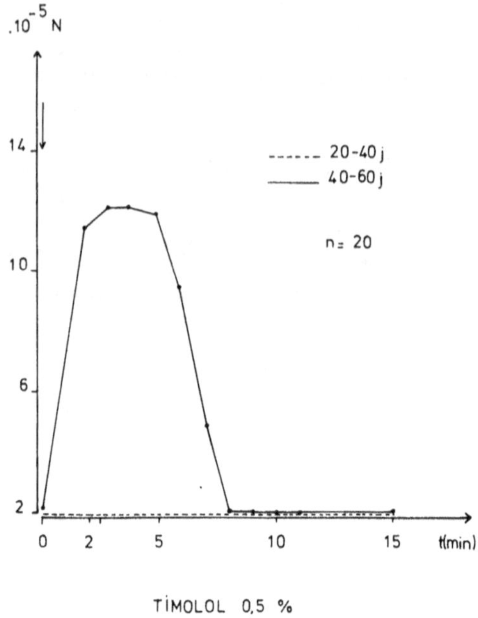


Fig. 11. Time dependent sensitivity profile at 6 h position as measured for Timolol

maximum of the sensitivity loss amounts to $13 \times 10^{-5}$ N. The normalization takes a little bit longer than determined for Timolol 0,5%, nearly the same as in Timolol.

*5. Dose-dependency*

In case of Timolol and Metipranolol additionally a dose-dependent fact was

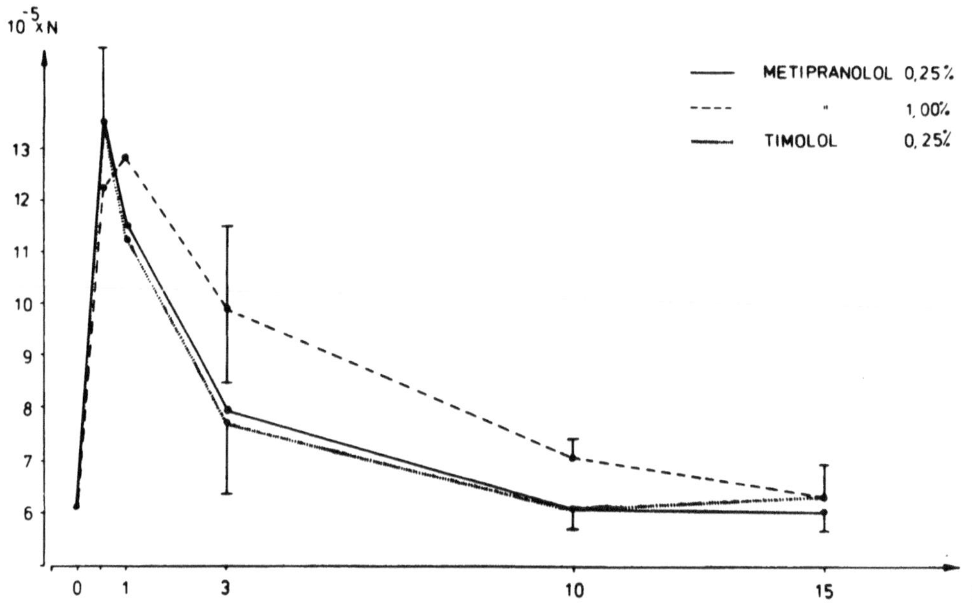


**Fig. 12.** Dose dependent corneal sensitivity threshold-curves for 6 h position as measured for Metipranolol 0,25% and 1,0%

observed. Comparison of Timolol 0,25% with 0,5% solution shows that the local anaesthetic effect enters for both concentrations immediately at the same level. Only for the high concentration the intensity of the effect lasts a few minutes longer (Fig. 12).

A similar effect is also observed for Metipranolol, where identical maximum values are achieved, although the threshold of the corneal sensitivity at the high concentration is clearly slowed down.

## Discussion

All the investigated beta-receptor-blockers exhibit a measurable local anaesthesia as side effect. However for Timolol and Metipranolol it is clearly much lower as has been observed for Propanolol and Bupranolol. Both the last named drugs, which are currently time dependent in use, lead to a loss of corneal sensitivity which is both, dose- and time-dependent. The degree of the sensitivity loss remains obviously uninfluenced at higher concentrations.

Depending on the local anaesthetic effect of Timolol and Metipranolol it is probable that a long-term treatment would lead to substantial trophic injury to the cornea. However the patient should be aware of the fact that due to the induction of hyposensitivity immediate instillation of the eye-drops a foreign body may remain unperceived. The contactlens-wearers therefore should be precautions!

A different observation on which we have previously reported, was found in the case of 4 probands (Buhr-Unger et al. 1980). In these cases the local anaesthesia was more pronounced and also the effect was obviously prolonged. This was the case specially for a 33 years old patient (Fig. 13).

Thus the increase in the sensitivity threshold for Propanolol amounted to $1000 \times 10^{-5}$ N. The normal sensitivity was regained only 20 minutes after instillation.

This deviation in behaviour could be explained from some possible enzyme-defects. Considering these so-called responders (at least for a part of the population) the unwanted local anaesthetic effects of the betareceptor-blockers is not to be ignored. In case of such outstanding sensitivity disturbances severe side effects for individual patients cannot be excluded with certain. A simple examination of the corneal sensitivity profile at the onset of the treatment could sort out such pre-disposed patients and this avoids the unexpected risk.

In summary the local anaesthetic potential of those beta-receptor-blockers, which

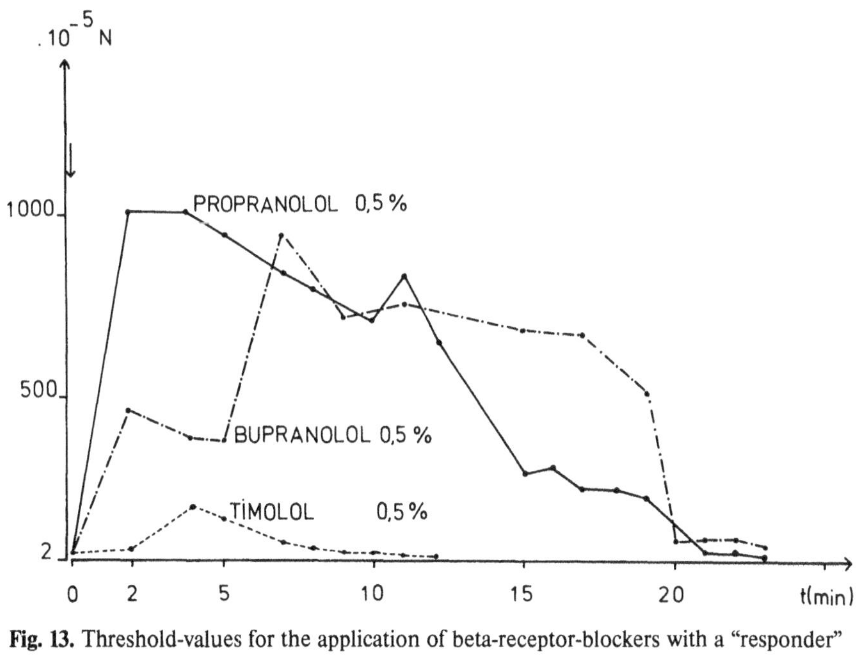


**Fig. 13.** Threshold-values for the application of beta-receptor-blockers with a "responder"

currently are in use in the therapy of glaucoma, could be considered as unserious side-effect.

## References


1. Buhr-Unger H, Draeger J, Lüders M (1979) Untersuchungen zur lokalanästhetischen Wirkung der Beta-Rezeptoren-Blocker. Ber deutsch Ophthalmol Ges 77:577–580
2. Frey M von (1894) Beiträge zur Physiologie des Schmerzsinns. Berichte über die Verhandlung der königl. 6. Ges. der Wissenschaften zu Leipzig. Mathematisch-Physische Classe. Leipzig, Hirtzel, pp 185–196
3. Kal'fa SF, Paramonov AF (1955) Vestn Oftal 34:33–37

Krieglstein G.K./Leydhecker W. (eds)
Glaucoma Update II


# Disc Haemorrhages - Forerunners of Chronic Glaucoma

C.E.T. Krakau, Lund

During the last decade a diagnostic sign overlooked for a long time, has attracted attention, namely hemorrhages (hh) in the optic disc. The importance of this sign was emphasized by Drance and collaborators, adducing evidence of increasing weight (Drance et al. 1970, 1971, 1976, 1977, 1979). The response to these efforts now come to the fore in several articles published also by other authors and devoted to the natural history of hh. During the last years the results have appeared from survey material and glaucoma follow up studies (Bengtsson et al. 1980, 1981; Holmin and Krakau 1981) and of retrospective investigations (Airaksinen et al. 1981, Gloster 1981).

We cannot claim that hh have not previously been observed. A connection between disc hh and glaucoma was recognized nearly a hundred years ago by Bjerrum (1889), who also pointed out that hh could be regarded as precursors or a first symptom in the development of a glaucomatous state.

Though Bjerrum's observations were published in Danish, it is amazing that an ominous and common sign like papillary hh could fall into oblivion for so long. To some extent this may be attributed to the use of miotics which, lowering the curtain, conceal what may be enacted in the posterior pole.

Drance's observations have essentially been confirmed by subsequent authors and there is full agreement on several points. Hh are mainly located on the rim of the papilla, more often near the poles than elsewhere. They emanate from the capillary network of the tissue, are deep or superficial, and appear rounded or splinter-shaped. They may even be flame-shaped, and bear a resemblance to a branch thrombosis. They remain observable for a few weeks, during which period they become thinner and diffuse and their existence appears doubtful. Photographs taken on different occasions are then of great value for the recognition of hh, establishing their appearance or disappearance beyond doubt. Many hh overlooked at ophthalmoscopy are detected on slides. It is hard to say if fundoscopy is superior to photographs at detecting the most minute hh, and possibly the observable size might be further reduced by use of a more advanced technique of observation.

The chance of finding a h increases with the number of observations. Hh are more common in glaucoma cases than in ocular hypertensions or glaucoma suspects. More than one third of glaucoma patients with field defects also show h at one time or another. Their capacity of precursors of glaucomatous defects is confirmed and they have also been associated with progression of field defects. There seems to be no reason to refer the glaucoma cases with hh to a separate group of glaucoma. A low IOP affords no protection against hh, on the contrary hh seem to be inclined to appear when the IOP is low, or prefer eyes with a low IOP (with the reservation that IOP at bleeding is unknown).

In the following discussion the results of investigations based on two materials will be dealt with. The first material is derived from the Dalby population survey, performed 1978-79. Among 1511 individuals aged between 55 and 70, 15 cases with field defects accepted as glaucomatous were detected by means of an automatic perimeter (Competer) (Bengtsson and Krakau 1979). These cases represented early stages of glaucoma since there were no subjective complaints, the IOP values were centered around 21 mmHg and the field defects generally small. Papillary substance defects of modest size were also found corresponding to the field defects. Among these field defects there were seven cases with disc h and a further five cases without defect but with h.

Both the cases with defects and those with hh were reexamined on several occasions during a follow-up period. New hemorrhages

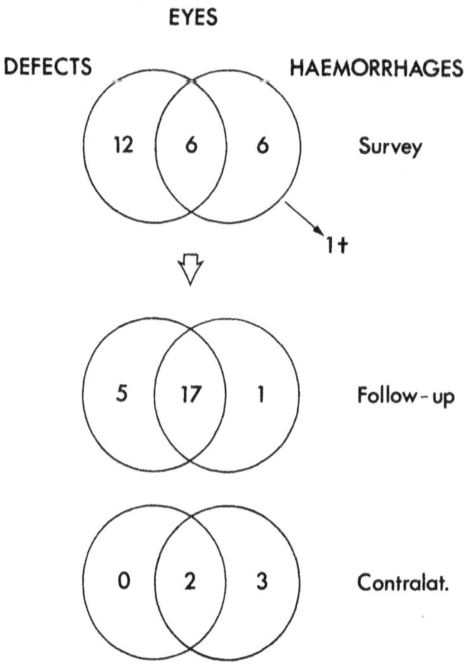


**Fig. 1.** Venn-diagram of eyes with field defects, haemorrhages and with both defects and haemorrhages detected at survey and after follow up (h seen at least once). During follow up another 5 eyes with hh, 2 also with h defects, were detected on contralateral eyes

were then observed both among the eyes with defects and among those with h only. Also new hh and defects appeared in previously unaffected contralateral eyes (Fig. 1).

## A Statistical Model

The occurrence of hh is conceived as a series of events, occurring apparently at random intervals. We have no detailed knowledge of the stability of the parameters which characterize the series. Hh may occur frequently or sporadically, and "wet" periods may alternate with "dry" ones. Possibly the frequency changes during the development of the glaucomatous state, and there may be great differences between different "bleeders". In spite of this lack of knowledge the discussion of a simple statistical model may help us to "fix the ideas". A process "without memory" seems appropriate. Many occurrences, e.g. radioactive disintegration, are adequately described by such a process. Whatever the number of events (hh) during a period (0, t) the probability that during (t, t + d) a h occurs is $\lambda d + 0$ (small term), where $\lambda$ is a parameter. It is assumed that only one h can appear in such an interval. A Poisson process derives from these postulates. It may be shown, for instance, that the probability of no h appearing during the time interval of length t is $p_h(t) = e^{-\lambda t}$, and that of exactly one h is $p_h(t) = \lambda t\, e^{-\lambda t}$.

A h remains observable during a certain period, S. So if we make an examination on an arbitrary occasion within a time T, of long duration in comparison to S, the probability that a h is found is $p_h = t_h/T$, where t is the total time during which at least one h is observable. Since the observable periods may overlap, $t_h = n.\,S\text{-}C$ where n is the number of hh within the period T. Our knowledge about the time S - probably very variable with the size of h etc - is insufficient and we will not proceed with estimates of the effect of overlapping (C), since this is not pertinent in the following conclusions. When we make repeated examinations at intervals $>$S and find either no h or at least one h, a binomial distribution is generated. By repeating the examinations on the same or on different hemorrhagic eyes (which we presume are statistically equivalent) we arrive at an estimate of the probability $p_h$ (1) to find at least one h at a single examination. This probability is not complicated by the overlapping mentioned above.

The probability p can be interpreted as the conditional probability of finding a h when the eye is known to be a haemorrhagic one. If we examine a number n′ of such eyes at a survey $n'.p_h$ eyes with h can be expected.

Recalling the results of the Dalby survey, there were 6 with h among the eyes with defects at the initial examination. (If we count from the other end of the series, taking the last examination as the initial one, 4 hh were detected). If the group of bleeders could be spotted by some sign, more constant than hh, subsequent examinations of this group should reveal an increasing number of eyes with at least one h. during follow-up.

In fact, eyes with glaucomatous field defects seem to form such a group. These cases, which were followed by examinations at intervals of about 3 months, showed an increasing prevalence of hh (Fig. 2) with the number of examinations. The probability of

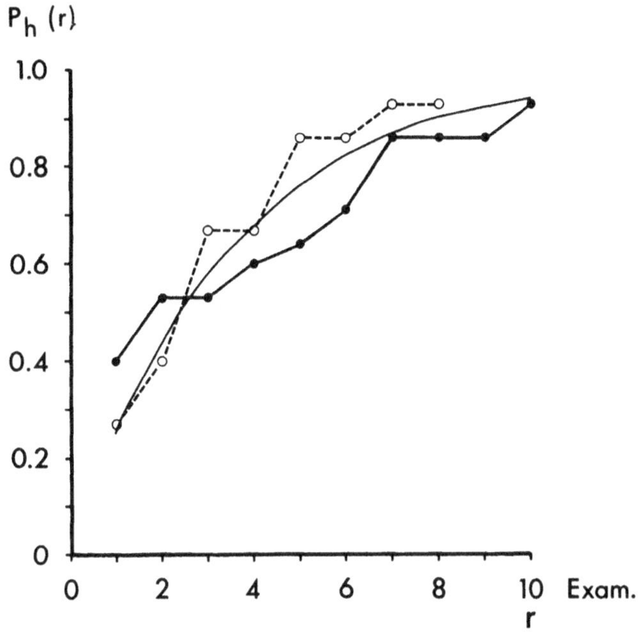


**Fig. 2.** Probability of finding at least one haemorrhage in *r* examinations. *Smooth curve:* theoretical values. *Irregular curves:* observed values among the eyes with defects, counted from start or from end

finding a h is estimated as the ratio between the total number of examinations with hh observed and the number of all examinations of the group of eyes with a field defect and showing a h at least once. The number of hh in the group of eyes with a field defect was 31 and the total number of examinations 121, giving the probability $p_h(1) = 0.26$ of finding a h at one random examination. In the five eyes with hh at survey but without defect we similarly find $p(1) = 15/52 = 0.29$. With an increasing number of examinations the proportion of eyes with at least one h increases (Fig. 2).

But it is also possible to deduce from $p_h(1)$ the probability $p_h(r)$ of at least one h in r examinations, assuming independent examinations. By a simple reasoning we get $p_h(r) = 1-(1-p_h(1))^r$. The correspondence between observed and calculated values (Fig. 2) is acceptable and supports the basic assumptions of our model. Thus we can reasonably assume that early glaucoma cases with field defects have also hh to a very great extent. The quantity of hh found in the defect group corresponds to what might be predicted from the number of hh found at a single survey, assuming that eyes with defects are also bleeding eyes.

*Five eyes with h, without defects*, were also detected at the survey. Since we have estimated the chance of detecting a h at one survey $p_h(1)$, we find $n = p_h(1)\, n'$ = the number of h eyes detected (where n′ is the total number of h eyes). That is, a total of about 17 hh (without defect) should exist in the population, which means that there should be another undetected 12 hemorrhagic eyes.

This prediction is to some extent confirmed during the follow up of eyes with h and with defects (Fig. 1), by the fact that five new h eyes were found among contralateral eyes, two of them became associated with defects. Accepting the idea that hh are generally precursors of defects (it is not known whether some h eyes never develop defects) there must be an incidence of hh and a transfer of hh cases to cases with both defects and h. Conjecturing that practically all defects are preceded by hh there should, on an average, be the same incidence of h as transfer of h to cases with defects though with a delay between the appearance of h and of defect. The following reasoning affords a very rough estimate of this delay.

Let us assume, in the absence of more precise estimates, that the incidence of defects is constant during the period between 55 and 70 years of age. The total prevalence during this period is estimated at 15 eyes. The number of eyes with h without defect is about the same.

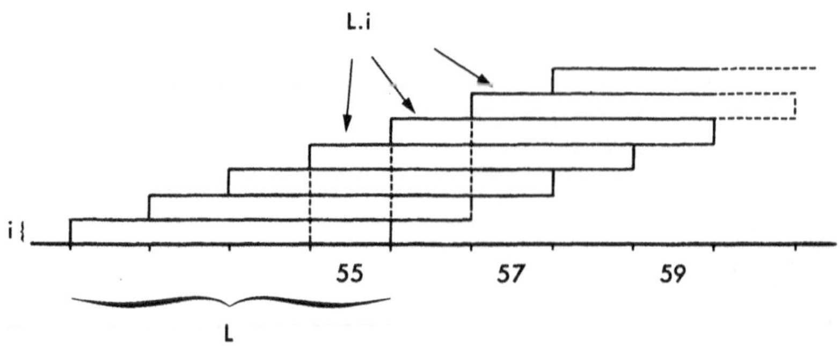


**Fig. 3.** Prevalence of eyes with haemorrhages, without field defects. *i*: incidence of h. *L:* average latency between appearance of h and field defect

We may assume that all of them develops defects in due time, and since we reckon with steady state, the incidence of eyes becoming hemorrhagic and the incidence of defects should be similar but with a delay between the onset of h and of defect. If the incidence i of defects per year in each one-year group is constant (and the age distribution uniform) from 55 years of age and zero before that age, i can be estimated from the total number of eyes with defects in the age group between 55 and 70 years by $N_d = \int_0^{15} i.t.\, dt = 15$, which gives $i = 2/15$. This means that another two eyes with defects per year can be expected in this population. (This estimate is in good agreement with the number of new eyes with defects found at a renewed survey of the Dalby population, pers. comm. Dr. B. Bengtsson). Assuming the same incidence for hh and an average period of "latency" L before an eye with h becomes an eye with h and defect, we get (Fig. 3) L.i. 15 = 17, where 17 is the estimated number of existing h eyes in the 55–70 age group. L is then 8.5 years.

The examination at which a h eye is detected may occur at any moment during L, and presumably with constant probability during this period. On an average the time between detection of a h and of a defect should then be L/2 or about 4 years.

The predictions of the incidence of hh and the latency before defects appear are derived from a crude model which can only be expected to indicate magnitudes. There are, however, observations of a long delay between the appearance of hh and of the field defects (Airaksinen 1981).

The estimate of nosological sensitivity (the number of eyes with hh and defect to the number of eyes with field defects) is high (0.77) and so is the diagnostic specificity (the number of eyes with defect and hh to the number of eyes with hh = 0.94).

*A follow-up study of a glaucoma material (Lund)* comprising 160 eyes (133 with field defects) in 90 patients (aged 48 to 83 years, mean 70 years) was performed with at least 5 separate examinations (minimum interval 2 months). The observation period ranged from 13 to 23 months. In all patients the treatment was unchanged (or there was no treatment) throughout the period of observation, the aim being conventional, namely to keep the IOP well controlled. At least one disc hh was found in 30 patients (39 eyes) during the follow up period. Six patients from the Dalby survey were included.

Routine taking of fundus photographs or use of fundoscopy at every examination could not be carried through to the full extent in this material. In some patients the risk of inducing an acute pressure attack by administration of mydriatics was found imminent, in others the miotic pupill did not respond to dilatation efforts. A few cases with lens opacities, blurring inspection and photography were found in the present material, which was on an average 5 years older than the survey material.

*The frequency of hh* was low as compared to that in the Dalby material, which may to a considerable extent be explained by the above mentioned difficulties at inspection. A stratification of the material according to treatment supported this assumption: the lowest frequency was found among the eyes treated with miotics (18 per cent, n = 77) and significantly higher values were found among the untreated ones (63 per cent, n = 19). The latter group also differed from the rest by having in general a less abnormal pressure, and was therefore untreated. The mean IOP was 19.6 mmHg in the untreated group, which is 2 mmHg lower than the mean of the treated group.

In the Dalby survey hh were an almost obligatory sign in glaucoma and, indeed, eyes with hh did develop glaucomatous field defects in a high percentage. The hypothesis that these observations have a general validity cannot be refuted on the basis of the Lund material. Defects remain but hh are transitory, they may have appeared at an earlier stage even in cases which now are "dry".

The high incidence of hh in glaucoma cases with defects and v.v. forces us to accept hh as an integral part of the glaucomatous destruction. However, difficulties present themselves when we want to involve an increased IOP as an etiological factor in the process. We have seen that *hh* occur especially at *low pressure* levels. The incidence of h was highest in the group with max IOP 11–20 mmHg in Glosters material (1981), in that from Lund in the group with IOP (mean) 18–20 mmHg. In the earliest stages, when hh but no field defects are detected, the pressure distribution is still like that of non-glaucomatous cases.

If we conjecture that *hh* is a sign which is suppressed by an increased *IOP*, a logical question is whether this occurs with or without retardation of the glaucomatous process. In the first case one might also expect a high IOP to retard the progression. This, however, is unsupported by experience.

An *immediate* association between the appearance of *hh and progression* of glaucomatous defects found no support in our material. Eyes with hh showed a decay of performance but so, to a similar extent, did the cases without detected h. The regr. coeff. were -2 (0 h), -1.7 (1–2 hh) and -1.9 (>2 hh) and not significantly different. On the other hand, a relation, though not immediate, exists between the appearance of hh and the glaucomatous destruction. The hh are undoubtedly precursors of field defects, often by several years, as has already been discussed. They keep their role as forerunners also when defects have appeared; their localization in the disc tissue indicates where substance and field defects can be expected (Bengtsson et al. 1981). But the time lag between hh and detectable defects is still great and this may be the reason why no immediate relation between the detection of a h and the performance decay was found.

It seems probable that this time lag has to be allowed for whenever the relations between hh, progression and IOP are considered.

Concerning pathogenesis the hh indicate a disturbance of circulation. According to several authors (a.o. Hayreh and Walker 1967, Spaeth 1975) the capillary network of the disc is reduced. Impaired circulation in one or several capillaries means insufficient nutrition in some small part of the optic nerve. The fibres in the disc are myelinized and have a lower metabolism than cell bodies or unmyelinized nerve fibres, and the effects of malnutrition may be retarded. The fluctuations of the threshold level, characteristic of the developing field defect, may indicate lacking reserve capacity and a function easily disturbed by occasional impairment of circulation - an impairment which normally passes without detection.

Finally the functional impairment is completely irreversible. In analogy with the delay between the first morphological signs and the functional damage one might guess that the response to treatment is similarly delayed. Even if the process damaging the small vessels were arrested, an immediate effect on the visual field decay would be surprising. Naturally, until long term follow up studies are available the role of the latency in various relations remains hypothetical.

**Abstract.** During follow up glaucoma cases with field defects spotted at a population study, show a high frequency of disc haemorrhages and those with haemorrhages develop field defects in high percentage. Conclusions are drawn from a statistical model. The prevalence of eyes with haemorrhages without defects in a population is estimated to be similar to the prevalence of eyes with field defects, or about 1 per cent in the age group 55–70 years. The average latency between the onset of bleeding and the appearance of defects is probably several years. This delay might be relevant in an evaluation of the relations between IOP, haemorrhages, progression of defects and therapeutic effects.

## References

1. Airaksinen J, Mustonen E, Alanko H (1981) Optic disc haemorrhages precede retinal nerve fibre layer defects in ocular hypertension. Acta Ophthalmol (Copenh) 59:627–641
2. Begg IS, Drance SM, Sweeney VP (1970) Haemorrhage on the disc - a sign of acute ischaemic optic neuropathy in chronic glaucoma. Can J Ophthalmol 5:321–330
3. Begg IS, Drance SM, Sweeney VP (1971) Ischaemic optic neuropathy in chronic simple glaucoma. Br J Ophthalmol 55:73–90
4. Bengtsson B, Krakau CET (1979) Automatic perimetry in a population survey. Acta Ophthalmol (Copenh) 57:929–937
5. Bengtsson B, Holmin C, Krakau CET (1980) Characteristics of manifest glaucoma in the early stages. Glaucoma 2:351–358
6. Bengtsson B, Holmin C, Krakau CET (1981) Disc haemorrhage and glaucoma. Acta Ophthalmol (Copenh) 59:1–14
7. Drance SM, Fairclough M, Butler DM, Kottler MS (1977) The importance of disc haemorrhage in the prognosis of chronic open angle glaucoma. Arch Ophthalmol 95:226–228
8. Gloster J (1981) Incidence of optic disc haemorrhages in chronic simple glaucoma and ocular hypertension. Br J Ophthalmol 65: 452–456
9. Kottler MS, Drance SM (1976) Studies of haemorrhage on the optic disc. Can J Ophthalmol 11:102–105
10. Hayreh S, Walker W (1967) Fluorescent fundus photography in glaucoma. Am J Ophthalmol 63:982
11. Holmin C, Krakau CET (1982) Regression analysis of the central visual field in chronic glaucoma cases. Acta Ophthalmol 60:267–274
12. Spaeth G (1975) Fluorescein angiography. Trans Am Ophthalmol Soc 73:491
13. Susanna R, Drance SM, Douglas GR (1979) Disc haemorrhages in patients with elevated intraocular pressure. Occurrence with or without field changes. Arch Ophthalmol 97: 284–285

## Discussion

**Hayreh to Krakau:** The true nature and mechanism of disc splinter haemorrhages in eyes with open angle glaucoma and low-tension glaucoma is not fully understood, although frequently seen in these eyes. These haemorrhages are indistinguishable from those seen in eyes with anterior ischemic optic neuropathy. I feel that the splinter disc haemorrhagic represent recurrent acute minute ischemic episodes in the optic nerve head. The neural damage by each episode is so minute so as to be clinically undetectable but over a period of years these produce collectively enough damage to produce clinically detectable optic disc and visual field damage. Thus, multiple recurrent minute acute ischemic episodes in the optic nerve head in glaucoma and low-tension glaucoma, when reviewed over a period of years, give an erroneous impression of chronic continuous ischemia instead of a step ladder phenomenon of acute ischemic damage.

Dr. Phelps showed me stereoscopic pictures of one eye in which the superficial splinter disc haemorrhage could be seen to be continuous deep into the prelaminar region. It is possible that in the majority of eyes the superficial hemorrhage masks its deeper connection.

**Spaeth to Krakau:** Can Dr. Krakau enlighten me as to the exact location of the disc haemorrhage. I have seen several cases with choroidal crescents in which the "disc haemorrhage" did not actually appear on the disc but rather at the edge of the choroidal crescent, well separated from the disc.

Krieglstein G.K./Leydhecker W. (eds)
Glaucoma Update II


# Hemorrhage on the Disc – A Risk Factor in Glaucoma

S.M. Drance, Vancouver

In a study done in Vancouver in 1969, to evaluate the relationship between intraocular pressure and other factors as a cause of chronic open angle glaucoma, all patients were found to have either a pressure high enough to explain the damage or alternately there were other abnormalities with appeared to account for the damage at the relatively low intraocular pressure. There remained two patients in whom neither pressure, nor other findings satisfactorily explained the glaucomatous damage. One of the two patients was noted to have two flame shaped hemorrhages on the optic nerve, but the significance of these was not immediately understood. Soon after that, an elderly man followed for chronic open angle glaucoma was found to have a small hemorrhage on the optic nerve head. The patients was quite unaware of any symptoms, but occurring so soon after the first patient, his findings alerted us to a possible relationship with chronic open angle glaucoma. A third patient showed the appearance of a fresh nerve fibre bundle defect, in a previously normal area of the visual field in association with a hemorrhage at the optic nerve head. This patient was described in a case report in 1970 [1].

In 1970 [2] we also encountered four patients in whom the occurence of a hemorrhage on the optic nerve head was associated with progression of visual field damage and by 1971 [3] we were able to report a number of patients with previously elevated intraocular pressure without field defect in whom following or accompanying a disc hemorrhage, a characteristic nerve fibre bundle defect occurred. At that time we had therefore realized the significance of these hemorrhages in chronic open angle glaucoma patients. We had described the progression of existing field defects in glaucoma patients associated with hemorrhages of the disc, and seen the development of field defects in preglaucoma patients, associated with or preceded by hemorrhages at the optic nerve head. In a review of patients with low tension glaucoma in 1972 [4], we reported that in six out of twenty-nine patients with low tension glaucoma, a linear splinter shaped disc hemorrhage on the optic nerve head had been seen. In 1976 [5], Chumbly and Brubaker reported linear hemorrhages in eight out of seventy-seven patients suffering from low tension glaucoma which confirmed our findings.

If splinter shaped hemorrhages are of significance in chronic open angle glaucoma, then their prevalence ought to be higher in patients with fully developed disease, compared to those who only had an elevated pressure without damage. In 1979 [6], we showed a statistically significant higher incidence of disc hemorrhage among patients with chronic open angle glaucoma, as compared to those whose pressure were elevated alone. By 1980 [7], Bengtson showed a 70% probability of a nerve with a disc hemorrhage having a glaucomatous visual field defect, which was very much higher than the probability of finding a glaucomatous field defect as judged by en enlarged cup alone, or from an intraocular pressure level above 21 mm, of mercury. He also showed a 47% probability of having a disc hemorrhage in a patient suffering from chronic open angle glaucoma which in his study was the same as the probability of having an elevation in intraocular pressure. In 1981 [8] Gloster studied 1 315 photographs of 617 eyes in 320 patients with glaucomatous field defects and disc changes. He found that the presence of disc hemorrhages increases with the number of photographs examined. In his series, 16.9% of glaucoma patients had hemorrhages on the disc. He showed a considerably greater prevalence of disc hemorrhages among those patients who had glaucoma as compared with glaucoma suspects. He also demonstrated a rising prevalence of hemorrhages the greater the vertical cup disc ratio and greater prevalence among those with low tension glaucoma, as opposed to those with chronic open angle glaucoma. Glaucoma patients with lower levels of intraocular pressure had more hemorrhages than those whose pressures were higher. Airaksinen in 1981 [9] reported that hemorrhages at the nerve head often followed localized defects of the retinal nerve fibres, followed by localized disturbance of the optic nerve head and only then the development of visual field defects. Rigby Slight [10] examined all patients in a general ophthalmic practice between 1974 and 1980 for the presence of disc hemorrhages. He reported in 1981 that of 36 patients with hemorrhages, 70% had glaucoma, low-tension glaucoma, elevated intraocular pressure, secondary glaucoma or suspicious discs, 16% had a posterior detatchment alone and the remaining 14% had systemic vascular disease. This paper gives the only overall review of the causes of such hemorrhages.

It has recently been shown that Bjerrum described cases of chronic open angle glaucoma with some hemorrhages at the optic nerve head and the retina in the 1898 Danish literature. While some of his cases looked like partial vein occlusions, some of the others were probably the sort of hemorrhages which we found again in 1970.

It would appear, therefore, that the splinter shaped hemorrhage is a frequent event in chronic open angle glaucomas and can be used to predict the subsequent damage to retina, optic nerve and visual field. It is a transient event, and therefore the estimates which show its presence in 36.9% of chronic open angle glaucoma patients is very likely to be an underestimate. The question has been raised as to whether hemorrhages occur in all patients suffering from glaucomatous visual field defects. It is too early to make such a statement with the evidence that is currently available. More than one hemorrhage can be present in an eye at the same time and a number of bilateral hemorrhages have appeared. We have so far seen a patient who has had 15 separate episodes of hemorrhages on one nerve head with a gradually deteriorating visual field. Hemorrhages may occur in areas of the nerve that have already been severely damaged with an absolute nerve fibre bundle defect. The hemorrhages may be splinter shaped, but may occasionally be blotchy and can occur in the depth of the cup. They are unaccompanied by hemorrhages elsewhere in the fundus from other ocular disease. In one of our studies [11] of other associated factors, vascular hypertension was the only positive association with hemorrhages. In a step-wise discriminant analysis of factors which would best differentiate between patients with glaucoma and those who have not suffered from the disease, the presence of a disc hemorrhage was picked out as one factor helping in the correct separation of these two groups of individuals.

It appears therefore, that a hemorrhage at the optic nerve head, though as yet of unexplained origin, appears to be a significant event both for the early recognition of open angle glaucoma, and the prediction that a patient with glaucoma is progressing. In ischemic optic neuropathy, small hemorrhages identical in appearance, are usually accompanied by mild oedema of the nerve head. Those patients however, are recognized because of altitudinal field defects or central scotomas, and therefore suffer from major ischemic changes while the chronic open angle glaucoma patients are unaware of any symptoms at the time when a hemorrhage is seen. It is therefore likely by analogy that the hemorrhages accompany small infarcts of the optic nerve.

## References


1. Drance SM, Begg IS (1970) Sector hemorrhage. A probably acute ischemic disc change in chronic simple glaucoma. Can J Ophthalmol 5:137
2. Begg IS, Drance SM, Sweeney VP (1970) Hemorrhage on the disc – a sign of acute ischaemic optic neuropathy in chronic simple glaucoma. Can J Ophthalmol 5:231
3. Begg IS, Drance SM, Sweeney VP (1971) Ischemic optic neuropathy in chronic simple glaucoma. Br J Ophthalmol 55:73
4. Drance SM (1972) Some factors in the production of low-tension glaucoma. Br J Ophthalmol 56:229
5. Chumbley LC, Brubaker RF (1976) Low-tension glaucoma. Am J Ophthalmol 81:761
6. Susanna R, Drance SM, Douglas GR (1979) Disc hemorrhages in patients with elevated intraocular pressure. Arch Ophthalmol 97: 284

7. Bengtson B (1980) Findings associated with glaucomatous visual field defects. Acta Ophthalmol (Copenhagen) 58:20
8. Gloster J (1981) Incidence of optic disc hemorrhages in chronic simple glaucoma and ocular hypertension. Br J Ophthalmol 65:452
9. Airaksinen J, Mustonen E, Hannu A (1981) Optic nerve hemorrhages precede retinal nerve fibre layer defects. Acta Ophthalmol (Copenhagen) 59:627
10. Slight Rigby J (1981) The significance of disc hemorrhages. Trans Pac Coast Otoophthalmol Soc Annu Meet 62:25–33
11. Kottler M, Drance SM (1976) Studies of hemorrhages on the disc. Can J Ophthalmol 11:102–105

## Discussion

**Bengtsson to Drance:** In order to stress the importance of the case reported by Drance. I would like to add a similar one found in Dalby.

At the initial examination in September 1978 a man born 1908 was considered to have enlarged cups in spite of the fact that his IOP was 13 in both eyes. When re-examined in November 1981 he had a disc haemorrhage in the left eye and a paracentral scotoma in the right eye. The IOP was 12 in both eyes. In March 1982 he had a disc haemorrhage in the right eye and paracentral scotomas in both eyes. The IOP was 13 in both eyes.

This case was one of ten cases with "new" glaucomatous visual field defects found at the re-examination of 1300 persons born 1907–21. This and similar cases with repeated disc haemorrhages and very low pressures have led us to consider the possibility that glaucoma often is initiated in eyes with low - but soon slowly rising - pressures.

**Spaeth to Drance:** I had a remarkably similar patient, but with a remarkable difference. I first examined a patient with similar symptoms and findings, in fact amazingly similar, in 1973. I did not believe that the patient had glaucoma and therapy was not started. The patient developed progressive visual field loss in both eyes so that by 1976 dense acurate scotomas were now present in both eyes. During this period of time the patient was having recurrent disc hemorrhages. In 1976 treatment with pilocarpine and epinephrine was started with a decrease in intraocular pressure from around 15 to around 12 mm of Hg as an average. The point is that there was a definite lowering of intraocular pressure associated with the start of the treatment. From 1976 till 1982 the patient had no further disc hemorrhages, nor did the patient have further progression of visual field loss. Thus in this patient in whom there had been progressive visual field loss and recurrent disc hemorrhages the institution of treatment was associated with a change in the level of intraocular pressure and a change in the clinical course so that there were no longer recurrent disc hemorrhages and there was no longer progressive visual field change. Please note that the duration of this lack of change of condition, that is to say the duration of the stability has been six years whereas in the three years prior to the initiation of treatment there was a marked change in one eye and a dramatic deterioration in the other eye, both eyes being untreated at that time.

Krieglstein G.K./Leydhecker W. (eds)
Glaucoma Update II


# Regression of Optic Nerve and Visual Field Defects in Glaucoma

G.L. Spaeth, Philadelphia

It is now generally agreed that the glaucomatous optic nerve of the infant or child will show remarkable improvement in appearance and function following lowering of intraocular pressure. While similar cases have been reported in adults, the phenomenon appear to be much rarer; indeed, its very existence is doubted by many.

The purpose of this paper is to document the occurrence in adults of improvement in the appearance of the optic nerve head and the visual field. The pathogenesis of such changes will be discussed (Table 1A, B). There is good evidence to support a variety of different mechanisms - including returning toward normal of blood flow, transient edema, and reversal of the mechanical posterior bowing of the lamina cribrosa caused by the elevated intraocular pressure.

**Table 1a.** Mechanisms of reversible cupping of the optic disc

1. Mechanical rearrangement of the tissues
2. Change in intracellular fluid content
   A. Related to axoplasmic transport
   B. Direct mechanical effect
3. Change in extracellular fluid content
4. Change in intravascular volume
5. Tissue loss or generation

**Table 1b.** Mechanisms of improvement in the visual field

1. Spurious improvement
   A. Poor standardization of test
   B. Change in refraction
   C. Etc
2. Real improvement in the visual field but not due to improvement in optic nerve function
   A. Clearer cornea
   B. Larger pupil
   C. Etc
3. Real improvement in optic nerve function
   A. Improved function of damage neurons

One phenomenon not previously reported is the differential improvement in visual fields that may occur; specifically, badly damaged areas of the visual field may show progression at the same time that less damaged areas show improvement. This supports the clinical contention that the damaged optic nerve is more sensitive to intraocular pressure elevation than is the less damaged optic nerve.

The major reason why improvement in the disc and field have not been observed frequently in the past include the following: 1. The failure to be looked for; 2. Associated decrease in visual acuity and visual function caused by the method by which the intraocular pressure is lower, the visual deterioration thus masking the real improvement in optic nerve function; 3. Inadequacy of methods of documentation of the nature of the optic disc and visual field.

## References

Greve EL et al. (1977) Pre- and post-operative results of static perimetry in patients with glaucoma simplex. Doc Ophthalmol 42:335-351

Hetherington J Jr et al. (1975) The Disc in Congenital Glaucoma. In: Etienne R, Paterson GD (eds) International Glaucoma Symposium (Albi 1974), Diffusion Generale de Librairie, Marseille, pp 127-143

Neumann E, Hyams SW (1973) Intermittent glaucomatous excavation. Arch Ophthalmol 90: 64-66

Quigley HA (1977) The pathogenesis of reversible cupping in congenital glaucoma. Am J Ophthalmol 84:358-370

Read RM, Spaeth GL (1974) The practical clinical appraisal of the optic disc in glaucoma: the natural history of cup progression and some specific disc-field correlations. Trans Pa Acad Ophthalmol Otolaryngol 78:255-274

Shiose Y, Kanda T (1974) Quantitative analysis of optic cup and its clinical application. II. Considerations on clinical cases. Jpn Source, pp 367–374

Spaeth GL et al. (1980) The pathogenesis of transient or permanent improvement in the appearance of the optic disc following glaucoma surgery. Doc Ophthalmol 22:111–126

Von Jaeger E (1869) Ophthalmoskopischer Hand-Atlas. Druck und Verlag der K.K. Hof- und Staatsdruckerei, Wien

## Discussion

**Schwartz to Spaeth:** We observed similar regression of optic disc cupping in glaucomatous patients who have been surgically and medically treated. At the meeting of the Association for Research in Vision and Ophthalmology in May of 1982, we presented our photogrammetric measurements of ocular hypertensive patients who were not being treated and who showed spontaneous decreases in cupping of the optic disc (Takamoto and Schwartz 1982). We have also used photogrammetry and computerized image analysis to do detailed serial studies of the optic disc of a nine-year-old girl who had a trabeculotomy for secondary glaucoma and showed reversibility of disc and visual field changes following the surgery. Our studies indicated, quantitatively, reversibility of cupping and pallor, not as a simple decrease, but in a biphasic mode. I wish to emphasize that the disc should not be viewed as a three dimensional rigid structure but as a dynamic one, which may change spontaneously and, certainly, in relationship to therapy.

Takamoto T, Schwartz B (1982) Optic disc cup volume chances in ocular hypertension. Invest Ophthalmol Vis Sci 22:129

Krieglstein G.K./Leydhecker W. (eds)
Glaucoma Update II


# Histology of Human Glaucoma Optic Nerve Damage Compared to Clinical Findings in the Same Eyes

H.A. Quigley, Baltimore

**Abstract.** Studies of 50 human eyes by histological methods and comparisons with clinical information available on the same eyes has added information about glaucoma optic nerve damage. Early optic disc cup size enlargement prior to detectable field loss is a result of nerve fiber loss undetected by present perimetric methods. The site of damage to axonal fibers is the level of the sclera at the optic nerve head (scleral lamina cribrosa). Actual optic nerve fiber counting in eyes with glaucoma before and after field loss shows a selectively greater loss at the vertical poles of the nerve, corresponding to vertical pole notching of disc rim and the positions of arcuate area ganglion cell axons. This selective susceptibility appears to derive from the less dense structural connective tissues in the more vulnerable zones of the nerve head. By the stage of moderately advanced field loss, so many axons are gone that further loss of fibers is more apparent in clinical testing; this may help to explain why damage appears to progress more rapidly later in the course of the disease. Compression of the scleral lamina cribrosa structure occurs in many eyes prior to the field loss stage and must be considered a potential first step in the pathogenesis of nerve damage.

## Introduction

A number of clinical observations regarding glaucomatous optic nerve damage have been consistently made, but until recently the precise meaning and/or significance of these findings lacked corroborative histological data. While primate experimentation with glaucoma models is able to help to answer some of these questions, the most convincing possible evidence for the nature of the glaucoma damage process would, of course, come from human glaucoma eyes. In 1976, while working in Miami, Douglas Anderson allowed me to participate in the examination of two eyes from a patient cared for by Ralph Kirsch with glaucoma and field loss. I evolved from this experience a set of examination techniques for histological study of material obtained from the Florida Lions Eye Bank, and more recently the Medical Eye Bank of Maryland and the Eye Pathology Laboratory, Wilmer Institute. In large part, we have obtained such eyes in two ways. First, all eye bank eyes donated in our state are screened by history taken from the family and by gross and microscopic examination. In those with signs of glaucoma, W. Richard Green and his staff notify me and ophthalmic information is sought. Second, surgical enucleations are occasionally performed on eyes with secondary glaucoma (e.g. iris melanoma) or on glaucoma eyes that suffered irreparable trauma. It is this material that forms the basis of this report.

## Why Does Cupping Precede Field Loss?

It has been repeatedly observed that the vast majority of eyes undergo enlargement of the optic disc cup prior to the detection of perimetric abnormality. Two previous explanations for this phenomenon suggested that early cup enlargement could precede field loss because the cup change was not due to axon loss, but to either 1) loss of astrocytes (glia) of the nerve head or 2) enlargement of the whole disc canal itself. Both the examination of human glaucoma eyes and studies of chronic experimental glaucoma in monkeys has now convinced me that astrocytes do not suffer selectively more from chronically elevated pressure-if anything, they are less bothered by it than nerve fibers (Quigley, 1979, 1980a, 1981a). Recently, I have been able to measure the diameter of the optic disc canal through the sclera in 24 human glaucoma eyes of adults. Their mean diameter, 1.77 mm in the vertical dimension, is identical with an age-matched group of normal eyes. Interestingly, children's eyes do undergo an enlargement of the canal in glaucoma, just as their eyes suffer corneal enlargement and buphthalmos. Thus, there seemed no other choice but that early cup enlargement represented axon loss. This hypothesis has now been confirmed by estimates of the number of nerve fibers remaining in optic nerves of eyes from patients with elevated intraocular pressure but normal field testing during their life. Briefly, the method for nerve counting involves measurement of the area of the cross-section of the optic nerve, distinguishing nerve bundle area from connective tissue septa area. Then, in 64 randomly selected locations, the number of nerve fibers per unit area is directly counted. By multiplying this figure by the neural area, an estimate of the total number of fibers is obtained. While it would be ideal to count every fiber in every nerve, this is quite impractical for any large number of nerves. Furthermore, in the method described, from 4% to 50% of all fibers (depending on the number remaining) are counted, and, much like a public opinion poll, error estimates by replication counting have shown that the total numbers obtained are probably in error by only 5%. Normal nerve counts were established by counting several age-matched nerves from eyes with no ocular abnormality clinically and/or histologically.

In five eyes of glaucoma suspects with elevated pressure but normal Goldmann-performed fields, four of those counted had significantly lower than the normal number of fibers. In three eyes of two patients in this category, the mean loss was 37% of the normal nerve count (about 600,000 fibers instead of the normal one million) (Quigley, 1982 and unpublished observations). One other suspect eye was indistinguishable from the normal number and another was just outside the normal range. While this may be an overstatement of the number of glaucoma suspects with normal fields who are already significantly damaged, it cannot be doubted that some minority of the nerve disappears in some suspects without psychophysical detection by present methods. An almost unspoken presumption in much recent writing about glaucoma is the idea that until field loss is confirmed, damage is not established, and in fact the diagnosis of glaucoma is not made. Since it is now more apparent than ever that glaucomatous optic nerve damage is occurring prior to demonstrable perimetric abnormalities, it is untenable to define glaucoma as present only when there is field loss (or to act as if the patient with elevated pressure but normal perimetry has a different disease or diagnosis). As we search for better methods of detecting optic nerve damage, the time at which typical field defects first appear will continue to be an important milestone in the process, but will be recognized as a later stage of glaucoma damage. This data raises the possibility that all patients (or more than we suspect) are losing optic nerve fibers from the start of their entry to the elevated pressure phase. Presumably, the optic nerve has considerable reserve functional capacity with which the early loss of fibers is masked. Our present clinical and laboratory efforts are directed at uncovering means to measure this early loss of function.

### Where is the Site of Damage to Ganglion Cell Axons?

While there was some controversy until recently about this point, the initial acute experiments of Anderson and Hendrickson (1974) demonstrated that the optic nerve head at the level of the sclera is the site at which elevated eye pressure injures axons. Subsequent primate and human data have confirmed this location (Quigley, 1980a, 1981a). As discussed below, this allows detailed studies of the pathogenesis of damage to concentrate on the relevant features of this site for clues.

### Why Disc Rim Loss at Vertical Poles and Arcuate Area Field Loss?

One characteristic of glaucomatous optic nerve damage is the apparently preferential loss of fibers serving the arcuate area. Since these fibers enter the vertical poles of the disc, and under favorable circumstances, this leads to highly localized loss of disc rim tissue at this site (vertically oval cupping or local vertical notch), I have been quite interested to search for potential factors leading to this feature. First, it was important to confirm that such a selective loss indeed is demonstrable in the histological examples we obtained. In fact, in every glaucoma nerve studied, where detectable loss of fibers was statistically proven, the loss was greater in the superior and/or inferior quadrant (Quigley, 1982). It must be pointed out, however, that this is not an *exclusive* loss in these areas, but the damage is often quantitatively greater there. Therefore, in some eyes with a lesser degree of selective susceptibility of the vertical zones, highly localized loss of upper or lower disc rim would not be expected, and the disc cup clinically would enlarge in a generally symmetrical fashion (Pederson and Anderson, 1980). The greater susceptibility of superior and inferior quadrant fibers and the development of arcuate area field defects appears to correlate with a feature of optic nerve head anatomy.

Some years ago, Jared Emery and coworkers (1974) published views of nerve head tissues by scanning electron microscopy after all neural and glia cells had been digested away with trypsin. Using both this method and a detergent digestion method devised in our laboratory, I studied the detailed structure of the normal lamina cribrosa (Quigley, 1981b). It was clear that one could easily distinguish the vertical poles of the tissue from the nasal and temporal zones, since the poles had less connective tissue per unit area. To put it another way, the pores for nerve bundles were larger at the vertical poles. Thus, it appeared plausible that when the nerve head was subjected to intraocular pressure-induced stress, the zones most likely to "give" first would be those least well supported by structural connective tissue - the vertical poles. The areas of lesser connective tissue appear to form an hourglass-shaped area in the disc, and this same shape represents the maximum loss of fibers in our quantitative nerve counts of glaucoma eyes. Therefore, it seems that the characteristic field loss pattern of glaucoma derives from an inherent feature of nerve head anatomy interacting with elevated intraocular pressure. Radius and Gonzales (1981) have confirmed this feature of regional structure of the human nerve head by a different method.

To place this finding in proper perspective, I must add that the capillaries that nourish nerve fiber bundles in the lamina cribrosa are only found within the connective tissue septa that were analyzed above. So, while it is likely that a physical distortion of the nerve head tissues is occurring early in the glaucoma process, it need not be inevitably concluded that this leads to mechanical compression of nerve fibers, and that this is the only possible mechanism of damage. While an initial mechanical step appears likely, the capillaries within the distorting laminar sheets could then be compressed, and the blood supply injured. Recent laboratory evidence does not suggest such a decrease in blood supply at the lamina cribrosa with acute intraocular pressure elevations in primate and cat eyes (Geijer and Bill, 1979; Sossi and Anderson, 1982). Nor were we able to reverse acute pressure-induced axon damage by eliminating the possibility of anoxia in the nerve head in experimental primates (Quigley, 1980b). While the laboratory investigations in young animals may be inexact copies of human glaucoma, it has been difficult to find data to support vascular compromise as a participating feature of glaucoma damage.

Our studies of human eyes with ocular disease have now extended to clinicopathologic correlations of toxic amblyopia, ischemic optic neuropathy, papilledema, and chiasmal syndromes. Each of these has individual features providing tantilizing clues to pathogenesis (Quigley, 1982; Levin, 1982). Suffice it to say that the pattern of glaucoma damage in the optic nerve is not mimicked by any of the other optic neuropathies examined thus far.

### Why do Advanced Glaucoma Eyes Seem to Deteriorate Rapidly?

A final feature of our quantitative data that has important relevance to clinical glaucoma management is in the eyes with advanced field loss. It was quite striking to realize that those eyes with dense scotomas, but still retaining reading acuity may have lost 80–90% of all optic nerve fibers by actual count. Many glaucomatologists have noted that at this stage the eye seems to slip into further functional loss quite easily, even at barely elevated pressures. This lead to the presumption that advanced disc change rendered the remaining axons more susceptible to damage. While this idea may have validity, one must consider as well that with the vast majority of the nerve gone, the loss of any further fibers will be much more noticeable than at the early stage where fiber loss is undetected due to reserve fibers serving the same area. The practical point for management is the same, however; extreme vigilance and vigorous pressure lowering are indicated for such eyes.

## References


Anderson DR, Hendrickson A (1974) Effect of intraocular pressure on rapid axoplasmic transport in monkey optic nerve. Invest Ophthalmol 13:771–783

Emery JM, Landis D, Boniuk M, et al. (1974) The lamina cribrosa in normal and glaucomatous human eyes. Trans Am Acad Ophthalmol Otol 78:290–297

Geijer C, Bill A (1979) Effects of raised intraocular pressure on retinal, prelaminar, laminar, retrolaminar optic nerve blood flow in monkeys. Invest Ophthalmol Vis Sci 18:1030–1042

Levin P, Newman S, Quigley HA, Miller NR (1982) Quantitative study of optic nerve fibers from patients with chiasmal syndromes. (in preparation)

Pederson JE, Anderson DR (1980) The mode of progressive disc cupping in ocular hypertension and glaucoma. Arch Ophthalmol 98:490–495

Quigley HA, Green WR (1979) The histology of human glaucoma cupping and optic nerve damage: clinicopathologic correlation in 21 eyes. Ophthalmology 86:1803–1827

Quigley HA, Addicks EM (1980a) Chronic experimental glaucoma in primates. II. Effect of extended intraocular pressure elevation on optic nerve head and axonal transport. Invest Ophthalmol Vis Sci 19:137–152

Quigley HA, Flower RW, Addicks EM, et al. (1980b) The mechanism of optic nerve damage in experimental acute glaucoma. Invest Ophthalmol Vis Sci 19:505–517

Quigley HA, Addicks EM, Green WR, Maumenee AE (1981a) Optic nerve damage in human glaucoma. II. The site of injury and susceptibility to damage. Arch Ophthalmol 99:635–649

Quigley HA, Addicks EM (1981b) Regional differences in the structure of the lamina cribrosa and their relation to glaucomatous optic nerve damage. Arch Ophthalmol 99:137–143

Quigley HA, Addicks EM, Green WR (1982) Optic nerve damage in human glaucoma. III. Quantitative correlation of nerve fiber loss and visual field defect in glaucoma, ischemic neuropathy, papilledema, and toxic neuropathy. Arch Ophthalmol 100:135–146

Radius RL, Gonzales M (1981) Anatomy of the lamina cribrosa in human eyes. Arch Ophthalmol 99:2159–2162

Sossi N, Anderson DR (1981) Axonal blockage in the cat: use of $I^{125}$ iodoantipyrine for the estimation of regional blood flow in response to raised intraocular pressure and effect of varying the blood pressure on the axonal blockage. Invest Ophthalmol Vis Sci (Suppl) 20:82 (also accepted for publication, Arch Ophthalmol, 1982)


## Discussion

**Schwartz to Quigley:** At the recent meeting of the Association for Research in Vision and Ophthalmology in May, 1982, we presented our findings on the stereological analyses of normal and glaucomatous optic discs and nerves (Schwartz and Sakimoto 1982). Our findings generally support Dr. Quigley's observations on his studies of the optic nerve. In the optic disc and the optic nerve we have observed a significant decrease in the volume of axons in glaucomatous eyes compared to normal eyes. In addition, we have not observed change in the glial tissue in the optic disc, but have found a significant decrease in the volume of vascular tissue, both in the optic disc and optic nerve in glaucomatous individuals compared to normal subjects. In contrast to Dr. Quigley's observation of the possible compression of the scleral lamina in the optic disc, we have found an increase in the volume of connective tissue in the scleral lamina cribrosa in glaucomatous individuals compared to normal subjects. The increase in volume of connective tissue is particularly striking; further studies will be needed to determine whether it is a primary or secondary phenomenon.


Sakimoto G, Schwartz B (1982) Stereological analysis of optic disc and nerve in normal and glaucomatous eyes. Invest Ophthalmol Vis Sci 22:257


**Hayreh to Quigley:** The histopathological studies and clinicopathological correlation presented by Dr. Quigley provide very useful information. For over 15 years I have advocated all along that in eyes with raised intraocular pressure, by the time the visual field loss can be detected by perimetry, a fair amount of nerve fiber loss has already taken place (Hayreh SS (1978) In: Heilmann K, Richardson KT (eds) "Glaucoma: Conceptions of a disease." Thieme, Stuttgart, p 133), and that rapid progression of visual field loss in advanced glaucoma cases is simply due to a markedly reduced population of nerve fibers. Dr. Quigley's studies provide us with proof of that. However, a number of statements are made in the paper which either lack definite proof or, I feel, are misleading, and these include the following:

Firstly, the author stated: "The pattern of glaucoma damage in the optic nerve is not mimicked by any of the other optic neuropathies." One of the optic neuropathies examined by him was "Anterior Ischemic Optic Neuropathy" (Arch Ophthalmol 100:135–146, 1982). A careful review of that paper reveals that only one patient with a dubious diagnosis of anterior ischemic optic neuropathy was examined by them. The patient was first seen at the age of 64 years with a history of sudden painless loss of *vision 25 years before.* The authors admit that the diagnosis of anterior ischemic optic neuropathy was presumptive because of inferior altitudinal visual field defect; incidentally, this type of field defect is *not* always due to anterior ischemic optic neuropathy. Thus, making a dogmatic statement based on *one dubious case of anterior ischemic optic neuropathy* is unwarranted. I have about 400 eyes with anterior ischemic optic neuropathy in my files and we find that almost all eyes with anterior ischemic optic neuropathy due to temporal arteritis develop optic disc cupping; I have just shown you that the optic disc cupping seen in these eyes with anterior ischemic optic neuropathy is indistinguishable from that seen in glaucoma. At this stage it may be appropriate to point out that neural ischemia is not an "all or none" phenomenon - a highly mistaken notion prevalent among ophthalmologists. The ischemia may be acute or chronic, and the acute ischemia may be transient or permanent; the severity of neural ischemia may vary over a wide spectrum - from subclinical to severe ischemia. Each type of ischemia would produce a different type of pathology. Lack of appreciation of these facts is responsible for a good deal of confusion.

Secondly, Dr. Quigley has stated that "The site of damage to axonal fibers is the level of the sclera at the optic nerve head (scleral lamina cribrosa)" because the lamina cribrosa is much more compact in eyes with glaucomatous optic nerve head damage. I feel that we do not have definite proof as yet about the changes in the lamina cribrosa being primary or secondary, because loss of neural tissue *per se* can produce compact lamina cribrosa. We need much more proof to decide one way or the other.

Thirdly, Dr. Quigley stated that optic disc cupping is essentially due to loss of axons and that loss of glial tissue is not of much importance. I find this hard to accept in the typical optic disc cupping seen in the vast majority of glaucoma cases. If loss of axons only is the cause of optic disc cupping, then why does not a similar cupping develop in various types of optic atrophy with loss of axons?

Finally, Dr. Quigley refers to his experimental studies in monkeys where they found that hyperbaric oxygen did not protect the axons from acute pressure induced damage (Invest Ophthal Vis Sci 19:505–517, 1980). I find the conclusion is not justified, because the acute rise of intraocular pressure arrests the circulation in the optic nerve head by compression of blood vessels, and that prevents any oxygen reaching the tissues in spite of breathing hyperbaric oxygen. It is like putting a man in a hyperbaric oxygen chamber and strangulating him with a rope, and then concluding that the man did not die from lack of oxygen because he was in a hyperbaric oxygen atmosphere.

Krieglstein G.K./Leydhecker W. (eds)
Glaucoma Update II


# The Mechanisms of Damage of the Optic Nerve

D.R. Anderson, Miami

## Introduction

I would like to review the evolution of thought that has led to a new hypothesis, for which there is as yet no compelling evidence, but which is interesting none-the-less. The hypothesis is suggested by some recent experimentation and is compatible with nearly all relevant scientific observations to date. I hope some of those assembled at this meeting can devise methods to explore this hypothesis in detail, for if the hypothesis is true, it may be possible (1) to devise clinical tests to predict those individuals who are at risk of developing nerve damage and (2) to devise therapeutic measures that can be directed at factors other than intraocular pressure that pertain to the pathophysiologic process by which the optic nerve is damaged in glaucoma.

## Ischemic and Mechanical Mechanisms

For a long time, the idea that intraocular pressure damages the optic nerve by diminishing its blood supply has been attractive (Hayreh, 1969; Phelps, 1972). However, the most recent (and seemingly accurate) studies show that there is quite an efficient autoregulation of circulation in the optic nerve head, just as in the retina, so that the blood flow is not impaired very much until the intraocular pressure approaches the diastolic blood pressure (Geijer and Bill, 1979; Sossi and Anderson, 1982a). The disappointment is that compared to the effect on the retinal circulation, the effect on the optic nerve head circulation is not striking enough to explain the fact that in glaucoma the optic nerve head can be very severely affected while the retina is not affected at all.

The absence of convincing evidence that intraocular pressure produces ischemia in the optic nerve head has made more attractive the alternate hypothesis that intraocular pressure might produce its damage by some mechanical means that acts specifically at the optic disc. For example, axonal transport might be impaired by the pressure gradient between intraocular pressure and the tissue pressure in the nerve behind the eye (Barany, 1975, 1978; Hahnenberger, 1978). Alternatively, posterior distension of the lamina cribrosa might block axonal transport by kinking the axons (Emery et al. 1974; Minckler et al., 1977, 1978; Maumenee, 1977, 1981; Quigley et al., 1981) or might pinch the arterioles that feed the optic disc.

However, the relevance of these mechanical factors has not been shown. The demonstrated posterior displacement of the lamina cribrosa (Levy et al., 1981) would be an expected mechanical occurance whether or not the distortion was harmful to the axons. The demonstrated impairment of orthograde and retrograde axonal transport (Anderson and Hendrickson, 1974; Minckler et al., 1977, 1978) could well be the result of ischemia. In fact, the expected result of a pressure gradient or partially compressed axon might be an impairment of slow axonal flow (as occurs in papilledema) (Radius and Anderson, 1981) instead of the blockage of rapid axonal transport that occurs when intraocular pressure is elevated. A particular problem is to explain "low-tension glaucoma" (optic nerve damage with intraocular pressures in the normal range), since there is no pressure-induced distortion of the lamina cribrosa.

## What Do You Think of This?

Although there are some puzzling facets (such as, what is the distinction between ischemic papillitis and ischemia due to glaucoma), the notion that intraocular pressure damages the optic nerve by producing ischemia still seems an attractive notion. It is hard to ignore the clinical observation that alterations in blood pressure and hemodynamics can accelerate glaucomatous visual field loss (Drance, 1972; McLean, 1957; Francois and Neetens, 1970; Reese and McGavic, 1942; Johnson and Drance, 1968; Lobstein und Herr, 1966; Ekbom, 1973; Harrington 1959, 1961) or by itself produce glaucoma-like damage to the optic nerve (Drance et al., 1973).

The fact that in the laboratory an elevated intraocular pressure does not produce ischemia except when severely elevated means that autoregulation (maintenance of blood flow) is the normal physiologic response to elevation of intraocular pressure. This corresponds to the fact that the optic nerve is usually not damaged in acute angle-closure glaucoma (Douglas et al., 1975, 1975; Radius and Maumenee, 1977) and that most individuals with chronic elevation of intraocular pressure suffer little harm except at an older age.

The problem then, is to determine if individuals that are susceptible to damaging effects from elevated pressure have a deficient autoregulation, how such an autoregulatory deficiency might arise, why the autoregulatory deficiency occurs only at the optic disc, on what basis the susceptibility increases with age, on what basis the damage is more localized to a certain region of the optic nerve in some individuals but in others is more diffuse, and on what basis some regions of the optic disc are more susceptible than others.

A new insight resulted from a recent experiment in which we sought to show that elevated blood pressure induced by angiotensin might protect the optic nerve from adverse effects of intraocular pressure on axonal transport (Sossi and Anderson, 1982b). Unexpectedly, the experiments seemed to show that axonal transport was blocked to a greater degree in animals receiving angiotensin, despite the higher blood pressure. Seeking to explain the results, we wondered if angiotensin might have caused a tonic constriction of the disc vessels, not allowing them to relax as an autoregulatory response when challenged by elevation of intraocular pressure. Such a microvascular spasm in the disc is plausible if angiotensin diffuses into the disc from the choroid, just as fluorescein and small proteins do, while the retinal vessels do not constrict because they are protected by the blood-retinal barrier.

Since this experiment, I have been intrigued with the possibility that the normally present circulating vasoconstrictors and vasodilators may affect the autoregulatory ability of optic disc vessels. The autoregulation might become deficient whenever a sufficient amount of vasoconstrictors diffuses into the extracellular space of the disc. The profile and quantity of circulating vasoconstrictors may change with the physiologic state or during minor hemodynamic crisis, producing times when there is less autoregulatory reserve in the optic nerve head than at others. Episodic progression of visual field loss may occur when autoregulatory deficiency coincides with a spike of elevated intraocular pressure. If a change in the profile of circulating vasoactive substances occurs with age, with an increase in diffusable vasoconstrictors, the greater susceptibility of the optic nerve to pressure-induced damage with age might be explained. The glaucoma-like "shock-induced optic neuropathy" (Drance, 1973) may result from the combination of low blood pressure and the emergency outpouring of vasoconstrictive substances that may diffuse into the disc. One sector of the disc might be more susceptible to glaucomatous damage than another if it has a greater area of contact with the choroid. individual variation in the anatomical relationships at the disc may explain why damage occurs in one sector of the disc in one person but in another sector in another person.

To date we have not been able to demonstrate this proposed pathophysiologic process with additional laboratory observations. I have noted with interest that the disc is surrounded by an extensive peripapillary halo in many patients with low-tension glaucoma. Is it possible that individuals with large congenital haloes are susceptible to low-tension glaucoma because a large area of the choroid is exposed to the disc tissue? Or is the halo an acquired peripapillary change that develops along with the excavation?

## References

Anderson DR, Hendrickson A (1974) Effect of intraocular pressure on rapid axoplasmic trans-

port in monkey optic nerve. Invest Ophthal 13:771-783
Barany E (1975) Experiments on axoplasmic flow. In: Etienne R, Patterson GD (eds) International Glaucoma Symposium (Albi 1974), Diffusion Generale de Librairie, Marseille, pp 83-84
Barany E (1978) Ability of retrograde axoplasmatic flow to overcome pressure gradients: preliminary communication. Docum Ophthal, Proc Ser 16:215-219
Douglas GR, Drance SM, Schulzer M (1974) The visual field and nerve head in angle-closure glaucoma. Can J Ophthalmol 9:404-407
Douglas GR, Drance SM, and Schulzer M (1975) The visual field and nerve head in angle-closure glaucoma. A comparison of the effects of acute and chronic angle closure. Arch Ophthalmol 93:409-411
Drance SM (1972) Some factors in the production of low tension glaucoma. Br J Ophthalmol 56:229-242
Drance SM, Morgan RW, Sweeney VP (1973) Shock-induced optic neuropathy. A cause of nonprogressive glaucoma. N Engl J Med 288: 392-395
Ekbom KA (1973) Scotoma due to arterial hypotension. Acta Ophthalmol 51:375-382
Emery JM, Landis D, Paton D, et al. (1974) The lamina cribrosa in normal and glaucomatous human eyes. Trans Am Acad Ophthalmol Otolaryngol 78:290-297
Francois J, Neetens A (1970) The deterioration of the visual field in glaucoma and the blood pressure. Doc Ophthalmol 28:70-132
Geijer C, Bill A (1979) Effects of raised intraocular pressure on retinal, prelaminar, laminar, and retrolaminar optic nerve blood flow in monkeys. Invest Ophthalmol Vis Sci 18:1030-1042
Hahnenberger RW (1978) Effects of pressure on fast axoplasmic flow. An in vitro study in the vagus nerve of rabbits. Acta Physiol Scand 104: 299-308
Harrington DO (1959) The pathogenesis of the glaucoma field. Clinical evidence that circulatory insufficiency in the optic nerve is the primary cause of visual field loss in glaucoma. Am J Ophthalmol 47/II: 177-185
Harrington DO (1961) Pathogenesis of the glaucomatous visual field defects: individual variations in pressure sensitivity. In: Newell FW (ed) Glaucoma. Transactions of the Fifth Conference, Princeton, NJ, 1960. New York, Josiah Macy, Jr Foundation p 259-310
Hayreh SS (1969) Blood supply of the optic nerve head and its role in optic atrophy, glaucoma and oedema of the optic disc. Br J Ophthalmol 53:721-748
Johnson DG, Drance SM (1968) Some studies on the circulation in patients with advanced open angle glaucoma. Can J Ophthalmol 3:149-153
Levy NS, Crapps EE, Bonney RC (1981) Displacement of the optic nerve head: response to acute intraocular pressure elevation in primate eyes. Arch Ophthalmol 99:2166-2174
Lobstein A, Herr FJ (1966) L'ophthalmodynamometrie dans le glaucome. Ann Oculist (Paris) 199:38-69
Maumenee AE (1977) The pathogenesis of visual field loss in glaucoma. In: Brockhurst RJ, Boruchoff SA, Hutchinson BT, Lessell S (eds) Controversy in Ophthalmology. Philadelphia, WB Saunders Co, pp 301-311
Maumenee AE (1981) Visual field loss in glaucoma. In: Symposium on Glaucoma. Transactions of the New Orleans Academy of Ophthalmology. St. Louis, CV Mosby Co, pp 160-171
McLean JM (1957) Management of the primary glaucomas. Am J Ophthalmol 44:323-334
Minckler DS, Bunt AH, Johanson GW (1977) Orthograde and retrograde axoplasmic transport during acute ocular hypertension in the monkey. Invest Ophthalmol Vis Sci 16:426-441
Minckler DS, Bunt AH, Klock IB (1978) Radioautographic and cytochemical ultrastructural studies of axoplasmic transport in the monkey optic nerve head. Invest Ophthalmol Vis Sci 17:33-50
Phelps CD (1972) The pathogenesis of optic nerve damage in glaucoma: a review of the vascular hypothesis. In: Blodi FC (ed) Current Concepts in Ophthalmology, vol. 3. St. Louis, The CV Mosby Co, pp 142-161
Quigley HA, Addicks EM, Green WR, Maumenee AE (1981) Optic nerve damage in human glaucoma. II. The site of injury and susceptibility to damage. Arch Ophthalmol 99:635-649
Radius RL, Maumenee AE (1977) Visual field changes following acute elevation of intraocular pressure. Trans Am Acad Ophthalmol Otolaryngol 83:61-68
Radius RL, Anderson DR (1981) Morphology of axonal transport abnormalities in primate eyes. Br J Ophthalmol 65:767-777
Reese AB, McGavic JS (1942) Relation of field contraction to blood pressure in chronic primary glaucoma. Arch Ophthalmol 27:845-850
Sossi N, Anderson DR (1982a) Effect of elevated intraocular pressure on blood flow. Occuence in cat optic nerve head studied with $^{125}$I-iodoantipyrine. Arch Ophthalmol 101:98-101
Sossi N, Anderson DR (1982b) Blockage of axonal transport in the optic nerve induced by elevation of intraocular pressure. Effect of arterial hypertension induceed by angiotensin I. Arch Ophthalmol 101:94-99

## Discussion

**Hayreh to Anderson:** I was very much interested in the hypothesis put forward by Dr. Anderson. In this connection some of our observations are relevant:

*1. Individual variations in blood supply of the optic nerve head:* There prevails a universal impression that the pattern of blood supply of the optic nerve head in all eyes is almost identical, and that all lesions are explainable on one standard vascular pattern. My findings on the subject have clearly demonstrated that this is a fundamental mistake, because the pattern of blood supply to the optic nerve head shows a marked inter-individual variation, so that each optic nerve head has its own vascular pattern, as different as our finger prints. In a grossly simplified pattern, we find the optic nerve head is supplied by the posterior ciliary arteries, mainly via the peripapillary choroid (by direct branches to the prelaminar region and the recurrent branches to the retrolaminar region) and by direct branches to the lamina cribrosa. There are usually 2 posterior ciliary arteris and the area supplied by each posterior ciliary artery varies markedly, so that the watershed zone situated between the 2 posterior ciliary arteries may be located anywhere between the fovea and nasal peripapillary choroid; (Hayreh SS (1981) Arch Neurol 38:675–678) there is a tremendous variation in the location of the watershed zone in different eyes. The location of the watershed zone is very important in determining the optic nerve head changes because whenever the perfusion pressure in the intraocular vascular bed supplied by the posterior ciliary arteries falls, the watershed zone is the first to show filling defects. We have observed that an acute marked fall in the perfusion pressure, resulting in non-filling of the watershed zone passing through the optic disc region, produces anterior ischemic optic neuropathy. In eyes with 3 posterior ciliary arteries, a Y-shaped watershed zone may involve the optic nerve head differently from that seen in eyes with 2 posterior ciliary arteries. In the literature there are a large number of fluorescein fundus angiographic studies in ocular hypertension, open angle glaucoma and low tension glaucoma, almost all of them showing vascular filling defects in the optic disc and choroid. The location of the watershed zone in the choroid would be of great importance in determining the extent of the optic disc involvement and degree of changes in glaucoma and allied disorders.

*2. Angiotensin and optic nerve head circulation:* We have produced experimental renovascular malignant arterial hypertension in about 40 rhesus monkeys by clamping the renal artery. In these animals the renin-angiotensin-aldosterone system plays an important role in the production of malignant arterial hypertension. In these animals plasma renin activity, angiotensin II concentration and aldosterone concentration are raised (J Endocr (1979) 81:69P–78P). It is well known that angiotensin is a powerful vasoconstrictor. In our monkeys, the majority of the eyes developed signs of anterior ischemic optic neuropathy and a few even showed cupping of the optic disc-similar to that seen in glaucoma. Our studies also clearly demonstrated that the choroidal vascular bed is most extensively involved in these animals and is the first to show changes, because widerspread focal retinal pigment epithelial infarction was the first of the fundus lesions seen in these animals, and serous retinal detachment in the macular region (due to retinal pigment epithelial ischemia) was also frequently one of the early signs. Thus the ischemic changes in the retinal pigment epithelium and optic disc seen at an early stage, indicate early choroidal vascular involvement. This lends further support to Dr. Anderson's observations. Angiotensin can cause optic nerve head ischemia not only by its direct diffusion into the prelaminar region (as suggested by Dr. Anderson) but also from its vasoconstrictive effect on the peripapillary choroid (as suggested by fluorescein fundus angiographic studies in our animals). Evidently the question arises, why the choroidal vascular bed is more susceptible to ischemic changes than the retinal vascular bed. The answer is that the latter has a good blood-retinal barrier but no such barrier exists in the choriocapillaris, so that the vasoconstrictor agents leak freely into the choroidal fluids, and lead to choroidal vasoconstriction.

*3. Autoregulation of optic nerve head circulation:* The basic premise of Dr. Anderson's hypothesis is that the impairment of autoregulation causes optic nerve head ischemia resulting in glaucomatous damage. The normal vascular pattern of the optic nerve head, however, does not support the presence of autoregulation, because the main source of blood supply is from the peripapillary choroid and its recurrent branches to the retrolaminar optic nerve. These arteries do not have autoregulation, since it is well-established that the choroidal arteries do not have autoregulation. Even if one presumes that autoregulation is present in the optic nerve head, there is plenty of evidence that vascular autoregulation in a tissue does not always effectively protect the tissues. For example, it is well-established that the blood vessels in the central nervous system have a very good autoregulation but transient ischemic attacks in the event of a fall of perfusion pressure are well known indicating that the autoregulation failed with the fall of perfusion pressure. Similarly in ordinary non-arteritic anterior ischemic optic neuropathy, with a segmental involvement of the optic nerve head, the evidence points to the fact that the acute ischemia is mostly due to transient collapse of circulation due to a fail of perfusion pressure - mostly during sleep. This would indicate that, if autoregulation exists in the optic nerve head, it does not protect the optic nerve head in such a fall of perfusion pressure. A similar mechanism of a mild, chronic type could be going on in glaucoma and low-tension glaucoma. I feel that the splinter hemorrhages of the optic disc seen so frequently in glaucoma and low-tension glaucoma represent minute ischemic lesions. Thus the optic nerve head damage in glaucoma and low-tension glaucoma represents recurrent acute minute ischemic episodes in the optic nerve head, but give an erroneous impression of chronic continuous ischemia.

*4. Peripapillary halos in glaucoma and low-tension glaucoma:* Dr. Anderson postulated that it is possible that individuals with large congenital peripapillary halos are susceptible to low-tension glaucoma because a large area of the choroid is exposed to the disc tissue. All the available evidence strongly suggests that this is not the case. I discussed the subject of peripapillary choroidal atrophy (i.e., peripapillary crescent or halo) in glaucoma in detail elsewhere (Hayreh SS (1978) In: Heilmann K, Richardson KT (eds) Glaucoma: conceptions of a disease. Thieme, Stuttgart, pp 110–112). Such halos have been described by a large number of authors. For example, Primrose (Br J Ophthalmol (1971) 55:820–825, found peripapillary halo in 94% of his glaucoma cases and found it was twice as likely to occur in glaucomatous eyes as in non-glaucomatous eyes. Also Wilensky et al. (Am J Ophthalmol (1976) 81:341-345) found the halo significantly ($P < 0.01$) more in glaucomatous eyes than in non-glaucomatous eyes. On fluorescein fundus angiography, a large number of investigators have shown peripapillary choroidal vascular filling defects in eyes with ocular hypertension, open angle glaucoma and low-tension glaucoma. Our studies in eyes with anterior ischemic optic neuropathy have shown that these eyes develop a similar peripapillary crescent or halo after the acute changes have resolved (Hayreh SS (1964) Br J Ophthalmol 58:964–980), thus suggesting that the peripapillary halo is an acquired ischemic lesion. All these observations indicate that the peripapillary crescent or halo seen in eyes with various types of glaucoma is an acquired lesion, secondary to peripaillary choroidal ischemia, and not a congenital lesion. Moreover, all cases with peripapillary crescent, as for example, seen in myopes, do not necessarily develp glaucomatous optic disc and visual field changes.

**Anderson to Hayreh:** In response to the discussion of Dr. Hayreh, may I just make one point. I don't want to imply that angiotension is necessarily the pertinent vasoactive factor. Angiotension happens to be the compound we used in our experiment. But, any number of circulating vasoconstricters and vasodilators might be involved.

It should be said also that this concept has certainly not been proven. It is simply an hypothesis that occurred to us after an experiment, but an hypothesis that seems interesting enough, at least to me, to warrant some exploration through further clinical and experimental observations.

Krieglstein G.K./Leydhecker W. (eds)
Glaucoma Update II


# Is Glaucoma Therapy Useless?

W. Leydhecker, Würzburg

**Summary**: Publications in recent years indicated that high IOP is not necessarily an indication for treatment in ocular hypertension. It was claimed furthermore that even in glaucoma treatment is not more than "a tradition based on obsolete ideas and never shown to be justified by any positive effect" (Bengtson, 1981), and that the "pressure theory has lost most of its meaning and has become almost completely useless" (Krakau, 1981). In contrast to these ideas, it is shown in this paper that high IOP produces the same damage as it is known from glaucoma in experimental animal studies, in otherwise healthy persons with secondary glaucoma, or in steroid-induced glaucoma, and that it produces arcuate scotoma in healthy volunteers. It is further shown, that normalization of the IOP prevents in most cases any further functional loss, especially so in early cases. Other diagnostic parameters are uncertain. A close correlation between disc and field changes exists only in the late cases. The usual kinetic perimetry with Goldmann's perimeter leaves every 3rd beginning field defect in glaucoma undetected, which is found with the computerized Octopus perimeter. For therapy, the IOP can usually be rather easily influenced, while additional risk factors (family history, vasosclerosis, large cupping, haemorrhages near the disc, late phase of glaucoma, low general blood pressure) cannot or only scarcely be influenced by therapy. It is concluded that

1. high IOP is the most important damaging parameter in glaucoma
2. that is the only one which is relatively easy to influence
3. the "normal" in the sense of the most frequent value in the healthy population is an IOP of 15-16 mmHg,
4. that normalization of IOP prevents further damage,
5. and that the advise of no treatment in glaucoma with high IOP has ethical implications which must be clearly understood.

## High Intra-Ocular Pressure and the Concept of Glaucoma

The concepts of glaucoma swing between exclusive emphazis of high IOP and disregard of the pressure theory. At present we are facing a swing of the pendulum of academic glaucoma concepts towards the neglect of high IOP. This is not so new. A look into medical history shows that the hardness of the eye was mentioned by Bannister in 1621/22, and rediscovered by Mackenzie in 1830 as a characteristic of glaucoma, but that the pressure concept of glaucoma was lost later on, even by Mackenzie himself, until von Graefe explained the excavation of the disc in 1857 as the consequence of high IOP. However, Treitel (1876), Deutschmann (1879) and especially Schnabel (1885-1902) described caverns of the optic nerve as characteristics of glaucoma which they supposed to be independent from IOP and of a "primary" nature.

In contrast to the concept that glaucoma was closely associated with high IOP and damage was the consequence of high IOP (the "mechanistic" theory), a very vague concept was stressed, predominantly in the 3rd and 4th decade of this century in France, describing glaucoma as a neuro-vascular disease supposed to be the local sign of an unknown general disease. Most of these papers did not explain anything about the way in which a general disease caused glaucomatous damages. A dysfunction of a hypothetical mid-brain center supposed to be pressure regulating, hormonal disturbances or swelling of the vitreous were erroneous hypothesis which received much attention in this century. Most ophthalmologists think at present that glaucoma is characterized by visual field defects and optic nerve atrophy which are in most cases the consequence of high IOP, in contrast to some authors who stress that high IOP is not the chief characteristic of glaucoma. A few authors even think that pressure is not important.

## Hypertension Without Glaucoma

The existance of ocular hypertension without damage of the optic nerve is known for long. Elschnig coined in 1924 the expression hypertension without glaucoma. There is no exact number separating normal from abnormal pressures because population studies showed that the distribution of IOP is not exactly normal but skewed at the upper end. The IOP shows seasonal and diurnal variations. It becomes slightly higher in old age. There are differences from sex and race. In mass screening IOPs over 21 mmHg are found in approximately 20% of the population. All this does not mean that the upper end of the distribution of normal IOP is without any limit. The Framingham study showed the 95% empirical limits for males and females below the age of 65 years to be 11-23 mmHg. This is not much different from my earlier statements of 21 mmHg (Leydhecker, 1958). All authors agree that IOP below 25 mmHg is well tolerated in most eyes for periods of 5-13 years. Only some 3% of the eyes below 23 mmHg in the glaucoma collaborative study developed field defects (Phelps, 1980). Eyes with IOP over 23 mmHg developed field defects in 8.4%. With IOPs of 26-30 mmHg a sharp rise of the frequency of field defects occurs.

David et al. (1977) report 12% with 26-30 mmHg and 41.2% with pressures over 30 mmHg, and similarly Schappert-Kimmijser 12.8% with IOPs of 22-30 mmHg, but 41.7% over 30 mmHg. There is no magical number which holds good for each individual, but there is definitely a region of increasing danger with IOPs over 26 and more so over 30 mmHg for most individuals.

## Glaucoma Without Hypertension

It is difficult to define "hypertension" if we insist that there is no upper limit of the normal distribution. However, usually glaucoma without hypertension signifies a condition with IOPs below 21 mmHg but field defects and disc changes as in glaucoma. A diurnal curve should make sure that there is never hypertension. Postural pressure rises which might induce hypertension by night should be excluded. How then can such conditions be in accordance with the pressure theory of glaucoma?

It should be pointed out first that I do not favor a pure pressure theory, but there are numerous other risk factors to be regarded which will be discussed below. However, the increased IOP is the main and most frequent factor damaging the field. The pressure distributions of 20 000 eyes, which 3 described in 1958, is showing in Fig. 1. The upper end is

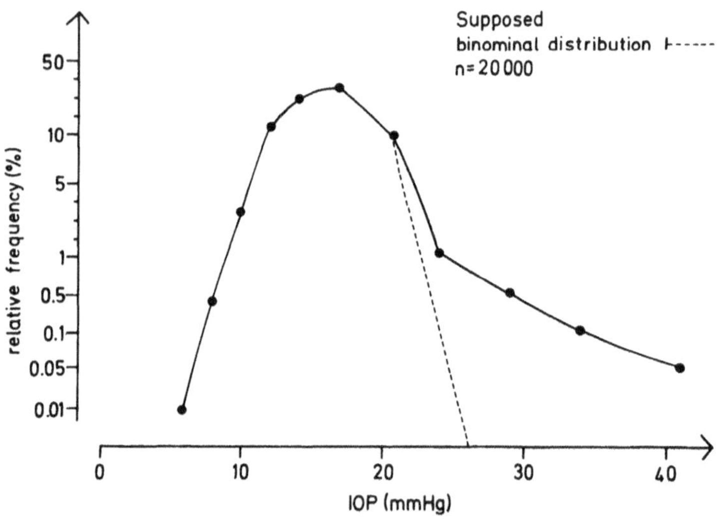


**Fig. 1.** Distribution of IOP (Schiötz) in 20 000 eyes of persons without subjective eye symptoms (Leydhecker et al. 1958). *Dots*, measured values; *Note*, lowest value approximately 8 mmHg; Mean 15-16 mmHg

skewed, as was also found by subsequent observers. It was suggested that the skew represents a second, not-normal distribution, the glaucomas, overlapping the normal distribution of healthy eyes. This suggestion has been debated since the healthy eyes do not necessarily have to show a normal distribution. The lower end of the curve are tonometric results and independent from arguments. The lowest IOPs of normal eyes were between 7–8 mmHg. This in accordance with the Framingham study showing the lowest pressure in 95% of the population to be 11 mmHg. If an eye with originally 10 mmHg suffers an increase of IOP of 11 mmHg it is still within the supposed "normal" limits of 21 mmHg but is has individually 11 mmHg over its individually normal condition. This will have the same consequences as an IOP of 31 mmHg would have to an eye with originally 20 mmHg. We must stop to think that 21 mmHg is a magic number below which everything is normal, and that pressure induced field defects are impossible within this "normal" ranges. 21 mmHg is not "normal" but is near the upper end of the normal distribution. Normal in the sense of the most frequent value in healthy eyes is 15 mmHg.

## Other Risk Factors Besides IOP

There is general agreement on risk factors for field loss in eyes with ocular hypertension such as glaucoma in the other eye, a family history of glaucoma, a large cup, pallor of the rim, haemorrhages near the disc, vasosclerosis, diabetes, thrombosis, acquired low blood pressure, a bad compliance of the patient.

Some of these may cause field loss similar to true glaucoma even in IOPs between 10–15 mmHg as was published from our hospital (Knapp 1968). Risk factors for the rate of progression in established glaucoma are, besides the elevated IOP, especially the phase of the disease. When the field loss has progressed considerably it will easily progress further at an accelerated rate. Van Heuven (1950) described further field loss in early cases in 7%, in late cases in 93% after normalization of the pressure, and Kopp et al. (1956) found progression of field loss in early cases in 10%, in late cases in 86%. Similar experiences were reported by Wilson et al. (1982). In addition to the early or late stage, the above mentioned risk factors will affect the prognosis.

## Effect of High IOP on Eyes Undisposed for Glaucoma

In animal experiments high IOP caused the same type of optic nerve destruction as in glaucoma in men. In rabbits 60 mmHg over 2 weeks increase the excavation (Erdmann, 1907), in young dogs 80 mmHg can cause complete cupping and atrophy with 8–13 days, 64–74 mmHg within 15 days (Ishikawa, 1930). In man, an experimental increase of IOP by dynamometer compression or suction cup below the systolic pressure of the ophthalmic artery produced the same type of arcuate scotoma in healthy eyes as they exist in glaucoma (Suda, 1952–1965, Goldmann, 1957).

While these experimental scotomas were reversibel, steroid induced glaucoma causes irrversible field defects of the same type as found in primary glaucoma. The field decay in other forms of secondary glaucoma follows the same pattern as in primary glaucoma. It is indeed difficult to understand why the high IOP in primary glaucoma should be unimportant if its destructive effect has been shown in experimental animal studies, in healthy volunteers, in secondary glaucoma and in steroid induced glaucoma.

## The Effect of Normalization of IOP on the Visual Fields in Glaucoma

I have shown in 1966 that normalization of IOP stops further field loss in glaucoma. Seven years after the mass-screening of 1958, I re-examined all patients with field defects who volunteered to accept the examination. I had prescribed miotics to all of them, but some had not applied the eye drugs and their IOP was above 21 mmHg. 12 out of 13 showed a progression of field loss after 7 years, while only 1 out of 9 with normalized pressure did so. A recent retrospective study (Krieglstein et al., 1982) showed no further field loss in 98% of 236 eyes which were observed for over 10 years with normalized pressure. Only 5 eyes had field loss and they were late cases. This is in accordance with the above mentioned results of Van Heuven, who found no further field loss in 93% of the early cases after normalization of pressure, and Kopp et al. who did so in 90%.

**Useless Therapy?**

There are a few papers suggesting that therapy is useless in glaucoma. Usually the effect of therapy was insufficiently monitored. Perkins (1978) reported that therapy does not prevent blindness, but 27.5% of his patients were late presentations and half of those were over the age of 80, with many patients having mental and physical handicaps. The IOP was not monitored. The conclusion to be drawn from his study is that handing over a prescription to old and handicapped people does not prevent blindness. David et al. (1977) reported that the initial pressure is very important for the development of field loss, but less so the fact whether or not the patient was treated. They advise glaucoma therapy in patients over the age of 70 years with IOP in excess of 26 mmHg. The only prospective study from Shin et al. (1976) in ocular hypertensive eyes showed in contrast to the previous findings progression of the optic nerve head cupping in 53% of the untreated and only 11% of the treated eyes. None of the eyes with IOPs below 24 mmHg developed glaucomatous functional loss, while 57% with 24 mmHg or over showed glaucomatous damage.

In recent years Krakau and his co-workers published that glaucoma is a disease independent from IOP, whatever high the IOP may be. Krakau (1981) stated that "the pressure theory has lost most of its meaning and has become almost completely useless", or, as Bengtson (1981) puts it: "What remains is, mainly a therapeutic tradition ... based on obsolete ideas and never shown to be justified by any positive effect". His hypothesis "that the optic neuropathy in glaucoma is due to small vessel disease and not to a low perfusion pressure, and that the increase of the IOP is an effect rather than the cause of glaucoma", is unproven and reminds to Schnabel's ideas 100 years ago. An IOP of 22 mmHg was chosen as the value separating normal from abnormal and to support the argument that therapy was useless (Holmin and Krakau, 1980), which was based on the finding that the field developed similarly with pressures below or above 22 mmHg. This is no support for the generalized statement that any IOP does not matter and that all therapy is useless. Why should there be a difference of field stability with IOP of 20 or 24 mmHg? There are differences with IOP below 15 mmHg or above 29 mmHg, but 22 mmHg is not the exact separating line and represents again the introduction of the so much debated magic number. If there are magic numbers they will be found in the region of 26–30 mmHg.

**Other Diagnostic Parameters**

Diagnostic parameters other than tonometry are very uncertain. For many years it was thought that a CDR over 0.3 is a symptom of glaucoma. Later on, longer and larger excavations were accepted as possibly normal. Gloster (1978) described a good correlation between excavation and field defects only with a CDR of 0.8 or over, which means that glaucoma can be diagnosed from this symptom only after the greater part of the optic nerve has died. The appearance of the disc is of little value for the early diagnosis and reliable only in the late stage – a phase of the disease with a bad prognosis which must be avoided. Other changes of the disc such as notching, pallor of the neuroretinal rim, haemorrhages, a bean pot phenomenon, can attribute to make the evaluation of the disc more certain, but again they are late signs not associated with beginning field defects but with a progressed decay of the visual field. Tests with experienced ophthalmologists have shown their considerable inter- and intraobserver variation in disc classification. Most interesting was the discrepancy between glaucoma specialists at Nara 1978, showing that some authors measure the excavation diameter from the beginning of the slope and some others refer to the bottom of the excavation, which gives completely different interpretations of CDR and throws a dubious light on previous publications on the diagnostic significance of the excavation.

The other diagnostic parameter, perimetry, is not always so reliable in its results as it is usually supposed. We have published (Gramer, 1979–1982) controlled studies comparing the results of the Goldmann perimeter, Woolf instrument, Friedmann, Competer, Fieldmaster and Octopus. It was shown, amongst other results, that with Goldmann kinetic perimetry every 3rd field in ocular hypertension is falsely classifield as normal in which the Octopus shows scotoma. Kinetic perimetry is greatly dependent upon observer influences and unsuitable for the diagnosis of early field defects in glaucoma.

## Conclusions

Functional loss typical for glaucoma can develop with an IOP below 21 mmHg. If this happens, it will occur within the upper limits of IOP (17-21 mmHg), but not so with low IOP (8-14 mmHg). Normal fields will usually be found with slightly elevated IOP (22-25 mmHg) and it does occur with IOP of 26-30 mmHg, but usually not beyond. It can be concluded that tonometries between 17-26 mmHg cannot serve by iself as a proof for or against glaucoma. An increase of the IOP over 26-30 mmHg is a most important factor in producing glaucoma functional loss in eyes with ocular hypertension or progression of field defects in eyes with established glaucoma. Pressures above 26 mmHg represent an increasing danger for the eye the higher they are. The destructive effect of high IOP has been shown in experimental animal studies, in experiments with healthy volunteers, in secondary glaucoma and in steroid induced glaucoma. An individual with bilateral glaucoma has usually the more constricted field on the eye with the higher IOP. Normalization of IOP to 15 mmHg or below will stop the further decay in almost all early cases and in many late cases. A general statement that the pressure does not matter or treatment does not help seems absurd and unjustified. High pressure destroys the optic nerve and treatment which lowers the IOP below the average of 15 mmHg prevents usually further destruction of the optic nerve.

We should not accept the negativistic-fatalistic attitude and neglect the only screw which we can turn to save vision in glaucoma. It is the only factor which we can influence easily. Other risk parameters such as the family history, age or vasosclerosis cannot be influenced and it is very difficult to raise the blood pressure without vasoconstriction which is contraindicated in glaucoma.

It must be clearly seen that there is an ethical responsibility of respected glaucoma clinicians and research workers, if they advise to leave high IOPs untreated or if they publish that treatment is useless. I know of untreated patients who turned up years later with one eye blind and the other eye in a late stage. The ophthalmologist who works in his own practice and who is not doing glaucoma research himself will possibly follow the advise to "sit back, to wait and watch the patient" who, however, will often not turn up again for regular controls, if he gets the impression that he is not really in danger. Thus the advise of no treatment can have ethical implications, and the responsibility of such publications must be clearly understood.

## References


Bengtsson B (1981) Aspects of the epidemiology of chronic glaucoma. Acta Ophthalmol [Suppl] (Copenhagen) 146:1-48

David R, Livingston DG, Luntz MH (1977) Ocular hypertension - a longterm followup of treated and untreated patients. Br J Ophthalmol 61:668-674

Elschnig A (1924) Glaukom ohne Hochdruck und Hochdruck ohne Glaukom. Z Augenheilkd 52:287-296

Erdmann P (1907) Über experimentelles Glaukom nebst Untersuchungen am glaukomatösen Tierauge. Albrecht Von Graefes Arch Klin Exp Ophthalmol 66:325-435

Gloster J (1978) Quantitative relationship between cupping of the optic disc and visual field loss in chronic simple glaucoma. Br J Ophthalmol 62: 665-669

Goldmann H (1957) Probleme der heutigen Glaukomforschung. In: Streiff EB, Babel J (Hrsg.) Moderne Probleme der Ophthalmologie. Karger, Basel

Gramer E, Pröll M, Krieglstein GK (1979) Die Perimetrie des blinden Flecks. Ein Vergleich zwischen kinetischer und computergesteuerter statischer Perimetrie. Ophthalmologica, Basel 179:201-208

Gramer E, Krieglstein GK, Leydhecker W (1980) Die Automation der Perimetrie. Z prakt Augenheilkd 1:5-26

Gramer E, Pröll M, Krieglstein GK (1980) Die Reproduzierbarkeit zentraler Gesichtsfeldbefunde bei der kinetischen und der computergesteuerten statischen Perimetrie. Klin Monatsbl Augenheilkd 176:374-384

Gramer E, Steinhauser B, Krieglstein GK (1982) The specificity of the automated supratheshold perimeter Fieldmaster 200. Albrecht Von Graefes Arch Klin Exp Ophthalmol (in press)

Gramer E, Gerlach R, Krieglstein GK (1982) Zur Sensitivität des Computerperimeters Competer bei frühen glaukomatösen Gesichtsfeldausfällen. Eine kontrollierte, klinische Studie. Klin Monatsbl Augenheilkd 180:203–209

Van Heuven JA (1950) Trephinig operations. Am J Ophthalmol 33:1387–1391

Holmin C, CET Krakau (1980) Visual field decay in normal subjects and in cases of chronic claucoma. Albrecht Von Graefes Arch Klin Exp Ophthalmol 213:291–298

Ishikawa F (1930) Experimentelles Glaukom beim Hunde mit besonderer Rücksicht auf Sehnervenerkrankungen. Albrecht Von Graefes Arch Klin Exp Ophthalmol 124:387–443

Knapp E (1968) Glaukom ohne Hochdruck bei Mutter und Tochter. Klin Monatsbl Augenheilkd 153:669–673

Kopp IF, Zatz LB (1956) Glaucoma cases in special dispensaries. Vestn Oftalmol 1:8–16 (1956); ref. Ophthal. Lit. 10, 513 (1956)

Krakau CET (1981) Intraocular pressure elevation – cause or effect in chronic glaucoma? Ophthalmologica 182:141–147

Krieglstein GK, Leydhecker W (1979) Glaucoma Update. Springer-Verlag Berlin Heidelberg New York

Krieglstein GK, Schrems W, Gramer E, Leydhecker W (1981) Detectability of early glaucomatous field defects. A controlled comparison of Goldmann versus Octopus perimetry. Greve EL, Verriest G (eds) Doc Ophthalmol (The Hague) Proc Series, vol 26. bv Publishers

Krieglstein GK, Glaab E, Gramer E (1981) Das Computerperimeter Fieldmaster 200. Eine vergleichende, kontrollierte klinische Studie zur Sensitivität und Spezifität in der Glaukomperimetrie. Klin Monatsbl Augenheilkd 179: 340–345

Krieglstein GK, Helmbold C, Leydhecker W (1982) Zur Prognose des chronischen Glaukoms. Eine epikritische Studie. Z prakt Augenheilkd 3:17–24

Krieglstein GK, Schrems W, Gramer E, Leydhecker W (1982) Die Perimetrie beginnender, glaukomatöser Gesichtsfeldausfälle. Eine vergleichende, kontrollierte Studie mit dem Goldmann- und Octopus-Perimeter. In: Lund OE, Riedel K (Hrsg) Automation und neuere Technologie in der Ophthalmologie. Ferdinand Enke Verlag Stuttgart

Leydhecker W, Akiyama K, Neumann HG (1958) Der intraokulare Druck gesunder menschlicher Augen. Klin Monatsbl Augenheilkd 133: 662–670

Leydhecker W (1959) Zur Verbreitung des Glaucoma simplex in der scheinbar gesunden, augenärztlich nicht behandelten Bevölkerung. Doc Ophthalmol 13:359–388

Leydhecker W (1973) Glaukom. Ein Handbuch. 2. Aufl. Springer-Verlag, Berlin Heidelberg New York

Perkins ES (1978) Blindness from glaucoma and the economics of prevention. Trans Ophthalmol Soc UK 98:293

Phelps CD (1980) The "no treatment" approach to ocular hypertension. Surv Ophthalmol 25:175–182

Schappert-Kimmijser J (1971) A five-year follow-up of subjects with intraocular pressure of 22–30 mmHg without anomalies of optic nerve and visual field typical for glaucoma at first investigation. Ophthalmologica 162:289–295

Shin DH, Kolker AE, Kass MA, et al. (1976) Longterm epinephrine therapy of ocular hypertension. Arch Ophthalmol 94:2059–2060

Suda K (1952) Early diagnosis of glaucoma. Acta Soc Ophthalmol Jpn 56:933–958; ref. Ophthalmol Lit 6, p 2568

Suda K, Abe Y (1964) Variation of the angioscotoma caused by bulbar compression in normal and glaucomatous eyes. Acta Soc Ophthalmol Jpn 68:1104–1114; ref. Ophthalmol Lit 18, p 4497

Suda K, Abe Y, Gyotoku, K (1965) Comparison of angioscotoma in glaucoma with that in retinal angiosclerosis. Jap J Ophthalmol 19:261–269; ref. Zentralbl Ophthalmol (1966) 96:538

Wilson R, Walker AM, Dueker DK, Crick RP (1982) Risk factors for rate of progression of glaucomatous visual field loss. Arch Ophthal 100:737–741

## Discussion

**Krakau to Leydhecker:** I am greatly honoured by Prof. Leydhecker quoting me "verbatim", but had been even more so if I had been the author of the lines he attributes to me. This is however not the case. My criticism, perhaps somewhat more subtly formulated, is directed against obvious contradictions and logical weaknesses in the pressure theory. The point I want to make is that the conception of pressure as the generally valid cause of damage in chron. glaucoma is a hypothesis and not an established fact. It does not seem fruitful to remain "imprisoned" by the framework of the pressure theory and interpret every result from the point of view that it is an axiom. (That very high pressures are deleterious is of course beyond doubt.) Ad hoc hypotheses such as that of the "normative pressure", which may or may not be right, saves the theory but at the cost of its predictive value. It becomes "immune to falsification" if we claim that the pressure, however low it may be, is still too high whenever progression of defects continues.

Fortunately the theory is testable in the range of moderately increased pressures, where our interest is focused, by investigations designed to avoid common fallacy. Prospective randomized studies with and without treatment are suggested and are in fact in progress.

**Bengtsson to Leydhecker:** In a small swedish community (Dalby) with 20 000 inhabitants we have examined 1500 and re-examined 1300 out of 2000 persons born 1907–21 by automatic perimetry and disc photography - as well as a few hundred patients out of 1000 persons born before 1907 by ophthalmoscopy.

According to our findings there are 30 patients with manifest High Tension Glaucoma (HTG) and also 30 patients with manifest Low Tension Glaucoma (LTG) in Dalby. We are aware of 15 persons that have had disc haemorrhages but no glaucomatous visual field defects and we know that there has to be many more - probably about 60 - making a total of 75 "preglaucomas" of which according to the longitudinal studies of Armaly and Perkins about 80% should have "normal" pressures.

In this way we arrive at the conclusion that there are 45 HTGs and 90 LTGs in Dalby. If the LTGs have lost 50% of their nerve fibers (as Harry Quigley ment yesterday) they have already suffered more damage than the HTGs possibly can in the future.

And this is our main concern. We must seek better methods to prevent, detect and treat low tension glaucoma.

The damage caused by low tension glaucoma can not be defined away and the literature cited by professor Leydhecker offers no support to his opinion that we should concentrate on the high tension glaucomas.

David et al. (1977) in fact reported a greater incidence of glaucoma in treated than in untreated ocular hypertension - even after stratification of the material (table 3, page 672). Shin et al (1976) found an unexpectedly high incidence of vision loss in the control eyes after treatment of one eye in patients with ocular hypertension. The King's College Hospital glaucoma data used by Wilson et al. (1982) have earlier been reported to suggest "that if the entire population were treated successfully and all ocular hypertension removed, 99% of the glaucomatous visual field loss would still remain". (Daubs and Crick 1980).

**Spaeth to Leydhecker:** Approximately 70% of visual loss in glaucoma occurs prior to the time that the patients are first seen by physicians. The other side of the coin is that about 30% of visual loss in glaucoma occurs after the patient has come under the care of the physician. This is clearly disturbing. We do not appear to be doing our job as well as might possibly be the case. It is appropriate to try to determine why that 30% of continuing visual loss takes place. Some of it results from the complications attendant to improperly, or for that matter, properly performed surgery. But in my practice, at any rate, the overwhelming majority is the result of inadequate therapy of glaucoma. The ophthalmologists picks a lower figure of intraocular pressure, perhaps 18 mmHg as a satisfactory lever, and when the intraocular pressure reaches that level he believes that the patients is controlled. Unfortunately, the only way control can be defined is retrospectively. That is, when there is no progressive damage to the optic nerve or visual field, then the patient is controlled. One cannot determine prospectively what level of intraocular pressure will be adequate. Thus, one determines control by stabilizing the disc and field, and then retrospectively decides that that intraocular pressure is the intraocular pressure which is likely to be satisfactory for continuing control.

In summary, lowering the intraocular pressure can prevent progressive optic nerve damage in glaucoma. Where progressive damage occurs, the ophthalmologist must conclude: 1. The nerve damage is caused by some mechanism other than glaucoma, or 2. The neurons were so mortally wounded that regardless of what intraocular pressure is achieved, they will continue to deteriorate, or 3. The intraocular pressure is higher than the eye can tolerate, regardless of what that intraocular pressure is.

**W. Leydhecker:** 1. It is not logical to call the pressure theory a mere hypothesis, as Krakau did, or to refute it completely as Bengtson did. It is a fact and not a hypothesis that normalization of the IOP prevents in approximately 90 per cent of glaucoma cases a further deterioration of the visual field, expecially in early cases. This holds good for all forms of glaucoma, secondary as well as primary. Since these different forms have nothing in common except high IOP, it seems logical to recognize high IOP as the main nocive factor. Kronfeld and McGarry, 1948, found that normalization prevented further damage in 81–88 per cent of their cases, but that 100 per cent of the not normalized eyes lost field. More literature was quoted in my paper. Eyes which continue to lose their field even after normalization of IOP are mostly late cases. An adequate analysis shows that their functional loss is often caused by other factors than glaucoma, e.g. beginning cataract, macular degeneration or vascular disease of the fundus. In 236 glaucoma eyes which have been observed for over 10 years, we found only 5 (2,1 per cent) with a further glaucomatous field decay in spite of IOP below 21 mmHg (Krieglstein, G.K., Helmbold, C. and Leydhecker, W., Zeitschrift für praktische Augenheilkunde 1982, pp. 17–24).

I am in addition to this literature showing here

the data of glaucoma patients from my clientele who have been followed for 14-17 years and kept their field unchanged after normalization of their IOP, although they were in a late stage.

2. The pressure theory cannot explain the field loss in all glaucomas. The glaucomas with low IOP are rare in comparison with hypertensive glaucomas. They are caused by vascular diseases (diabetic, sclerotic) or diseases such as carotid insufficient with an abnormally low perfusion pressure of the optic nerve. In most glaucomas such vascular factors are combined with high IOP, and high IOP is the most important factor and the only one we can change for the better.

3. Normalization of IOP was usually not really achieved in patients who are quoted as having field decay in spite of "normalization". Tonometry was performed every few months only and briefly after the application of miotics, diurnal curves were not obtained, the patients were not instructed how to apply their eye drops, and they were not informed about any basic understanding of their disease and its treatment. These points came out in discussion with Luntz and collaborators after my lecture in South Africa in 1977. One cannot expect compliance from uniformed patients and one should not state that therapy is useless if there were insufficient tests on how and whether at all therapy was correctly applied. Simply handing over a prescription does not prevent blindness.

4. The range of normal IOPs is between 8–21 mmHg and in some eyes up to 25 mmHg. We have learned in the last decade that most no-risk eyes tolerate IOPs up to 25 mmHg for periods of ten or even more years. 21 mmHg is not a magic number. It does not strictly separate two groups, one which will lose field and another one which will not. However, in some papers this number is wrongly used in this sense in order to demonstrate that even "normalized" IOPs below 21 mmHg can be associated with a further loss of the visual field. I want to stress that 21 mmHg is somewhere near the upper limit, but not "normal" for all eyes. Normal in the sense of the most frequent IOP is 15 or 16 mmHg. Normalization means to bring the average IOP of an eye to 16 mmHg. It is therefore not always sufficient to bring the IOP to 20 mmHg, if there is already a glaucomatous field loss. Such eyes may further go down hill, especially if not their peak, but their mean IOP is just 20 and peaks will be considerably higher. (See fig. 5 in David, Livingston and Luntz, Br J Ophthalmol 1977.) Their conclusion from the observed field loss with 20 mmHg was that miotics are useless, but this is wrong. It only shows that 20 mmHg is not good enough. The observation that lowering IOP for 2,5 mmHg does not help much either (Levene, Trans Am Acad 1975), and it does certainly not allow the conclusion that therapy is useless.

5. I have been told in this meeting about glaucoma patients in Sweden who heard about the "useless" therapy on television and stopped their therapy. I urge authors to consider the consequences of their publications. The IOP is the only screw which we can adjust in glaucoma. We can do nothing to alter all the other factors, such as heredity, vascular factors, diabetes, the condition of the disc or the stage of the second eye. Please do not allow an intellectual play with hypotheses to cause blindness.

**Leydhecker to Bengtson:** I was not speaking about glaucoma without hypertension nor on ocular hypertension in contrast to glaucoma. My lecture referred to the most common form of glaucoma with high IOP, and my conclusion was that therapy which really normalizes IOP is indeed very useful and furthermore, the only thing we can do. The authors mentioned in my paper and quoted in Bengtson's discussion have drawn wrong conclusions from their material, as I showed in my paper.

**Leydhecker to Krakau:** The misquotation was taken from Bengtson's paper Acta Ophthalmol (1981) Suppl 146 p 4. I apologize for Bengtson's error.

Krieglstein G.K./Leydhecker W. (eds)
Glaucoma Update II


# Contrast Sensitivity and Glaucoma

C.D. Phelps and M.A. Motolko, Iowa City

In the past, our clinical methods of testing vision in glaucoma have, for the most part, been limited to routine light-sense perimetry in which we measure differential light sensitivity at selected loci in the field of vision. Such testing has disclosed that glaucomatous impairment of light sensitivity usually begins in the paracentral and nasal portions of the visual field and spares central and temporal vision until late in the disease.

At present, there is a growing interest in the investigation of other techniques for testing vision in glaucoma. The measurement of central contrast sensitivity is one of these new techniques. In this test, we determine how much contrast is required for the patient to perceive a series of centrally fixated grating targets that differ in spatial separation.

Several investigators [1–5] have tested contrast sensitivity functions in patients with glaucoma and have concluded that an impairment of central contrast sensitivity accompanies and may precede the onset of glaucomatous visual field damage. Other investigators have challenged these results because of the large overlap between glaucoma patients and age-matched controls [6–10]. The object of our study was to use patients with asymmetric glaucomatous optic nerve damage so that the patient's fellow eye could be used as a control.

## Methods

We have been testing contrast sensitivity on an instrument that uses the principle of laser interferometry to generate the target. A helium-neon laser beam is split into two beams that are both focused with a convergent lens in the patient's entrance pupil. Where the two beams diverge beyond their point of focus and overlap on the retina, the patient perceives a pattern of interference fringes. The fringes appear to the patient as alternating red and black stripes. The separation of the stripes can be varied from a wide separation (low spatial frequency) to a closely spaced pattern (high spatial frequency). The orientation of the stripes can also be varied from vertical to oblique to horizontal. The patient's task is to tell us if he can see the stripes and, if so, to describe their orientation as confirmation.

Laser interferometry with a high contrast grating has been widely used by many investigators for the measurement of central visual acuity. Perception of the gratings does not depend on the patient's refractive error, and the striped pattern can be perceived even through incipient cataracts. To modify the instrument for contrast sensitivity testing, we placed a laser polarizing beam-splitter in front of the laser, splitting off a portion of the main beam before it was subsequently again split to form the two beams that generated the interference fringes. The first beam was optically superimposed on the laser interference pattern, as seen by the patient. By rotating polarizers in front of the laser beams, we could vary the contrast of the fringes from zero to 100% while maintaining a constant average luminance.

The field size was five degrees, and the patient was allowed to fixate anywhere on the target. Contrast was gradually increased from zero percent until the patient first perceived the pattern. This was repeated at least four times, with vertical, horizontal, and oblique presentations, at each of several spatial frequencies. The reciprocal of the mean contrast threshold (i.e., the contrast sensitivity) at each spatial frequency was plotted and the results for the entire spatial frequency function were compared between the two eyes.

## Results

We examined 22 patients with unilateral

**Table 1.** Contrast sensitivity in different ocular conditions

| | Relative impairment of contrast sensitivity | | |
|---|---|---|---|
| | "Damaged" eye | "Normal" eye | No difference |
| Secondary glaucoma (3) | 3 | 0 | 0 |
| Ocular hypertension (5) | 4 | 0 | 1 |
| Low-Tension glaucoma (6) | 4 | 1 | 1 |
| Primary Open-Angle glaucoma (13) | 4 | 1 | 8 |
| | 15 | 2 | 10 |

visual field loss and five ocular hypertensive patients with asymmetric cupping. The results (Table 1) indicated that patients with asymmetric visual field loss usually had more impairment of contrast sensitivity in the damaged eye than in the fellow eye. This was true for all patients who had a strictly unilateral secondary glaucoma, but in some patients with asymmetric primary open-angle glaucoma there was either no difference in contrast sensitivity between the two eyes or, rarely, greater impairment of contrast sensitivity in the eye with the lesser amount of field loss.

Impairment of contrast sensitivity was distributed over a wide range of spatial frequencies (0.4 cycles/degree to 40 cycles/degree) but was most frequently present at 3 cycles/degree (visual equivalent of 20/200).

## Discussion

These results confirm that glaucoma impairs contrast sensitivity and, thus, alters central vision at a time when visual acuity is still normal and the visual field defects are away from fixation. Most of our patients with unilateral visual field loss had relative impairment of contrast sensitivity in the predicted direction, but in some with primary glaucoma the contrast sensitivity was symmetrical or even impaired in the unpredicted direction. Primary open-angle glaucoma and low-tension glaucoma, of course, are usually bilateral diseases, even though the visual field loss is often asymmetric, and it is possible that those patients in whom the asymmetry of contrast sensitivity did not match up with the asymmetry of field loss already had damage to the fellow eye. Examination of their optic discs seemed to confirm this. When the cupping was asymmetric, contrast sensitivity was impaired in the predicted direction. Only in patients with symmetric cupping was the contrast sensitivity symmetric or impaired in the opposite direction to the visual field impairment.

Overlap between elderly normals and glaucoma patients may limit the usefulness of contrast sensitivity testing as a diagnostic test, but in a patient suspected of having glaucoma, asymmetric contrast sensitivity may indicate early unilateral damage. Also, the observation that contrast sensitivity is impaired in early glaucoma, in addition to the loss of color discrimination that has been shown in other studies, requires that we reexamine our classical concepts of optic nerve damage in glaucoma, especially the concept that central vision is spared until late in the disease.

**Acknowledgment.** This work was partially supported by Research Grant EY-03330 from the National Eye Institute.

## References

1. Arden GB, Jacobson JJT (1978) A simple grating test for contrast sensitivity: preliminary results indicate value in screening for glaucoma. Invest Ophthalmol 17:23–32
2. Atkin A, Bodis-Wollner I, Wolkstein M, Moss A, Podos SM (1979) Abnormalities of central contrast sensitivity in glaucoma. Am J Ophthalmol 88:205–211
3. Atkins A, Wolkstein M, Bodis-Wollner I, Anders M, Kels B, Podos SM (1980) Interocular comparison of contrast sensitivity in glaucoma patients and suspects. Br J Ophthalmol 64:858–862
4. Tagami Y, Onuma T, Mizokami K, Isayama Y (1981) Comparison of spatial contrast sensiti-

vity with visual field in optic neuropathy and glaucoma. Doc Ophthalmol Proc Series 26: 147–154
5. Stamper RL, Hsu-Winges C, Sopher M (1982) Arden contrast sensitivity testing in glaucoma. Arch Ophthalmol 100:947–950
6. Derefeldt E, Lennerstrand E, Lundh B (1979) Age variations in normal human contrast sensitivity. Acta Ophthalmol 57:679–690
7. Sekular R, Hutman LP, Owsley CT (1980) Human aging and spatial vision. Science 209: 1255–1256
8. Skalka HW (1980) Effect of age on Arden grating acuity. Br J Ophthalmol 64:21–23
9. Sokol S, Domar A, Moskowitz A (1980) Utility of the Arden grating test in glaucoma screening: high false-positive rate in normals over 50 years of age. Invest Ophthalmol 19:1529–1533
10. Singh H, Cooper RL, Alder VA, Crawford EJ, Terrell A, Constable IJ (1981) The Arden grating acuity: effect of age and optical factors in the normal patient, with prediction of the false-negative rate in screening for glaucoma. Br J Ophthalmol 65:518–524

## Discussion

**Anderson to Phelps:** I was interested to see that in the patients that showed a unilaterally abnormal result on acuity perimetry, the Goldman field showed a depressed field compared to the other eye. In such a case, if each isoper is moved inward to the normal position of the next weakest stimulus, there is a generalized reduction of visual sensitivity of 0.5 log unit. So these cases do have a distinct reduction in visual sensation tested by standard perimetry, but we simply ignore this type of visual alteration (and pay attention mainly to nerve fiber bundle defects), because the generalized depression due to glaucoma can't be distinguished from the depression caused by age, small pupil size, media opacities, and other causes of biologic variation.

The point I wish to make is that there is a generalized depression of the visual field that is recognizable at times. Some automated perimeters that quantitate static threshold at a pattern of points (competer, Perifect, Octopus, for example), the visual field may be identified as abnormal because with each instrument has been determined a set of normal values for each age. When an abnormal result is obtained, the clinician must be careful to determine if the depression is due to the glaucoma or due to media opacity or other cause. Notice that a difference between these facts and Goldmann perimetry is in the interpretation – for when perimetry is performed with the Goldmann perimeter we usually simply discuss any generalized depression would be indistinguishable from non-glaucomatous cause, so we haven't bothered to define as precisely the range of normal isopter position and in effect have included any effect of media, pupil size, and age within our rather informally defined notion of a "normal" visual field.

Now, it could be done for the Goldmann perimeter, couldn't it. We could define those points that at a given age are normally always endrosed by the I = 2e isopter, etc. And then if the visual field is depressed, one must decide if the clinical findings (lens clarity, pupil size, examination of the disc) suggest what is the cause of the depression.

Now, the question. If this were done, would acuity perimetry show an abnormality before ordinary threshold perimetry? Is the acuity visual function really affected earlier than threshold function, or might threshold function be equally sensitive if the same care were taken to study and define the range of normal responses? And will acuity perimetry also be of imperfect specificity, being affected by media opacity and other disease?

My reason for raising this question is that visual threshold correlates with ganglion cell density also, perhaps just as well as visual acuity does. Dr. Robert Knighton has recently pointed out that if one compares two locations in the normal retina, one with half the ganglion cell density of the other other, there will be approximately a 0.5 log unit difference in visual threshold. This relationship is interesting in that we might consider a 0.5 log unit change in visual sensitivity to be about the magnitude that we would consider clinically detectable; and Dr. Quigley tells us that about 50% of the nerve fibers can be lost without producing a field defect. Actually, his fields may show a generalized depression, but it is simply that it can't be recognized given our difficulty in being certain that a diffuse reduction of visual sensation is pathological. Of course, if only 5% of the nerve fibers are lost, but all in one bundle, a well localized definite visual field defect may be present, and it is hard to accept the notion as it is always necessary to lose a large number of nerve fibers to get a field defect – it might depend on how diffuse or localized the axon loss is. This would be true of both standard threshold perimetry and acuity perimetry.

So, my point of discussion is that there is such a thing as generalized depression in glaucoma that is a real change, and in cases with generalized depression, it can't be said that there is no glaucomatous field defect. Any my question is, if two retinal locations are compared, one with half the number of ganglion cells of the other, what is the difference in acuity (for example, need the special frequence be halved): and how does this difference compare with the acuity change that could be reliability distinguished by acuity perimetry?

Krieglstein G.K./Leydhecker W. (eds)
Glaucoma Update II


# Abnormalities of the Visual System in Ocular Hypertension and Glaucoma: Seeing Beyond Routine Perimetry[1]

A. Atkin, S.M. Podos and I. Bodis-Wollner, New York

## Introduction

The more timely diagnosis of glaucoma may reasonably be pursued by looking for indicators of its earliest and possibly reversible visual consequences. Subtle abnormalities of foveal vision, detectable through sensitive psychophysical and electrophysiologic measurements, apparently occur in glaucoma before or in conjunction with classical defects. Discerning such early abnormalities may eventually permit the systematic detection of subclinical visual changes, prior to the development of frank scotomata.

Two main areas of glaucoma research suggesting foveal dysfunction will be reviewed: (1) color vision studies, and (2) measurements of spatial and temporal contrast sensitivity. In addition, available data from pattern ERG and VEP measurements will be discussed. Results from other relevant areas, such as pupillometry and unconventional (layer) perimetry, will also be surveyed.

## Psychophysical studies

### *Color Discrimination and Thresholds*

Several studies, most using the Farnsworth-Munsell 100 Hue test (but also the D-15 panel, anomaloscopic and other techniques: Koliopoulos 1979), have noted color vision defects in glaucoma patients (Fishman et al. 1974; Kalmus and Seedburgh 1974; Marmion 1978; Koliopoulos 1979), generally of blue-yellow discrimination. Some have also detected such defects in ocular hypertensive patients (Lakowski et al. 1972; Fishman et al. 1974; Marmion 1978; Koliopoulos 1979; Drance et al. 1981). It has been proposed that this kind of defect may be one of the earliest visual signs of elevation of intraocular pressure (Foulds et al. 1972, 1974; Koliopoulos 1979; Drance et al. 1981), and may be a useful predictor of glaucomatous visual field damage (Drance et al. 1981). In another type of study, reduced sensitivities of ocular hypertensive (OHT) and open-angle glaucoma (OAG) patients both to yellow and to blue-green targets were found during dark adaptation (Goldthwaite et al. 1976). Acquired blue-yellow discrimination defects are generally thought to indicate retinal rather than optic-nerve pathology (Francois & Verriest 1968). However, sensory impairment for blue can occur in diabetes, and also in cerebral acquired achromatopsia, e.g., from tumors or strokes.

### *Unconventional Perimetry Methods*

There have been several investigations of flicker fields. These earlier psychophysical observations noted diminished critical flicker fusion frequencies, which sometimes occurred in parts of the visual field that had seemed normal by kinetic perimety (Miles 1950; Campbell and Rittler 1959; Kozousek 1968).

Psychophysical deficits in glaucoma have also been reported within the past few years using several newer techniques. Those which have not been used perimetrically will be mentioned in a later section. However, one perimetric technique, termed layer-by-layer perimetry, has recently been used to examine "altered receptive field-like properties" (Enoch and Campos 1979). In essence, an incremental test flash is detected against a background target of varying diameter. The background can either be a static disc, or a rotating

[1] Supported in part by grants EY-01867 & EY-01708 from the National Institutes of Health, Bethesda, Maryland, and an unrestricted grant from Research to Prevent Blindness, Inc

windmill. Changes in both static and dynamic functions occur in various retinal disorders. Characteristic changes were noted in glaucoma, and these differed from the changes reported in anterior ischemic optic neuropathy (Enoch et al. 1980).

### *Spatial Contrast Sensitivity*

Gratings composed of black and white bars have been used since the eighteenth century to measure visual acuity. Acuity can be related to the contrast and spatial frequency (number of cycles - i.e., pairs of dark-and-light bars - per degree of visual angle) of a just-visible grating. In the past several years, sinusoidal gratings (gratings with sinusoidal luminance profiles) have been used increasingly in physiologic and pathophysiologic studies of the visual system (reviews: Bodis-Wollner and Bender 1973; Arden 1978; Bodis-Wollner and Camisa 1980). Sinusoidal stimuli provide the simplest means for testing input-output relationships in a complex sensory system. Visual losses can be measured with sinusoidal gratings in much the same way that pure, sinusoidal tones are used in audiology to characterize hearing losses.

Static gratings have been used to demonstrate reduced wide-field contrast sensitivity in glaucoma patients to coarse stimuli of low contrast (Arden and Jacobson 1978; Hitchings et al. 1981). Arden (1978) has developed a book of printed test-plates, each a grating of a different spatial frequency. The contrast of each pattern is very low at the bottom of the plate and increases continuously toward the top; as the plate is gradually uncovered from bottom to top, regions of progressively higher contrast are exposed, until the subject is able to detect the pattern. Arden noted that most glaucoma patients were unable to detect the grating until portions of the plate had been uncovered that had contrasts substantially higher than those required by normal subjects. However there has been some disagreement concerning the sensitivity and specificity of this method as a diagnostic and prognostic tool. Sokol and colleagues (1980) did a similar study, concluding that there was a large age effect which vitiated the test's usefulness for older patients. Singh and colleagues (1981) also reported a somewhat discouraging result.

### *Flicker Detection and Temporal Contrast Sensitivity*

Several of the foregoing approaches may have potential value for predicting eventual visual field damage in ocular hypertensive patients; however, flicker contrast sensitivity methods seem particularly promising on the basis of results already obtained (Atkin et al. 1979, 1980; Tyler 1981). Moreover, these methods can be very simple and fast. Techniques of sinusoidal flicker stimulation at variable modulation depths and over a range of temporal frequencies (deLange 1958) have provided information analogous, in the temporal realm, to the spatial resolution data summarized in a spatial contrast sensitivity curve (Bodis-Wollner and Camisa 1980). This method has been used with ocular hypertensive and glaucoma patients to demonstrate reduced central sensitivity to rapid flicker (Tyler 1981). A different but related method has shown impaired temporal resolution determined by a two-flash detection method (Galvin et al. 1976).

The early stages of glaucomatous visual damage are generally detected outside of the central 5-10 degrees of the visual field. As long as Snellen acuity remains good, it is ordinarily assumed that vision in the central field has not yet been affected by the disease process. However, as previously reported (Atkin et al. 1979, 1980), we found abnormalities of central vision in glaucoma patients who had normal Snellen acuities. These abnormalities occurred in a variable named the "dynamic response coefficient" (DRC), which is based on the contrast required for the detection of flickering patterns. Two types of stimuli (Fig. 1), a homogeneous flickering field, and a counterphase flickering grating of low spatial frequency, were presented on a screen subtending 4 degrees of visual angle. The average of the contrast sensitivities to these two stimuli (defined as the DRC) was consistently lower in glaucomatous eyes with characteristic extramacular field loss than in normotensive eyes (Fig. 2), and this difference was maintained after correction for age differences. The difference was highly significant statistically. DRC was also below normal in half the ocular hypertensive eyes (IOP $>$ 22 mmHg, without visual field damage in either eye). No relation between DRC and ocular medication or intraocular pressure at the time of testing

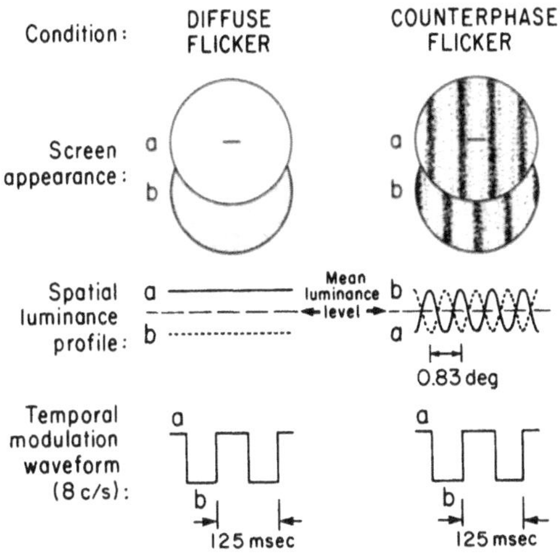


**Fig. 1.** Schematic representation of stimuli electronically generated on an oscilloscope screen. *Left:* Diffuse flicker condition. The overall luminance of a blank, evenly illuminated screen changed abruptly back and forth between two levels (level *a* and level *b*) at a rate of 8 Hz. *Right:* Counterphase flicker condition. The stimulus was a 1.2-cpd sinusoidal grating pattern which was temporally modulated at a rate of 8 Hz. The separation between adjacent *dark bars* of the grating was 0.83 degrees of visual angle. Sixteen times per second, each *dark bar* of the pattern changed abruptly into a *bright one*, and vice versa. The alternating gratings "*a*" and "*b*" were a half cycle out of phase. As the two patterns alternated at a frequency of 8 Hz, the *center of each stripe* was flickering in a manner identical to the flicker of the whole screen in the diffuse flicker condition. In diffuse flicker, the whole screen changed from darker to lighter every 125 msec; in counterphase flicker, the center of a given *bar* changed from darker to lighter every 125 msec. (From *Atkin* et al. 1979)

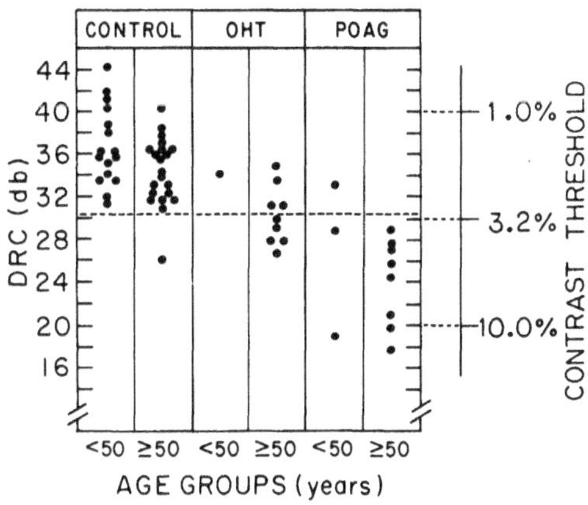


**Fig. 2.** Dynamic response coefficient (*DRC*) distributions for the control group (*left*), the ocular hypertension group (*OHT*) (*middle*), and the primary open-angle glaucoma group (*POAG*) (*right*). The *ordinate* is a logarithmic scale giving the mean of the 8 Hz contrast sensitivities for diffuse flicker and counterphase flicker. We named this mean value the dynamic response coefficient (*DRC*). A change of 20 db signifies a tenfold change of stimulus contrast. Three threshold levels of stimulus contrast, corresponding to three of the contrast sensitivity values of the *left ordinate scale*, are indicated by the *Contrast Threshold scale* on the *right*. In this plot, each group has been subdivided by age, as indicated at the bottom (younger than 50 years *on left*, older *on right*). (From *Atkin* et al. 1979)

was detectable. A clear relation of DRC loss to glaucomatous visual field defect and optic disc abnormality, but not to ocular medication or to the immediate intraocular pressure level, was confirmed through interocular comparisons (Atkin et al. 1980).

Recent work by Tyler (1981) lends further support to the appropriateness of this approach to a glaucoma-predictive test for OHT patients. He found a high incidence of flicker contrast-sensitivity abnormalities in the fellow eyes of patients with unilateral glaucoma. These eyes were considered ocular hypertensive because their intraocular pressures were elevated but they did not have visual field defects. However, the risk of future visual damage in such an eye, when the other eye already shows visual damage, is high (Harbin et al. 1976; Susanna et al. 1978). Therefore, the reported high incidence of flicker contrast-sensitivity abnormalities in these glaucoma-suspect eyes suggests that such abnormalities may have prognostic usefulness.

The ocular hypertensive patients in our study (Atkin et al. 1979) showed a much lower percentage of flicker (DRC) abnormalities than Tyler's (1981) study, but this difference can probably be accounted for by the different selection criteria. These studies suggest that flicker contrast-sensitivity methods can detect early visual changes associated with ocular hypertension, but neither study makes any direct test of predictive power. The prognostic value of visual psychophysical variables has not, till now, been tested in any prospective study of ocular hypertensive patients.

## Electrophysiologic Studies

The foregoing findings are consistent with the occurrence of a generalized reduction of visual sensitivity in glaucoma. Electrophysiologic indications of reduced visual sensitivity in glaucoma include changes in both electroretinographic (ERG) and visual evoked potential (VEP) characteristics. These have the advantage over psychophysical tests of being objective measurements.

ERG tests of glaucoma patients have usually been read as normal. However, some studies report decreased amplitudes, specifically lower photopic a-waves to single, diffuse flashes, and lower responses to diffuse flicker (Alvis 1966). Most recently, significant ERG abnormalities were shown in glaucoma using patterned stimuli which apparently evoke corneally recordable signals from the inner retinal layers (Fiorentini et al. 1981; May et al. 1982; Maffei et al. 1982).

VEP studies have shown abnormalities such as increased latencies and reduced amplitudes (Cappin & Nissin 1975; Bartl 1978; Huber and Wagner 1978). Reduction in steady-state VEP amplitudes measured by power spectral analytic techniques can also be an indication of glaucomatous damage (Maffei et al. 1982; Bodis-Wollner 1981; Towle et al. 1981).

We recently examined pattern VEP latencies in OHT and OAG patients and again found them to be abnormally large (Bodis-Wollner et al. 1982). The VEP stimulus was a 2.3 c/d sinusoidal grating, counterphase modulated at 1 Hz. Field size was 9 deg and mean luminance 1.7 log foot lamberts. The mean latencies of both patient groups were significantly different from normal ($p < .001$), as well as from each other (Table 1). As part of the same study, DRC values (contrast sensitivities to 8 Herz flicker of low spatial frequency targets: see above) were determined for 22 of the 32 patients, and this psychophysical measurement, previously found to be abnormal in glaucoma (Atkin et al. 1979), was significantly correlated with VEP latency ($r = -.66$, $p < .001$).

We conclude (1) that VEP latency, an objective measurement, may have prognostic value in glaucoma; and (2) that its relation to abnormal flicker sensitivity deserves further exploration.

## Pupil Light Reflex

Besides the above-mentioned psychophysical and electrophysiologic studies on visual effects of glaucoma, a very modest amount of research has made use of pupillography. The effects of open-angle glaucoma may include afferent pupillary defects, characterized by reduction of the reflex constriction to a luminance stimulus. These clinically detectable pupil abnormalities sometimes occur while perimetric defects are still mild (Kabak et al. 1976) or absent (Kohn et al. 1979).

Using quantitative pupillography, Lowenstein and Schoenberg (1944) described instances of reduced amplitudes and abnormally long latencies, but we know of no subsequent study. We have begun this type of investigation (Atkin et al. 1982). Pupil responses were measured to 0.4 sec flashes of light in patients not receiving antiglaucomatous medication but with intraocular pressures above 21 mmHg, using TV pupillography (Atkin et al. 1982). Amplitudes and

**Table 1.** Pattern vep in glaucoma

| Group | No. of patients | VEP latency[a] msec | No. of patients with abnormal VEP[c] (%) One eye abn. | Both eyes abn. | One or both |
|---|---|---|---|---|---|
| Normal | 37 | 107 ± 5.7 | 1 (3%) | 0 (0%) | 1 (3%) |
| OHT | 24 | 114 ± 9.2[b] | 5 (21%) | 5 (21%) | 10 (42%) |
| OAG | 8 | 129 ± 12.2[b] | 1 (12%) | 5 (62%) | 6 (75%) |

[a] Mean ± SD; [b] Difference of mean from the normal group mean is statistically significant ($p < 0.001$; one-tailed t-test). The difference between OHT and OAG group mean is also significant at this level; [c] Using, as the upper limit of normal, 119 msec, which is two standard deviations above the mean

latencies of responses as well as pre-flash diameters were obtained from 13 ocular hypertensive (OHT) patients, 7 open-angle glaucoma (OAG) patients, and from 27 control subjects with normal intraocular pressures. Both OHT patients and OAG patients showed very distinct patterns of pupil light response, different from normal, and different from each other. Specifically, it was noted that: (1) Pre-flash pupil diameters did not differ between groups. (2) Mean latencies were abnormally long in both patient groups. (3) Low amplitudes, similar to afferent pupillary defects noted clinically, occurred in some OAG patients. (4) The response amplitudes of most OHT patients were also abnormal but in the opposite direction - that is, they were abnormally large. (This was quite unexpected.) Using both latency and amplitude, OHT and OAG patients could generally be distinguished from normal (< 15–20% false negatives, < 15% false positives), and from each other. Pupillography may thus have potential usefulness both for unraveling the pathophysiology of visual changes in OHT and OAG, and as a diagnostic and possibly prognostic tool.

## Pathophysiology and Specificity

Most of the vision testing techniques touched upon above had been used to measure the effects of optic neuritis and demyelinating disorders before their application to glaucoma. With certain interesting exceptions, the defects observed in those disorders are similar to those of glaucoma.

1. Both kinds of disorder tend to increase the latencies of response. In fact, pattern VEP latency has been particularly sensitive in picking up subclinical visual effects of multiple sclerosis (Halliday 1977; Cant et al. 1978; Bodis-Wollner et al. 1979). Increased latency of the pupil light reflex has also been found in optic neuritis patients (Alexandridis et al. 1981).

2. Both kinds of disorder also produce generally similar losses of spatial contrast sensitivity and of flicker sensitivity (Brussel et al. 1982). Psychophysical testing of multiple sclerosis patients has revealed decreased contrast sensitivities not only at high but also at medium and low spatial frequencies (Bodis-Wollner et al. 1979; Regan 1981), as well as decreased temporal performance manifested by reduced CFF (Daley et al. 1979).

3. Finally, both affect color vision. As in OHT and OAG, color discrimination is impaired in optic neuritis and multiple sclerosis (Griffin and Wray 1978; Fallowfield and Krauskopf 1982).

However, some psychophysical methods appear to give contrasting results: (1) optic neuritis typically produces red-green color vision defects, whereas, as noted above, the color vision defects seen in OHT and OAG are in the blue-yellow region; and (2) the "flashing repeat static test" used by Enoch to test for fatigue-like decay of visual sensitivity shows such an effect in optic neuritis and multiple sclerosis patients but not in OHT/OAG patients (Enoch et al. 1980a, b). Rather, patients of the latter group showed changes typifying reduced lateral inhibition (Enoch and Lawrence 1975; Enoch et al. 1980). Thus, these differences between the usual defects of demyelinating disease and glaucoma imply that the latter may involve a significant retinal component, possibly at the receptor cell level, while the former does not. Taking the foregoing exposition all together, it seems reasonable to suppose that the visual alterations found in OHT and early OAG have more than one origin.

Care must be taken that the glaucomatous changes in psychophysical and electrophysiologic measures of vision are not confounded with normal aging effects. Aging changes have been observed in several flicker contrast sensitivity variables (Atkin et al. 1979; Sekuler et al. 1980), as well as in VEP latencies (Celesia & Daly 1977; Sokol et al. 1981) and pupil reflex latencies (Feinberg 1965). Our studies (Atkin et al. 1979) have demonstrated significant age changes in flicker sensitivity, which could not, however, account for the observed flicker contrast-sensitivity deficits in the group of glaucoma patients. The underlying mechanisms of these changes are unknown.

Visual thresholds and response latencies in general tend to rise with aging (McFarland 1963; Corso 1975), and such changes may be accounted for at least in part by an age-associated reduction of mean pupil diameter and increase in optical density of the ocular media (Corso 1975; Weale 1973), both of which lower retinal illumination. Based on static perimetry data on a photopic background, Dannheim and Drance (1971) concluded that there was "a gradual decrease in retinal sensitivity with age".

The great majority of the apparently disparate kinds of visual abnormalities observed in OHT and OAG might also be seen as manifestations of a generalized glaucomatous reduction of visual sensitivity, similar in effect to an overall lowering of luminance (as by a neutral density filter). For a normal eye, as luminance levels and stimulus intensities are reduced: (1) response latencies increase (Feinberg and Podolak 1965; Mansfield 1973; Cant et al. 1978); (2) contrast sensitivities and cut-off frequencies, both spatial and temporal, decline (Babel et al. 1969; Kelly 1971a, b); and (3) color discriminations, particularly blue-yellow, become poorer (Grigorovici and Aricescu-Savopol 1958).

One other result of a generalized reduction of retinal sensitivity would be "shrinkage" of the visual field (VF), defined as decreased area of Goldmann perimetric isopters. Such decreased sensitivity and VF shrinkage occurs not only with age (Drance et al. 1967; Wolf and Nadroski 1971; Chisolm et al. 1980), and with hypoxia (Wolf and Nadroski 1971), but also with ocular hypertension (Hart and Becker 1977; Hart et al. 1978; Chisholm et al. 1980), and with glaucoma (Hart et al. 1978).

Another type of support for a reduced sensitivity hypothesis may be found in color vision studies; color vision may be impaired by miosis (Lakowski and Oliver 1974; Grutzner and Schleicher 1972), which may elicit blue-yellow defects (Grutzner and Schleicher 1972). Furthermore, when the pupils of glaucoma patients are dilated, nearly all their blue-yellow anomalies disappear (Ourqaud et al. 1972). This effect of pupil diameter appears to be attributable to retinal illumination (Grigorovici and Aricessu-Savopol 1958; Ourqaud et al. 1972), as does the improvement of color vision after a glaucoma operation (Koliopoulos 1979).

Thus, with certain apparent exceptions (e.g., selective temporal frequency losses: Tyler 1981), each visual change looked at individually appears to be consistent with a generalized reduction of visual sensitivity that has effects like those of reduced stimulus intensity. But if such a single predominant factor underlies the different types of visual change, then they should be correlated with each other. This has been observed for color vision and VEP abnormalities in OHT and OAG (Towle et al. 1982), and for VEP and flicker CS (Bodis-Wollner et al. 1982), but few other studies have looked at such relationships so far.

The pathophysiology of this hypothesized underlying abnormality also remains unexplained. Evidence pointing to a loss of visual sensitivity casts initial suspicion toward the retinal receptors. This level of the visual system may be involved in hypoxic changes in rod visual thresholds with aging (McFarland 1963). Color vision abnormalities in OHT and OAG, mainly in the blue-yellow region (Francois and Verriest 1968; Foulds et al. 1972, 1974), may indicate dysfunction of the outer retinal layers - probably at the cone receptor level (Foulds et al. 1972, 1974). Recent animal experiments have demonstrated anatomical lesions in both the retinal pigment epithelium and the receptor cell layer of rabbits after acute IOP elevation for 3–4 hours (Melamed et al. 1981). These changes may have resulted from impaired choroidal circulation (Foulds et al. 1972, 1974; Takats & Leiszter 1979).

A central nervous system abnormality may also be considered. A possible locus of effect is the lateral geniculate nucleus. Damage to ganglion cells, the nerve fiber layer, the optic nerve head, and the optic nerve itself do not exhaust the possible kinds of dysfunction that might underlie the visual changes in OHT and in early OAG. Elevated intraocular pressure (or optic nerve hypoxia from other causes) impedes rapid anterograde axoplasmic transport (Hayreh 1978; Gaasterland et al. 1978; Quigley et al. 1979). Since there is evidence that this transport process brings neurotransmitter supplies to the axon terminal (Hayreh 1978), the impaired sensitivity and temporal responsiveness of the visual system in glaucoma, and the associated VEP and pupil response delays, could result from neurotransmitter depletion in axon terminals of the retinal ganglion cells. (VEP delays from synaptic dysfunction have recently been demonstrated in Parkinson's disease and in neuropharmacologically-manipulated rats: Bodis-Wollner and Onofrj 1981).

Finally, the possibility that the hypothalmic-pituitary-adrenocortical (HPA) axis plays a role in the visual changes of OHT and OAG is intriguing. The HPA axis has been implicated in glaucoma (Zondek and Wolfson 1947; Schwartz et al. 1978), and may affect IOP by neural as well as hormonal routes (Podos and Krupin 1977). Plasma levels of glucocorticoid hormone, as well as sensitivity to the hormone's effects, are abnormally high in glaucoma patients (Kass and Sears 1977). Glucocorticoids affect sensory processes both peripherally and centrally, altering sensory receptor thresholds, axonal conduction, and synaptic processes (Henkin 1970). It is possible, therefore, that some of the psychophysical, electrophysiologic and pupillary abnormalities we and others have found in OHT and OAG patients reflect direct retinal and neuronal effects of abnormal hormonal regulation by the HPA axis.

## References


Alexandridis E, Argyropoulos TR, Kratel H (1981) The latent period of the puil light reflex in lesions of the optic nerve. Ophthalmologica 182:211-217

Alvis DL (1966) Electroretinographic changes in controlled chronic open-angle glaucoma. Am J Ophthalmol 61:121-131

Arden GB (1978) The importance of measuring contrast sensitivity in cases of visual disturbance. Br J Ophthalmol 62:198-209

Arden GB, Jacobson JJ (1978) A simple grating test for contrast sensitivity: preliminary results indicate value in screening for glaucoma. Invest Ophthalmol Vis Sci 17:23-32

Atkin A, Bodis-Wollner I, Wolkstein M, Moss A, Podos S (1979) Abnormalities of central contrast sensitivity in glaucoma. Am J Ophthalmol 88:205-211

Atkin A, Herman P, Paz J (1982) Pupil light reflex in ocular hypertension and glaucoma. Invest Ophthalmol Vis Sci ARVO Suppl 22(3):96

Atkin A, Wolkstein M, Bodis-Wollner I, Anders M, Kels B, Podos S (1980) Interocular comparison of contrast sensitivities in glaucoma patients and suspects. Br J Ophthalmol 64: 858-862

Babel J, Rey P, Stangos N, Meyer J-J, Guggenheim P (1969) The functional examination of the macular and perimacular region with the aid of flicker-fusion thresholds. Doc Ophthalmol 26:248-256

Bartl G (1978) Das Elektroretinogram und das evozierte Sehrindenpotential bei normalen und an Glaukom erkrankten Augen. Albrecht Von Graefes Arch Klin Exp Ophthalmol 207: 243-269

Bodis-Wollner I (1981) Differences in low and high spatial frequency vulnerabilities in ocular and cerebral lesions. In: Maffei L (ed) Pathophysiology of the Visual System. The Hague, Junk, pp 195-204

Bodis-Wollner I, Atkin A, Podos S, Wolkstein M, Mylin L, Nitzberg S (1982) VEP latency in ocular hypertension and glaucoma. Invest Ophthalmol Vis Sci ARVO Suppl 22(3):95

Bodis-Wollner I, Bender MB (1973) Neuroophthalmology: electrophysiology and psychophysics of acuity and contrast detection. Prog Neuro Psychiatr 38:93-115

Bodis-Wollner I, Camisa JM (1980) Contrast sensitivity measurement in clinical diagnosis. In: Lessell S, van Dalen JTW (eds) Neuro-Ophthalmology, Excerpta Medica, Princeton, pp 373-401

Bodis-Wollner I, Hendley CD, Mylin LH, Thornton J (1979) Visual evoked potentials and the visuogram in multiple sclerosis. Ann Neurol 5:40-47

Brussel EM, White C, Mustillo P, Overbury O (1982) Multiple sclerosis only indirectly affects spatial contrast sensitivity. Invest Ophthalmol Vis Sci ARVO Supl 22(3):224

Campbell CJ, Rittler MC (1959) Diagnostic value of flicker perimetry in chronic simple glaucoma. Trans Am Acad Ophthalmol Otolaryngol 63:89-97

Cant BR, Hume AL, Shaw NA (1978) Effects of luminance on the pattern visual evoked potential in multiple sclerosis. Electroencephalogr Clin Neurophysiol 45:496-504

Capin JM, Nissim S (1975) Visual evoked responses in the assessment of field defects in glaucoma. Arch Ophthalmol 93:9-18

Celesia GG, Daly RF (1977) Effects of aging on visual evoked responses. Arch Neurol 34: 403-407

Chisholm IA, Stead S, Tan L, Melenchuk JW (1980) Prognostic indicators in ocular hypertension. Can J Ophthalmol 15:4-8

Corso JF (1975) Sensory processes in man during maturity and senescence. In: Ordy JM (ed) Neurobiology of Aging Plenum Press, New York, pp 119-143

Daley ML, Swank RL, Ellison CM (1979) Flicker fusion thresholds in multiple sclerosis. Arch Neurol 36:292-295

Dannheim F, Drance SM (1971) Studies of spatial summation of central retinal areas in normal people of all ages. Can J Ophthalmol 6:311-319

DeLange HD (1958) Research into the dynamic nature of the human fovea-cortex systems with intermittent and modulated light. I. Attenuation characteristics with white and colored light. J Opt Soc Am 48:777-784

Drance SM (1975) Visual defects in glaucoma. In: Symposium on Glaucoma. Transactions

of the New Orleans Academy of Ophthalmology. C.V. Mosby, St. Louis, pp 190–209
Drance SM, Berry V, Hughes A (1967) Studies on the effects of age on the central and peripheral isopters of the visual field in normal subjects. Am J Ophthalmol 63:1667–1672
Drance SM, Lakowski R, Schulzer M, Douglas GR (1981) Use of 100-hue test and Pickford anamoloscope as predictors of glaucomatous field change. Arch Ophthalmol 99:829–831
Enoch JM, Campos EC (1979) Analysis of patients with open-angle glaucoma using perimetric techniques reflecting receptive field-like properties. Doc Ophthalmol Proc Series 19:137–149
Enoch JM, Fitzgerald CR, Campos EC, and Temme LA (1980a) Different functional changes recorded in open-angle glaucoma and anterior ischemic optic neuropathy. Doc Ophthalmologica 50:169–184
Enoch JM, Fitzgerald CR, Campos EC (1980b) Quantitative Layer-by-Layer Perimetry: an extended Analysis. Grune & Stratton, New York
Enoch JM, Lawrence B (1975) A perimetric technique believed to test receptive field properties: sequential evaluation in glaucoma and other conditions. Am J Ophthalmol 80:734–758
Fallowfield L, Krauskopf J (1982) Selective impairment of color perception in patients with demyelinating disease. Invest Ophthalmol Vis Sci ARVO Suppl 22(3):17
Feinberg R, Podolak E (1965) Latency of pupillary reflex to light stimulation and its relationship to aging. In: Welford AT, Birren JE (eds) Behavior, Aging, and the Nervous System. Charles C Thomas, Springfield, Ill pp 326–338
Fiorentini A, Maffei L, Pirchio M, Spinelli D, Porciatti V (1981) The ERG in response alternating gratings in patients with diseases of the peripheral visual pathway. Invest Ophthalmol Vis Sci 21:490–493
Fishman GA, Krill AE, Fishman M (1974) Acquired color defects in patients with open-angle glaucoma and ocular hypertension. Mod Probl Ophthalmol 13:335–338
Foulds WS, Chisholm IA, Reid HCR (1972) The effects of raised intraocular pressure on visual function. In: Cant JS (ed) The Optic Nerve. Kimpton, London, pp 323–330
Foulds WS, Chisholm IA, Bronte-Stewart JM (1974) Effects of raised intraocular pressure on hue discrimination. Mod Probl Ophthalmol 13:328–334
Francois J, Verriest G (1968) Nouvelles observations de deficiences acquises de la discrimination chromatique. Ann Oculist (Paris) 201: 1097–1114
Gaasterland D, Tanishima T, Kuwabara T (1978) Axoplasmic flow during chronic experimental glaucoma. 1. Light and electron microscopic studies of the monkey optic nerve head during development of glaucomatous cupping. Invest Ophthalmol Vis Sci 17:838–846
Galvin RJ, Regan D, Heron JR (1976) Impaired temporal resolution of vision after acute retrobulbar neuritis. Brain 99:256–268
Goldthwaite D, Lakowski R, Drance SM (1976) A study of dark adaptation in ocular hypertensives. Can J Ophthalmol 11:55–60
Griffin JF, Wray SH (1978) Acquired color vision defects in retrobulbar neuritis. Am J Ophthalmol 86:193–201
Grigorovici R, Ariscescu-Savopol I (1958) Luminosity and chromaticity in the mesopic range. J Opt Soc Am 48:891–898
Grutzner P, Schleicher S (1972) Acquired color vision defects in glaucoma patients. Mod Probl Ophthalmol 11:136–140
Halliday AM, McDonald WI, Mushin J (1977) Visual evoked potentials in patients with demyelinating disease. In: Desmedt JE (ed) Visual Evoked Potentials in Man: new Developments Clarendon Press, Oxford, pp 438–449
Harbin TS, Podos SM, Kolker AE, Becker B (1976) Visual field progression in open-angle glaucoma patients presenting with monocular field loss. Trans Am Acad Ophthalmol Otolaryngol 81:OP253–257
Hart WM, Becker B (1977) Visual field changes in ocular hypertension. Arch Ophthalmol 95: 1176–1179
Hart WM, Yablonski M, Kass MA, Becker B (1978) Quantitative visual field and optic disc correlates early in glaucoma. Arch Ophthalmol 96: 2209–2211
Hayreh SS (1978) Fluids in the anterior part of the optic nerve in health and disease. Surv Ophthalmol 23:1–25
Henkin RI (1970) The neuroendocrine control of perception. In: Perception and Its Disorders (Res Publ Assoc Res Nerv Ment Dis, vol XLVIII). Baltimore, Williams & Wilkins, pp 54–107
Hitchings RA, Powell DJ, Arden GB, Carter RM (1981) Contrast sensitivity gratings in glaucoma family screening. Br J Ophthalmol 65:515–517
Huber C, Wagner T (1978) Electrophysiological evidence for glaucomatous lesions in the optic nerve. Ophthalmol Res 10:22–29
Kaback MB, Burde RM, Becker B (1976) Relative afferent pupillary defect in glaucoma. Am J Ophthalmol 81:462–468
Kalmus H, Luke I, Seedburgh D (1974) Impairment of colour vision in patients with ocular hypertension and glaucoma. Br J Ophthalmol 58:922–926
Kass MA, Sears ML (1977) Hormonal regulation of intraocular pressure. Surv Ophthalmol 22: 153–176

Kelly DH (1971a) Theory of flicker and transient responses. I. Uniform fields. J Opt Soc Am 61:537-546
Kelly DH (1971b) Theory of flicker and transient responses. II. Counterphase gratings. J Opt Soc Am 61:632-640
Kohn AN, Moss AP, Podos SM (1979) Relative afferent pupillary defects in glaucoma without characteristic field loss. Arch Ophthalmol 97: 294-296
Koliopoulos JX (1979) Acquired color vision deficiency in open-angle glaucoma. Glaucoma 1(3): 155-161
Kozousek V (1968) L'importance de la frequence critique de fusion subjective pour le pronostic de la destruction du champ visuel. Ann Oculist (Paris) 201:1126-1140
Lakowski R, Bryett J, Drance M (1972) A study of colour vision in ocular hypertensives. Can J Ophthalmol 7:86-95
Lakowski R, Oliver K (1974) Effect of pupil diameter on colour vision test performance. Mod Probl Ophthalmol 13:307-311
Lowenstein O, Schoenberg MJ (1944) Pupillary reactions of the seemingly unaffected eye in clinically unilateral simple glaucoma. Arch Ophthalmol 31:392-398
McFarland RA (1963) Experimental evidence of the relationship between aging and oxygen want: in search of a theory of aging. Ergonomics 6:339-366
Maffei L, Bodis-Wollner I, Harnois C, Bobak P, Podos S (1982) A preliminary study of pattern VEP and ERG in glaucoma and RBN. Invest Ophthalmol Vis Sci ARVO Suppl 22(3):258
Mansfield RJW (1973) Latency functions in human vision. Vision Res 13:2219-2234
Marmion V (1978) The colour vision deficiency in open-angle glaucoma. Mod Probl Ophthalmol 19:305-307
May JG, Ralston JV, Reed JL, Van Dyk HJL (1982) Loss in pattern-elicited electroretinograms in optic nerve dysfunction. Am J Ophthalmol 93:418-422
Melamed S, Ben-Sira I, Ben-Shaul Y (1981) Acutely elevated ocular pressure on rabbit retinal pigment epithelium and photoreceptors. Glaucoma 3(1):59-66
Miles PW (1950) Flicker fusion fields. III. Findings in early glaucoma. Arch Ophthalmol 43:661-677
Onofrj M, Bodis-Wollner I (1982) Dopaminergic deficiency causes delayed visual evoked potentials in rats. Ann Neurol 11:484-490
Ourgaud A, Vola J, Jayle G et al. (1972) A study on the influence of the illumination level and pupillary diameter on chromatic discrimination in glaucomatous patients. Mod Probl Ophthalmol 11:141-144
Owsley C, Sekuler R (1982) Spatial summation, contrast threshold, and aging. Invest Ophthalmol Vis Sci 22:130-133
Podos SM, Krupin T (1977) Central nervous system control of aqueous humor dynamics. Doc Ophthalmol Proc Series 16:177-180
Quigley HA, Guy J, Anderson DR (1979) Blockade of rapid axonal transport: effect of intraocular pressure elevation in primate optic nerve. Arch Ophthalmol 97:525-531
Regan D (1981) Psychophysical tests of vision and hearing in patients with multiple sclerosis. In: Waxman SG, Ritchie JM (eds) Demyelinating Disease: basic and clinical electrophysiology. Adv Neurol 31:217-237
Schwartz B, Golden MA, Wiznia RA, Miller SA (1978) Differences of adrenal stress control mechanisms in glaucoma and normals. Invest Ophthalmol Vis Sci ARVO Suppl p 145
Sekular R, Hutman LP, Owsley CJ (1980) Human aging and spatial vision. Science 209:1255-1256
Singh H, Cooper RL, Alder VA, Crawford GJ, Terrell A, Constable IJ (1981) The Arden grating acuity: effect of age and optical factors in the normal patients, with prediction of the false negative rate in screening for glaucoma. Br J Ophthalmol 65:518-524
Sokol S, Domar A, Moskowitz A (1980a) Utility of the Arden grating test in glaucoma screening: high false-positive rate in normals over 50 years of age. Invest Ophthalmol Vis Sci 19:1529-1533
Sokol S, Domar ADD, Moskowitz A, Schwartz B (1980b) Pattern VEP latency and contrast sensitivity in glaucoma. Invest Ophthalmol Vis Sci ARVO Suppl 19:84
Sokol S, Moskowitz A, Towle VL (1981) Age-related changes in the latency of the visual evoked potential: Influence of check size. Electroencephalogr Clin Neurophysiol 51:559-562
Susanna R, Drance SM, Douglas GR (1978) The visual prognosis of the fellow eye in uniocular chronic open-angle glaucoma. Br J Ophthalmol 62:327-329
Towle VL, Moskowitz A, Sokol S, Schwartz B (1982) Abnormal color vision and visual evoked potentials in ocular hypertension and glaucoma. Invest Ophthalmol Vis Sci ARVO Suppl 11(3):258
Towle VL, Sokol S, Moskowitz A, Schwartz B (1981) The visually evoked potential in glaucoma: effects of check size, field size, and alternation rate. Invest Ophthalmol Vis Sci ARVO Suppl 20(3):22
Tyler CW (1981) Specific deficits of flicker sensitivity in glaucoma and ocular hypertension. Invest Ophthalmol Vis Sci 20:204-212
Weale RA (1963) On the eye. In: Welford AT, Birren JE (eds) Behavior, Aging, and the Ner-

vous System. Chas. Thomas, Springfield, pp 307–325

Wolf E, Nadroski AS (1971) Extent of the visual field: changes with age and with oxygen tension. Arch Ophthalmol 86:637–642

Zondek H, Wolfsohn G (1947) Primary glaucoma and the pituitary-diencephalic system. Am J Ophthalmol 30:596–600

## Discussion

**Schwartz to Atkin:** Dr. V.L. Towle, Dr. A. Moskowitz, Dr. S. Sokol, and I studied the changes in latency of the visually evoked potential in normal, glaucomatous, and ocular hypertensive subjects (Towle et al. 1982). Despite our findings of statistical differences on the basis of population between normal, ocular hypertensive and glaucomatous subjects, on an individual basis we found it very difficult to make exact correlations. For instance, we saw patients with open angle glaucoma and advanced visual field loss who showed normal latencies of their visually evoked potentials, rather than the increased latencies that can be shown on a population basis. In addition, we have made similar observations concerning color vision using the Farnsworth hue test (Towle et al. 1982). In groups of patients we found a good correlation between the latency of the visually evoked potential and the score on the Farnsworth hue test. However, individual patients with advanced glaucoma sometimes showed normal color vision.

1. Towle VL, Moskowitz A, Sokol S, Schwartz B (1982) The visual evoked potential in glaucoma and ocular hypertension: effects of check size, field size, and alternation rate. Invest Ophthalmol Vis Sci (in press)
2. Towle VL, Moskowitz A, Sokol S, Schwartz B (1982) Abnormal color vision and visual evoked potentials in ocular hypertension and glaucoma. Invest Ophthalmol Vis Sci 22:258

Krieglstein G.K./Leydhecker W. (eds)
Glaucoma Update II


# Colour Vision in Glaucoma

S.M. Drance and R. Lakowski, Vancouver

The management of patients with elevated intraocular pressure and no damage has undergone significant changes in the last 20 years. In the 1940's and 1950's the threat of slightly elevated intraocular pressure, was much exaggerated as compared to the evidence gleaned from population studies and follow-up. Elevated intraocular pressure remains an important risk factor in developing damage to the optic nerve but the small elevations in intraocular pressure are not universally treated. This change in philosophy has led to a great interest in the description of the earliest signs of damage of the disease as evidenced by subtle tissue changes at the optic nerve and psychophysical abnormalities. It is realized that in many patients the tissue changes precede the earliest disturbances in the visual field but it is also realized that disturbances in the field can occur prior to recognizable changes in the optic nerve. Attempts to study other psychophysical parameters which might show a disturbance earlier than the differential threshold measured in perimetry have therefore been made and reported.

Contrast sensitivity (1) and receptive field-like functions (2) have been reported to be abnormal in patients with elevated intraocular pressures but without visual field disturbance. In neither of these has a follow-up been reported to show that these disturbances precede nerve fibre bundle defects. A localized increased scatter (3) of the perimetric increment threshold has been shown to precede nerve fibre bundle defects. Colour vision disturbances have been reported to be abnormal in the glaucomas since 1883 and while some authors suggested red-green disturbances, the majority feel that the yellow-blue disturbances are more characteristic. It has been shown, that the degree of colour disturbance correlated with the degree of visual field disturbances, (4, 5 and 6), but while many patients with elevated intraocular pressure and no field defect show colour disturbances there are a number of patients with very advanced visual field defects of glaucoma whose colour vision remains normal.

The present study was carried out to see whether colour vision disturbances could be used to predict the subsequent visual field defects of chronic open angle glaucoma.

## Method

Forty-seven patients with elevated intraocular pressures who had their colour scores examined more than five years before and in whom visual field defects did not develop during that period were studied. Field defects developed in 22 other patients (24 eyes) during the course of the five-year follow-up. One randomly selected eye of each of the 47 patients who were followed up for more than five years and one eye of the 22 patients in whom open angle glaucoma developed were used to calculate the incidence of glaucoma in the group with normal colour discrimination and the group with poor colour discrimination, as measured by the 100-Hue test. Forty-five eyes with elevations of intraocular pressures and 20 of the glaucomatous eyes had anomaloscopic (Pickford Nicholson) assessment at that time and were similarly studied. The $\chi$ test was used to compare the incidence of visual field loss in the various groups of colour disturbance. Cox's method of logistic linear regression of the colour scores on the logarithm of the odds of the development of a field defect was used. All patients had repeated examinations, including visual acuity, IOP, examination of the optic nerve head and detailed visual field studies.

## Results

The scores of the 100-Hue test were arbitrarily divided into the following three groups: 0 to 100, 101 to 200 and greater than 201. Of those patients with 100-Hue test scores of 100 or less, visual field defects developed in only 19% (8/42) during a five-year period, whereas of those patients with scores greater than 200, a field defect developed in 77% (10/13) during the five-year follow-up. These differences were statistically significant ($P < .001$) (Table 1). The frequency distribution of the colour vision scores of the entire group of patients who were glaucoma suspects and who were followed up for more than five years and those patients in whom field defects developed is shown in Fig. 1.

When using Cox's method of logistic linear regression, the logarithm of the odds of visual field defects developing ($\lambda$), utilizing the information from the 100-Hue test, is equal to $-1.19 + 0.005\,(x - 133.53)$, where x represents the individual's score on the test. The slope is significantly different from 0 ($P < .0062$). The probability (P) that visual field defects will develop in a patient can be calculated from the following equation:

$$p^{\lambda} = e^{\lambda}/1 + e^{\lambda}$$

**Table 1.** 100-Hue Scores of patients in whom glaucomatous field defects developed and ocular hypertensive patients[a]

| | 100-Hue score | | | |
|---|---|---|---|---|
| | 0–100 | 101–200 | 201 | total |
| No field defects | 34 | 10 | 3 | 47 |
| Field defects | 8 | 4 | 10 | 22 |
| Total | 42 | 14 | 13 | 69 |

[a] Patients were followed up for five years. Differences in scores were statistically significant ($P < .001$; $x^2 = 15.43$)

### *Anomaloscope*

The incidence of visual field defects was not related to the red-green discrimination on the anomaloscope. The yellow-blue and green-blue scores on the anomaloscope were arbitrarily divided into scores of 0 to 40, 41 to 80, and greater than 81 just noticeable discrimination steps. For the yellow-blue equation, the incidence of subsequent visual field defects in patients with scores of 40 or less was 23%, whereas the incidence in those patients with scores of 80 or more was 80%. For the blue-green equation, the incidence in those patients with scores of 40 or less was 18%, whereas those patients with scores greater than 80 was 55%. These differences were statistically significant with a probability for the yellow-blue scores ($P < .05$) and for the green-blue scores ($P < .025$) (Table 2). The frequency distribution of these scores and the visual field defects subsequently developed are shown in Fig. 2 and Fig. 3.

With the use of Cox's method of logistic linear regression, the logarithm of the odds of a visual field defect developing for the red-green equation was $-1.22 - 0.024\,(x - 9.02)$, where x is the individual's score on this test. This slope is not statistically different from 0 ($P < .47$). For the yellow-blue equation, the logarithm of the odds was $-1.22 + 0.019\,(x - 39.36)$. This slope was significantly different

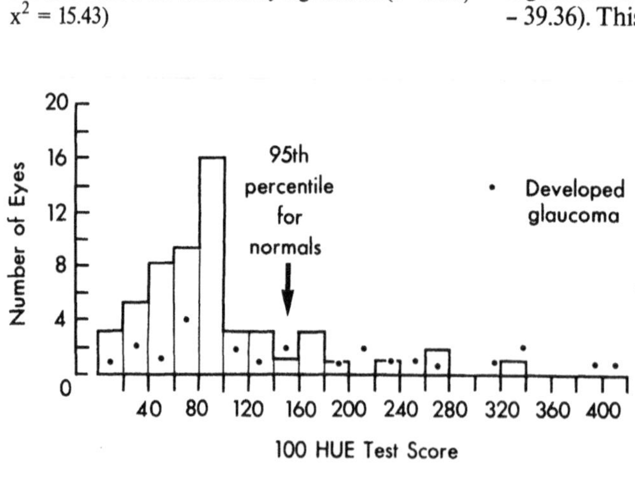


**Fig. 1.** Frequency histogram showing 100-Hue test scores in patients in whom field defects did not develop during five-year follow-up. Scores of patients in whom field defects developed are also shown. *Closed circles* indicate patients in whom glaucoma developed

**Table 2.** Anomaloscopic scores of patients in whom glaucomatous field defects developed[a]

| | Yellow-blue score | | | Blue-green score | | |
|---|---|---|---|---|---|---|
| | 0–40 | 41–80 | 81 | 0–40 | 41–80 | 81 |
| No field defect | 31 | 13 | 1 | 33 | 7 | 5 |
| Field defect developed | 9 | 7 | 4 | 7 | 7 | 6 |
| Total | 40 | 20 | 5 | 40 | 14 | 11 |

[a] Patients were followed up for five years. Differences were statistically significant for yellow-blue scores (P <.0,5; $x^2$ = 7.134) and for blue-green scores (P <.025; $x^2$ = 8.666)

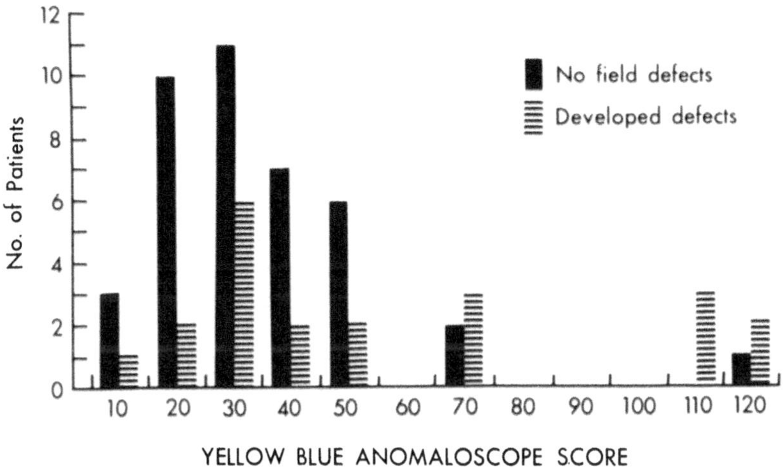


**Fig. 2.** Frequency histogram of yellow-blue scores in must noticeable discrimination steps of patients who showed no field defects during five-year follow-up and patients in whom field defects developed, for comparison

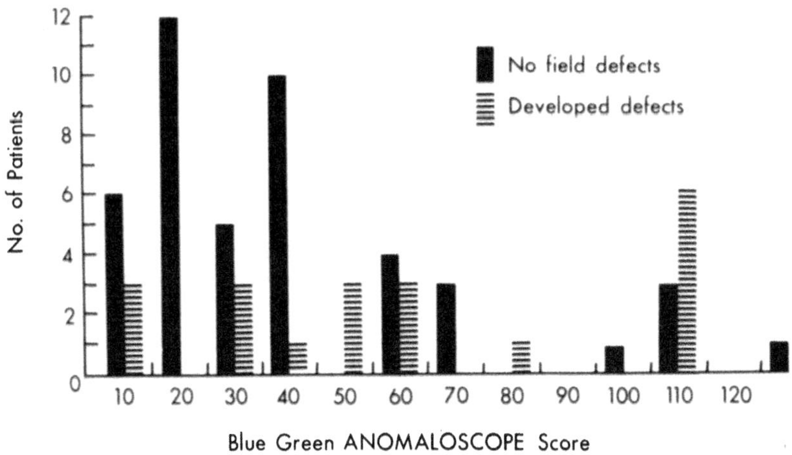


**Fig. 3.** Frequency histogram of blue-green scores in just noticeable discrimination steps of patients who showed no field defects during five-year follow-up and patients in whom field defects developed, for comparison

**Table 3.** Logistic linear regression of logarithm probability against colour vision[a]

| Test | Regression | Significance level of slope[b] |
|---|---|---|
| 100-Hue | $\lambda = -1.19 + 0.005\ (x - 133.53)$ | ≈ .0062 |
| Red-green | $\lambda = -1.22 - 0.024\ (x - 9.02)$ | ≈ .47 |
| Yellow-blue | $\lambda = -1.22 + 0.019\ (x - 39.36)$ | ≈ .0013 |
| Blue-green | $\lambda = -1.22 + 0.013\ (x - 42.38)$ | ≈ .0113 |

[a] Cox's logistic linear regression was used; [b] Coefficient of x

from 0 ($P < .0034$). For the green-blue equation, the logarithm of the odds was -1.22 + 0.013 (x - 42.38), and the slope was significantly different from 0 ($P < .0150$) (Table 3).

## Comment

The present study shows that after a long period of follow-up of patients who were glaucoma suspects and whose visual fields were perfectly normal at the time when their color vision was tested, those patients who had more severe disturbances in colour vision, both by the 100-Hue test and the anomaloscopic assessment, had a significantly higher incidence of subsequent visual field disturbances.

These differences were severe, and by using Cox's method of logistic linear regression, one can actually work out the probability of the development of a visual field defect from the colour vision scores. It would seem that disturbances of colour vision can precede nerve fiber bundle damage, and this may, in fact, denote an earlier change in visual function than the increment threshold, which is measured when the visual field is examined. The implications are important, because these other visual functions might be used in a predictive way before the visual field disturbances. They probably would correlate much better with the early changes at the optic nerve head and might, in fact, denote a stage of disturbance that is reversible with therapy. Although colour vision testing is carried out from the macula, this does not mean a disturbance of the papillomacular bundle of nerve fibers or disturbances of central receptor mechanisms per se, but rather a disturbance of the whole system, which happens to be measured at the fovea. Our laboratory studies suggest that the extra-foveal areas also have disturbed chromatic dark adaptation thresholds.

In patients with advanced glaucoma, whom we had previously described, there were some patients whose colour vision was still normal on the 100-Hue test and on the anomaloscope. However, in the majority of patients, the colour vision was disturbed; thus, if colour vision disturbances always preceded visual field defects, one would have expected the colour vision scores to be abnormal in all of the patients with severe disturbances of the visual field. A number of patients in whom a visual field defect developed during the five years in the present study had normal colour vision tests five years previously. It would be interesting to retest thc colour vision at the time when the visual field disturbance occurred, but this has not been done. In any case, it would seem that severe visual field defects in glaucoma can occasionally occur with normal colour vision, which suggests that there may be at least two mechanisms for developing a nerve fiber bundle defect in glaucoma. This fact should prompt research to explore if there are even more than two mechanisms of damage that might explain some of the conceptual difficulties that we have had in understanding this disease. Our study also suggests that the yellow-blue and blue-green colour-matching functions are disturbed in chronic open angle glaucoma, whereas the red-green colour matching function does not seem to be disturbed at all. In fact, the slope of Cox's logistic linear regression for the red-green equation was the only one that was normal and statistically not significant ($P < .47$).

## References

1. Atkin A, Bodis-Wollner I, Wolkstein M, Moss A, Podos S (1979) Am J Ophthalmol 88:205–211

2. Enoch JM, Campos EC (1978) Analysis of patients with open angle glaucoma using perimetric techniques reflecting receptive field-like properties. Doc Ophthalmol 173:137–149
3. Werner EB, Drance SM (1977) Early visual field disturbances in glaucoma. Arch Ophthalmol 95:1173–1175
4. Lakowski R, Drance SM (1979) Acquired dyschromatopsias: the earliest functional losses in glaucoma. Doc Ophthalmol Proc Ser 19: 159–165
5. Austin DJ (1974) Acquired colour vision defects in patients suffering from chronic simple glaucoma. Trans Ophthalmol Soc UK 94: 808–883
6. Poinoosawmyd Nagasubramanian S, Gloster J (1980) Colour vision in patients with chronic simple glaucoma and ocular hypertension. Br J Ophthalmol 64:852–857
7. Cox DR (1970) Analysis of Binary Data. London, Methuen Co. Ltd, 1970

## Discussion

**Drance**: There is a general excitment in the field of psychophysics in relationship to the glaucomas. It is disappointing to see obvious tissue changes at the optic nerve and yet not to find field defects but it should be remembered that in 15% of cases there are field defects without reliably recognisable disc changes. Even when there are early field defects we can not reliably reverse them although some do get better. We want to find the earliest psychophysical changes for these main reasons:

1. in order to get a better understanding of the pathophysiology of functions in glaucoma
2. to study glaucoma suspects and hopefully find abnormalities of visual function before field defects occur and preferably at a reversible stage
3. to find out in longitudinal studies whether these abnormalities have a predictive value for subsequent field defects.

We have shown that blue green and yellow blue green disturbances take place early in the disease and are related to the stages of the disease showing greater severity with increasing field defects but some patients with severe field defects still have good colour vision. If colour disturbances precede field defects than one would obviously expect all severe field defects to have colour disturbances. We have shown that glaucoma suspects with poor colour vision have a chance of developing field defects more than those with normal scores. This suggests a predictive value. We have also shown that colour vision can greatly improve after surgery for glaucoma although the field remains unchanges. In a series of asymetric discs with elevated IOP we have also shown that anonaloscopy anomalies are more frequent than prolongeol visual evoked response latencies. 100 Hue test anomalies and are almost univerally abnormal. It may also be time that in patients with normal IOP and abnormal colour scores in the absence of other disease one might predict low tension glaucoma but this should be investigated.

**Hart to Drance:** One of the problems that appears to have plagued the use of visual function testing in the study of glaucoma is that most such tests represent spatially averaged functions of the central visual field. Glaucomatous defects in vision are known to have a high degree of spatial specificity. Color vision in particular has been a lure to perimetrists, who have sought to meet visual defects for color perception. Such attempts have thus far been largely unsuccessful.

I recall that you and Dr. Lakowski have reported on anomaloscopic studies of color vision in the mid-periphery of the visual field, and I wonder if you can now tell us more about the nature of extrafoveal color perception on patients with glaucoma.

**Krakau to Drance:** When comparing the sensitivity in detecting functional defects in glaucoma by perimetry and by other methods it is inevitable to define the parameters carefully. The sensitivity may be radically changed by changing the procedure at perimetry. Thus points in areas of relative defects show a decay in sensitivity during a prolonged (30 min.) test session, whereas normal areas keep their sensitivity. It is likewise possible to provoke new defects or increase already detected ones by increasing the period of examination or by changing various parameters (such as shortening the exposure time for the test objects).

Krieglstein G.K./Leydhecker W. (eds)
Glaucoma Update II


# Visual Field Decay in Chronic Glaucoma

C.E.T. Krakau, Lund

In two important respects, computerization has increased the capacity of perimetry. The method has become objective in the sense that the influence exerted by the assistant is eliminated. The results are presented in numerical form, which opens up possibilities for consistent interpretation and statistical evaluation of changes in the visual field (Krakau 1978). Comparisons of actual results with previous examinations or with the outcome in normal or pathological groups require the construction of parameters which summarize the pertinent information. A very simple parameter intended to measure the total performance was used in the study of normals and glaucoma cases during a follow-up (Holmin and Krakau, 1980, 1982). After some properties of the performance value have been described the results of these investigations, supplemented by some further calculations and arguments, will be discussed in the present article.

## Performance Value

Perimetry was performed with an instrument, "Competer", which estimates the sensitivity at a number of points (64) in the central part of the visual field (inside 20 degrees). To obtain a value of performance, sensitivity values are added with equal weight ($P = \Sigma_1^{64}, p_i$). In normal adults, the value of P in the present set-up for routine examinations ranges between 600–700. The test levels are arranged with constant ratio (0.5) between the successive steps. An overall reduction of sensitivity by 50 per cent corresponds to a lowering by 64 units (minus ca. two for the blind spot) of the P value. Repeated determinations of the P value show a random variation which may conceal any slow trend which may prevail in a series of P values.

## Regression Analysis

The performance values describe a time series with a slow trend – linear for practical reasons – on which short term random variations are superimposed. Our aim in follow-up studies is to determine the trend in glaucoma cases and compare it with that found in normal subjects.

A standard procedure convenient for this purpose is to calculate the regression coefficient b considering time as an independent non random and P as a dependent random variable (Fig. 1).

$$b = \Sigma\,(t-\bar{t})\,(P-\bar{P})\,/\,\Sigma\,(t-\bar{t})^2$$

In order to test the significance of b we need the residual variance

$$S_{y}^2.x = \Sigma\,(Y-P)^2\ /\ n-2;\ Y = \bar{P} + b\,(t-\bar{t})$$

to obtain the variance of the regression coefficient b

$$S_{byx}^2 = S_{y.x}^2/\Sigma\,(t-\bar{t})^2$$

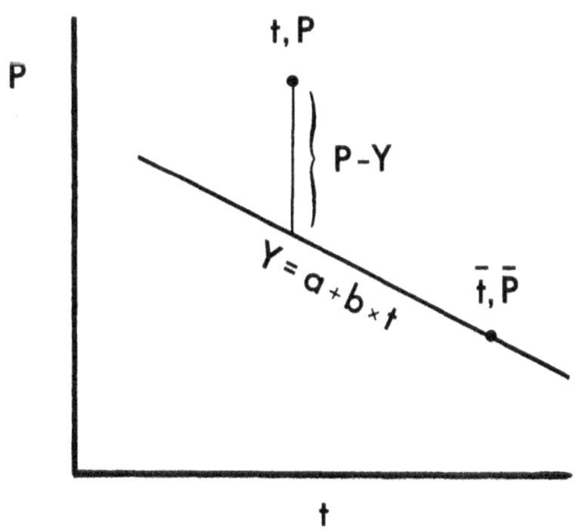


**Fig. 1.** (See text)

The confidence interval of b is found from the t-distribution

$$b \pm t_{2a} \cdot S_{byx};\ v = n\text{-}2 \leqslant 200.$$

## Short Term Variations

Some covariation between the P values of the two eyes has been observed (Holmin and Krakau, 1980), indicating that a general factor might be involved. General alertness is of some importance. So is the condition of the general circulation; e.g. the pulse rate (Holmin and Krakau 1982) is correlated to the P values. Seasonal and diurnal variations of moderate size have been traced in the materials from Dalby and Lund.

The random variation of the threshold sensitivity is higher in areas of relative scotomata than in normal parts of the field (Armaly 1969, Drance 1967). A similar difference also holds for the P values (Holmin and Krakau 1979). The s.d. of the residuals (Sy.x) was 18.0 in a group without defects and 29.6 in the defect group (Holmin and Krakau 1982).

## Detection of a Trend

The hazards in ascribing a trend to a time series containing a random component is shown in the simulation Fig. 2. P values was obtained every third month, and there is a random variation and a seasonal variation superimposed on a slow trend towards decay in a, but without decay in b. There is an obvious risk of mistakes in assessing stability (effect of therapy?) or decay if the estimate is based on few observations. In fact, a statistical trap is set if one suggests improvement by therapy at 2–2′ after a series of falling performance values (Holmin and Krakau 1981) in a series like (a). It can be shown, that the selection of a series of falling values from a random series makes likely an improvement of the subsequent value. A *trend* towards decay *in normal eyes* with age was noted by Goldmann (1945) and by Drance et al. (1967). In the material from a population survey comprising the age group 55 to 71 years the decay corresponded to a decrease in sensitivity of about 50 per cent in 20 years (Holmin and Krakau 1980). The decay in glaucoma cases has to be tested with reference to the normal decay.

## The Trend in Chronic Glaucoma Cases

A preliminary study of chronic glaucoma cases (54 eyes) indicated falling performance values both in well and in less well controlled cases. This material was extended and stricter inclusion criteria were adopted. 90 patients (160 eyes) with a visual field defect in one or

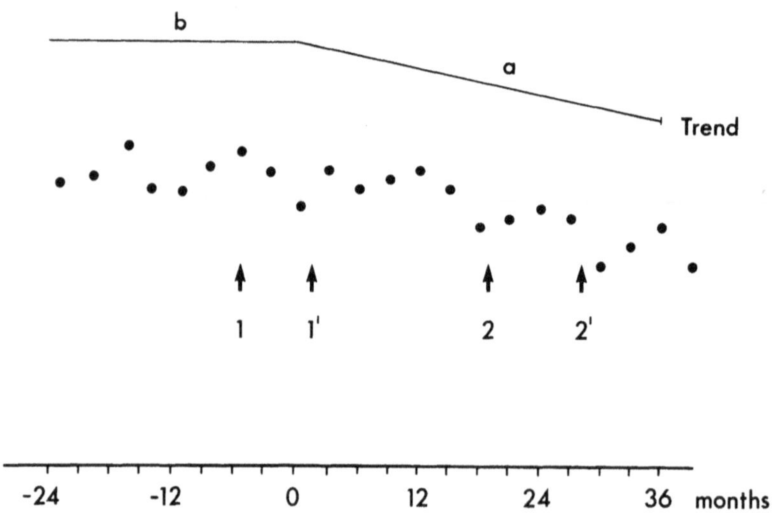


**Fig. 2.** Simulated series of P values without (*b*) and with (*a*) decay superimposed by random and seasonal variations. Short series are deceptive: *1-1* suggests decay, *2-2* stability

both eyes were included. In 27 eyes there were no defects. All patients were acquainted with the perimetry method before being included. Effects of training can therefore be neglected. At least five examinations at intervals of at least two months have been required. The average follow-up period was 18.6 months. The visual acuity of the eyes included was at least 0.3, mostly 0.9–1.0. No decay of acuity due to increasing cataract was included.

The glaucoma patients were treated conventionally, which means that therapy was instituted when necessary for keeping the IOP under control. 120 eyes recieved medical pressure reducing therapy, 9 had been operated. No change of therapy was made during the follow-up period, patients - very few - needing intensified therapy during this period were excluded from the series. In spite of the fact that IOP in this group was considered acceptably controlled, the mean decay was significantly higher (b = -1.9) than that in eyes without defects (b = -0.52) (Fig. 3). Obviously therapy did not stop the progression. No significant decay difference was found between the group with IOP below or equal to 21 mmHg and that with pressure above this value.

Stratification of the material according to age (above and below 69 years of age) and to sex did not reveal any significant difference in decay, nor did the separation of the material according to treatment. It should be noted, however, that the group of pseudoexfoliations (22 eyes) had a relatively high mean value (b = -2.55).

## Further Results and Discussion

The studies of the glaucoma group were continued in collaboration with Dr. C. Holmin. On an average there are now 8 sessions per eye (range 5 to 11). Some preliminary results from an analysis of this extended material are available.

The favourable effect of an increased number of observations on the dispersion of the b values is clearly demonstrated in Fig. 4. In A the b values are calculated from only three observations; in B from at least five (average 5.8) and in C from on an average 8.0 observations. The distributions derive their width partly from the dispersion of the regression coefficient $s_{byx}$ (cf def) which is substantially reduced with an increasing number of examinations. Part of the width is attributed to the proper distribution of the 'b' values.

The mean decay in the defect group was -1.62, which is slightly less than that found in the previous analysis. This is probably mainly due to the fact that several cases with extreme decay took more ordinary values in the latest analysis.

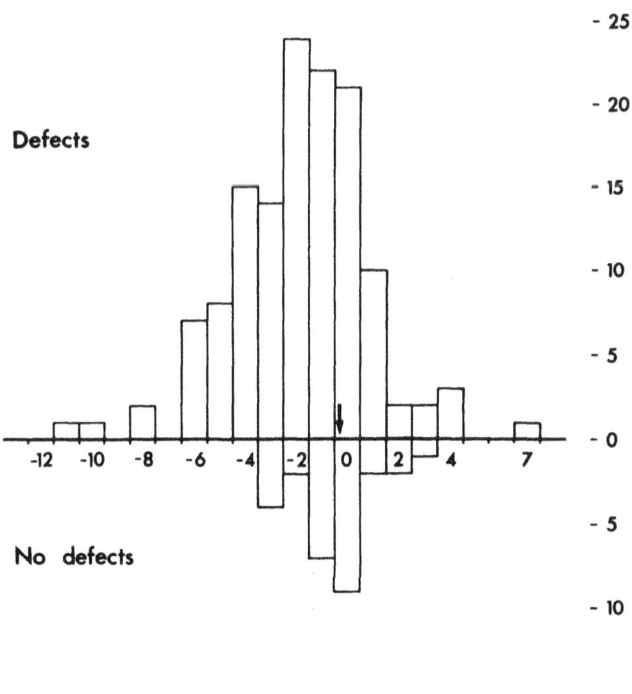


**Fig. 3.** The frequency distributions of 'b' for 133 eyes with a v.f.d. and for 27 normal fields. The *arrow* indicates the normal decay with age

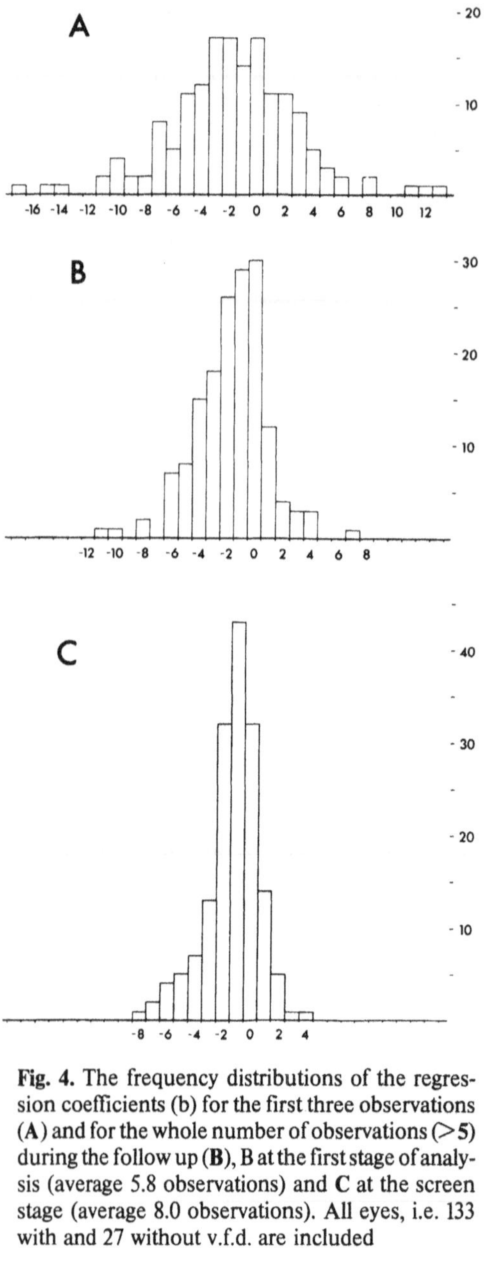


**Fig. 4.** The frequency distributions of the regression coefficients (b) for the first three observations (**A**) and for the whole number of observations (>5) during the follow up (**B**), B at the first stage of analysis (average 5.8 observations) and **C** at the screen stage (average 8.0 observations). All eyes, i.e. 133 with and 27 without v.f.d. are included

The frequency distributions of Figs. 3 and 4 can be regarded as the convolution integral of the proper distribution and the distribution due to the dispersion of the regression coefficient. For the dispersion of the latter, we accept the mean of $s_{byx}$. The proper distribution can in fact be calculated, since the two others are known. If we accept the approximation that all the distributions involved are normal, this task is highly simplified. Denoting the s.d. of the proper distribution $s_p$ and that of the observed distribution (Fig. 4) s, we have $s^2 = s_{byx}^2 + s_p^2$.

$s_{byx}$ was found to be 1.05 and s = 1.9, which gives $s_p = 1.6$.

The mean decay for the group with defects is -1.62, which is of the same magnitude as the s.d. for the frequency distribution proper. There is obviously a number of eyes whose regression coefficient lies near zero. The glaucoma group, in other words, includes cases which for a long period (about 2 years in this material) do not show an abnormal progression of field defects.

Stratification of the defect eyes with reference to various treatments revealed tendencies like those discerned in the previous analysis, only the trends were even more obvious. The decay in the groups with composite therapy was highest, in those with simple therapy (pilocarpine or timolol) it was lower, whereas the untreated group had the lowest decay values (Table 1). This trend may mirror the use of more effective pressure-reducing therapy in the more severe cases but the possible causal relation between therapy and decay is obscure.

Calculation of the regression coefficient for IOP versus b gave the value -0.12 which is not significant. This is in agreement with the lack of significant difference in decay between the low and high pressure groups mentioned above. Admittedly, the pressure distribution, which has the range 10–33 mmHg but covers 77 per cent of all eyes concentrated within 18–25 mmHg, is not ideal for a study of the correlation between IOP and decay. Supplementary cases are necessary in order to establish this relationship. Those with low pressures are likely to be available in due time, but cases in the higher range will probably remain exceptional.

Another argument in the discussion of this correlation is of a technical character. The maximal light output of the test lights puts a limit to lowest testable threshold sensitivity. The values for points with very low sensitivity is therefore truncated. There is no room for decay, and dispersions of P values might be reduced for eyes with large and deep defects. In fact, ten eyes had mean performance values below 200 and no doubt the low decay in this group (-0.57) can largely be attributed to truncation. Advanced glaucoma

**Table 1.** (See text)

| | n | Decay | SEM | $\overline{IOP}$ | $\overline{P}$ |
|---|---|---|---|---|---|
| Pilocarpin | 31 | -1.31 | 0.33 | 21.3 | 440 |
| Timolol | 23 | -1.32 | 0.42 | 20.5 | 443 |
| Miotics - tim | 24 | -2.18 | 0.36 | 23.4 | 435 |
| Miotics - Diamox | 12 | -2.0 | 0.60 | 19.8 | 323 |
| Miotics - adr | 7 | -2.1 | 0.72 | 20.4 | 509 |
| OP | 9 | -1.7 | 0.83 | 17.2 | 284 |
| O ter | 21 | -1.0 | 0.44 | 19.4 | 491 |
| O def | 23 | -0.33 | 0.25 | 22.6 | 614 |

cases with low P values and high IOP could in this way be prevented from fully contributing to a correlation high IOP with high decay. However, the IOP was not high in this group, on the contrary the mean IOP was 17.6 mmHg in this group with extensive defects (and 20–21 mmHg in all groups with performance values above 200). The low correlation IOP-decay is not likely to be an effect of truncation.

An *immediate* connection between IOP and performance should be discernible in a correlation between these parameters, calculated for each individual eye from the value pairs obtained at each examination. The effect of decay by using the residual performance values is allowed for, as is the variation caused by different hours of the day. The partial correlation coefficients calculated for all eyes separately showed a predominance of positive values in the frequency distribution (i.e. better performance connected with higher IOP and v.v.). This rather remarkable finding is not likely to be an effect by mere chance. The mean of the frequency distribution is significantly ($p < 0.01$) greater than zero. When grouped according to mean IOP correlation mean values with positive sign predominated in the lower range of IOP, whereas negative means were found in the higher range (Fig. 5).

In a study on the effect of timolol and placebo on the performance in short-term experiments on eyes with a mean IOP below 27 mmHg, there was on an average a slight reduction of performance associated with a lowered IOP (Holmin and Krakau 1982). Though insignificant statistically, the results are in agreement with the present observation.

Any inference from the relation between *instant* IOP-performance and the *long term* relation mean IOP-performance decay is still hypothetical. It is possible that an optimal IOP might exist where the decay is minimal. This gives rise to questions like the following: Are there eyes with glaucomatous defects and relatively low pressure, which are better off without or with a less efficient pressure reduction? Would it be possible, by establishing the

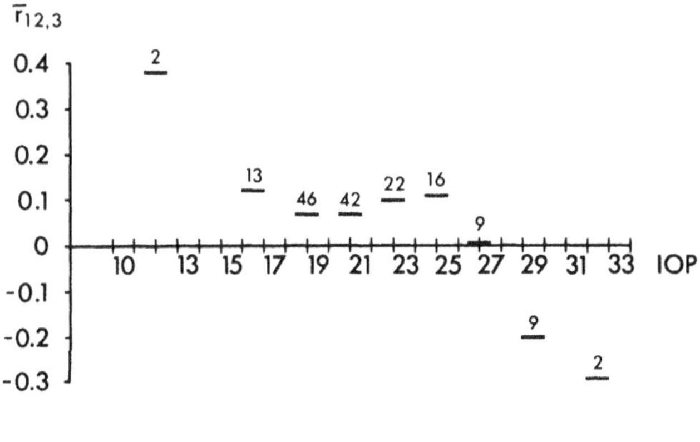


**Fig. 5.** Mean of partial correlation coefficients *IOP* – Performance versus mean *IOP*

correlation between performance and IOP to spot these cases (and also those which improve at reduced pressure)?

The question remains whether a more efficient pressure reducing therapy could have prevented the visual field decay. Supplementary cases with a low IOP are required in order to calculate the correlation between IOP and decay. As to the short term variations a more extensive material may elucidate the problem if they contain information bearing on decay or if they are only random noise, signifying nothing.

**Abstract.** A procedure for trend analysis of a series of visual field examinations, obtained by computerized perimetry, is described. The need for several consecutive examinations to establish a significant progression of field defects in the individual case is stressed. The method was applied to a group of 90 chronic glaucoma cases (160 eyes, 133 with defects). On an average, the group showed a decay corresponding to a reduction of sensitivity by 50 per cent over a period of about three years.

**Acknowledgment.** Fig. 3 and 4 from (Holmin and Krakau 1982) are reproduced with kind permission from Acta Ophthalmol (Copenh).

## References

1. Armaly MF (1969) The visual field defect and ocular pressure level in open angle glaucoma. Invest Ophthalmol 8:105–124
2. Drance SM, Berry V, Hughes A (1967) The effects of age on the central isopter of the normal visual field. Can J Ophthalmol 2:79
3. Goldmann H (1945) Grundlagen exakter Perimetrie. Ophthalmologica 109:57
4. Holmin C, Krakau CET (1979) Variability of glaucomatous visual field defects in computerized perimetry. Albrecht Von Graefes Arch Klin Ophthalmol 210:235–250
5. Holmin C, Krakau CET (1980) Visual field decay in normal subjects and in cases of chronic glaucoma. Albrecht Von Graefes Arch Klin Ophthalmol 213:291–298
6. Holmin C, Krakau CET (1981) Automatic perimetry in the control of glaucoma. Glaucoma 3:154–159
7. Holmin C, Krakau CET (1982) Regression analysis of the central visual field in chronic glaucoma cases. Acta Ophthalmol (Copenh) 60:264–267
8. Holmin C, Krakau CET (1982) Short term effects of timolol in chronic glaucoma. Acta Ophthalmol (Copenh) 60:337–346
9. Krakau CET (1978) Aspects on the design of an automatic perimeter. Acta Ophthalmol (Copenh) 56:389–405
10. Scientific Tables (1962) Documenta Geigy, sixth edn Konrad Diem JR Geigy S A. Basle
11. Werner EB, Drance SM (1977) Early visual field disturbances in glaucoma. Arch Ophthalmol 95:1173–1175

## Discussion

**Greve to Krakau:** The P-value of the competer is the sum of all the threshold of values. Thus it is a value that represents both general and local reduction of sensitivity. As these two reductions may be caused by different disease processes it may be necessary to separate them.

**Kitazawa to Krakau:** When we try to correlate IOP level and the progress of field defects, I think the time factor should be given a due consideration. In this connection I like to draw your attention to the recent study by Dr. Kosaki, Japan in that his group demonstrated that the change of field loss expressed in terms of a decrease in the area of isoptors correlated significantly with the product of time and IOP level but did not with the IOP level in chronic primary glaucomas.

**Spaeth to Krakau:** I would like to make a comment on methodology. It is important for all of us to recall that lack of demonstration of significance is a finding of limited value. For example, that Professor Krakau was not able to demonstrate a significant difference between the decay curves in the eyes that he has described does not mean that there was not a difference between the two groups. It may be that the measurements were not sufficiently accurate to notice a change, that the numbers were too few to make the calculation significant, etc. Similarly, the fact that Dr. Hetherington was unable to confirm the value of examining patients for nerve fiber bundle defects in the experimental settings he employed should not be taken to mean that nerve fiber bundle defects are not valuable signs of glaucoma. If Dr. Quigley is able to demonstrate this in a positive way this is a far more valuable indicator of reality than a negative investigation which may merely have missed the condition being sought.

Krieglstein G.K./Leydhecker W. (eds)
Glaucoma Update II


# The Value of the Retinal Nerve Fiber Layer Examination in the Diagnosis of Glaucoma

H.A. Quigley, Baltimore

**Abstract.** A major problem in glaucoma management is the lack of reliable, objective, and early indicators of the presence of optic nerve damage. The striated nerve fiber layer pattern demonstrates defects that precede detection of visual field damage in some eyes. The examination is objective, requires no patient response, is within the capacity of any physician to learn, and requires only standard clinical instruments. The definitive demonstration of its predictive value is now being tested in a large prospective trial. The method is not applicable to some lightly pigmented eyes.

## Introduction

Prospective studies following large numbers of eyes with elevated intraocular pressure suggest that only a small percent of such eyes will develop detectable field defects without therapy during several years of follow-up (Graham, 1968; Armaly, 1969; Perkins, 1973; Wilensky and Podos, 1975; to name a few). This intriguing finding has changed the approach to the initiation of glaucoma therapy. As in the past, patients judged to have optic nerve damage or those felt to have an unacceptable risk of damage still undergo attempted pressure lowering. But, in those judged not to have definitive evidence of damage, therapy is frequently not offered. The assumptions are that some or all of these eyes are not suffering damage below the level of detection despite abnormal pressure, or that if damage is occurring, it is slight, will be detected prior to serious functional loss, and pressure lowering at that time will halt further damage. The obvious advantage of avoiding the side-effects of medical therapy as long as possible are weighed against the physician's judgment of the risk of irreversible vision loss.

In most of the studies of glaucoma damage, the visual field test is usually utilized as the standard denoting the presence or absence of definitive optic nerve damage. Most glaucomatologists are aware, however, that physically visible changes in the optic disc often precede field loss, and that recently a number of other measures of visual function have been noted to be abnormal prior to the detection of field loss in some patients (afferent pupil defects, Kohn, 1979; Farnsworth-Munsell 100 Hue tests, Drance, 1981). I have been able to confirm that the early changes in optic disc cup size are due to loss of nerve fibers, and that significant losses of optic nerve axons can precede detectable visual field loss in actual counts of fibers performed histologically (Quigley, 1981, 1982a). Hence, it is becoming more obvious that "field loss" is not a firm boundary between those with glaucoma and those who do not have it, but rather a stage of damage that begins at some earlier time. As field testing improves and new psychophysical tests are devised, the definition of damage will hopefully move back closer to the start of the nerve fiber loss process. It is in the hope that the examination of the retinal nerve fiber layer will be a means of detecting damaged eyes earlier in the process that the studies to be described have been undertaken.

## Initial Nerve Fiber Layer Observations

The observation of nerve fiber bundles in the retina coursing toward the optic disc was probably first made in the last century. It was also noted during the same period that the use of a green light enhanced the ophthalmoscopic view of these striations. Hoyt (1973) pointed our attention to defects in the normal nerve fiber layer pattern in glaucoma patients. These defects were either localized or diffuse abnormalities. The local defects were dark zones, some narrower than retinal arterioles, found emanating from the optic disc in an arching shape over or under the macular area.

Diffuse nerve fiber layer atrophy was detected as a loss of the normal striated pattern over a broader zone and appeared in more damaged eyes. Several variations from the normal appearance were designated pseudodefects that needed to be distinguished from truly pathological atrophy of the nerve fiber layer. He and his co-workers noted that abnormalities in the nerve fiber layer appeared in some eyes prior to field defects on the Goldmann perimeter, and even prior to the recognition of abnormal disc cup size or shape in some eyes. Of course, it was recognized that such defects were not specific for glaucoma, since any disorder causing loss of ganglion cell axonal fibers might give rise to nerve fiber layer defects. However, by taking into account the known topographic anatomy of retinal ganglion cell fibers, it was possible to distinguish eyes with foveal fiber loss from eyes with hemianopia by nerve fiber layer exam alone.

**Presently Established Data**

Sommer (1977) carefully examined photographs taken during the Collaborative Glaucoma Study at the Wilmer Institute for the state of the nerve fiber layer. While these were color photographs centered on the optic disc (and therefore often less than optimally demonstrative of nerve fiber layer findings), a striking result was obtained by comparing the photographs with the patient histories and visual fields. Photos were read, of course, without knowledge of the clinical findings. Of 14 eyes with available photographs that developed visual field defects while being followed without therapy, all had been detected to have abnormal nerve fiber layer patterns in photographs taken prior to the field defect detection. In some eyes, abnormal fiber layers were seen as long as 5 years preceding field loss. This raised the possibility that nerve damage could potentially be detected earlier and patients be selected for therapy better.

There were still a number of questions left by Sommer's study. There were some false positive readings on the normals included as controls, and in quite a number of photographs the nerve fiber layer was not visible enough to evaluate. Furthermore, the disc and cup were not covered in the reading sessions, leaving open the possibility that the cup appearance unconsciously influenced the nerve fiber layer reading. In fact, it was not known whether the information obtainable from the nerve fiber layer was simply duplicating what could just as easily be learned from the standard disc exam.

In part, these questions have been addressed by further study. First, Sommer (1979a, b) compared the nerve fiber layer's sensitivity and specificity with that of the disc exam in the eyes of the previous study. More of the eyes had abnormal nerve fiber layer exam than abnormal discs by several standard criteria prior to field loss. But the remaining questions were at least partially addressed in a separate study (Quigley, 1980). While the latter did not have the advantage of using eyes with long follow-up that had developed field defects under observation, it combined much larger numbers of eyes (335) examined, optimal nerve fiber layer photography (Miller, 1978), masked discs during fiber layer readings, and further estimates of specificity, particularly as compared to disc cup exam. The findings of this study encouraged us to pursue the nerve fiber layer exam for several reasons.

First, we were able to see the striated pattern (or abnormalities) in almost 90% of eyes examined in a glaucoma referral office. While this does not correspond to an unselected population, it does have relevance for the population about whom we most need this information. Older patients and those with lightly pigmented fundi were more difficult to detect. This occurs because a dark background helps to bring out the inner retinal reflexes from the nerve fiber bundles. Melanin pigment absorbs the green illuminating light well and helps to provide such a dark backdrop. Note that this study was conducted on photographs, however; in some eyes the nerve fiber bundles are visible with the direct ophthalmoscope or the slit lamp (and green light) even though the pupil is small, but photography is impossible or unsatisfactory. Naturally, no test or examination will be possible on all persons. Not everyone can respond adequately for perimetry or a 100-Hue test. Enough patients can have their nerve fiber layers seen to be of value based on this study.

Second, the degree of field loss and the degree of nerve fiber layer abnormality were highly associated. In those with established field defects, 84% had nerve fiber defects. The 16% false negatives all had small paracentral defects. This figure compares quite well with the sensitivity of disc exams in detecting eyes with field loss (Drance, 1976), and the disc could *not be seen* by the examiner of the photos in this study. There were clearly cases in which the disc exam did not indicate an abnormal appearance but the nerve fiber layer did - illustrating that it can be an *added* help.

Third, the false positive rate appears acceptably low at 3%. Defects had to be distinguished from pseudo-defects as pointed out by Hoyt. True abnormal local defects most frequently are seen as narrow dark arcs heading for the disc and extending to within one disc diameter of the disc margin. More than a disc diameter out, the nerve fiber layer thins out and alternating light and dark zones are not uncommon in normal eyes. However, these do not come as near to the disc as delineated above.

Most interesting to us was the fact that 13% of eyes with elevated intraocular pressure but normal field testing in both eyes had nerve fiber layer defects. These were predominately local defects, the type we associate with earlier damage. In patients with field loss in one eye, the fellow eyes with normal field had more nerve fiber layer defects, 28% of this group. Since the fellow eyes of unilateral field loss patients have a greater chance of developing field loss themselves, this seems to provide further evidence that the greater the estimated damage (the closer to field loss) the more likely nerve fiber layer deficits were.

We have also conducted laboratory investigations of nerve fiber bundle atrophy in primates (Quigley, 1982b). While previous studies had demonstrated that the dark zones without striations did correspond to nerve fiber bundle loss (Radius, 1979), it had not been determined what percent of the thickness of the bundles needed to atrophy before it was clinically detectable. When fiber layer atrophy was produced in macaque monkeys by orbital optic nerve trauma, local and diffuse defects could be photographed and compared with the histological thickness of nerve fiber layer loss and the approximate number of nerve fibers damaged. The clinical detection of nerve fiber bundle thinning varied depending upon the thickness of the nerve fiber layer. In general, when 50% of the thickness of axons in an area had been lost, it could be seen by clinical exam and photography. In the zone temporal to the disc, where the nerve fiber layer is thinner, as little as 20 microns of thickness lost was detectable (50% of the normal 40 microns). In the thicker fiber layer of the superior and inferior poles of the disc, the 50% loss required for detection amounted to more absolute neural atrophy. Yet, highly localized defects comprised of relatively small percentages of the overall nerve fiber complement were visible. Therefore, the more closely grouped together are the fibers lost, the more likely their loss will be detectable.

## Conclusion

From the presently available data, it can be stated that the examination of the nerve fiber layer is of value in detecting nerve damage in some glaucoma patients. Its strong points are its simplicity, its objectivity, and the fact that one is looking for and detecting the nerve fiber loss itself, rather than some more indirect measure of damage. Whether this form of examination will prove to be highly predictive of early progressive damage in a significant number of glaucoma suspects awaits appropriate controlled observations underway at present at our Institute.

## References


Armaly MF (1969) Ocular pressure and visual fields: a ten year follow-up study. Arch Ophthalmol 81:25–40

Drance SM (1976) Correlation between optic disc changes and visual field defects in chronic open-angle glaucoma. Trans Am Acad Ophthalmol Otolaryngol 81:224–225

Drance SM, Lakowski R, Schulzer M, Douglas GR (1981) Acquired color vision changes in glaucoma. Use of 100-Hue test and Pickford anomaloscope as predictors of glaucomatous field change. Arch Ophthalmol 99:829–831

Graham PA (1968) The definition of pre-glaucoma, a prospective study. Trans Ophthalmol Soc UK 8:153–165

Hoyt WF, Frisen L, Newman NM (1973) Fundoscopy of nerve fiber layer defects in glaucoma. Invest Ophthalmol 12:814–829

Kohn AN, Moss AP, Podos SM (1979) Relative afferent pupillary defects in glaucoma without characteristic field loss. Arch Ophthalmol 97:294–296

Miller NR, George T (1978) Monochromatic (red-free) photography and ophthalmoscopy of the peripapillary retinal nerve fiber layer. Invest Ophthalmol Vis Sci 17:1121–1124
Perkins ES (1973) The Bedford glaucoma survey. I. Long-term follow-up of borderline cases. Br J Ophthalmol 57:179–185
Quigley HA, Miller NR, George T (1980) Clinical evaluation of nerve fiber layer atrophy as an indicator of glaucomatous optic nerve damage. Arch Ophthalmol 98:1564–1571
Quigley HA, Addicks EM, Green WR, et al. (1981) Optic nerve damage in human glaucoma. II. The site of injury and susceptibility to damage. Arch Ophthalmol 98:635–649
Quigley HA, Addicks EM, Green WR (1982a) Optic nerve damage in human glaucoma. III. Quantitative correlation of nerve fiber loss and visual field defect in glaucoma, ischemic neuropathy, papilledema, and toxic neuropathy. Arch Ophthalmol 100:135–146
Quigley HA, Addicks EM (1982b) Quantitative studies of retinal nerve fiber layer defects. Arch Ophthalmol 100:807–814
Radius RL, Anderson DR (1979) The histology of retinal nerve fiber layer bundles and bundle defects. Arch Ophthalmol 97:948–950
Sommer A, Miller NR, Pollack I, Maumenee AE, George T (1977) The nerve fiber layer in the diagnosis of glaucoma. Arch Ophthalmol 95:2149–2156
Sommer A, Pollack I, Maumenee AE (1979a, b) Optic disc parameters and onset of glaucomatous field loss. I. Methods and progressive changes in disc morphology; and II. Static screening criteria. Arch Ophthalmol 97:1444–1454
Wilensky JT, Podos SM (1975) Prognostic parameters in primary open angle glaucoma. In: Anderson DR, Drance SM, Galin MA, et al. (eds) Symposium on Glaucoma. CV Mosby Co, St. Louis, pp 7–30

## Discussion

**Kitazawa to Quigley:** The ease of detecting changes of retinal nerve fiber bundle defects is determined by a variety of factors including pupillary diameter, clarity of media and thickness of nerve fiber layer. Above all the retina is thinner in the myopes and the detection of nerve fiber changes is often very difficult in many of them at least by means of routine fundus photography or ophthalmoscopy. This seems to be of particular importance in the myopes who are less resistant to an elevated IOP and tend to develop field defects.

Keeping these in mind and in view of high detection rate of nerve fiber defects in your group I am interested to know how many myopes are in your groups.

**Spaeth to Quigley:** I would like to ask Dr. Quigley how he instructs his residents in examining patients so that they can detect nerve fiber layer defects.

Krieglstein G.K./Leydhecker W. (eds)
Glaucoma Update II


# The Earliest Finding of Primary Open-Angle Glaucoma (POAG) and the Mode of Progression

K. Iwata, Niigata-city

It is generally accepted that in early POAG the visual field shows spot-like deep scotomata or arcuate scotoma (Aulhorn, Bengtsson 1979) and disc cup becomes larger. In the earliest stage, usually any abnormal findings can not be recognized by routine examination. It is impossible, therefore, to distinguish the earliest POAG from ocular hypertension. The earliest diagnosis should be established by the earliest identification of optic nerve damage.

As Hoyt demonstrated (Hoyt et al. 1973), early attrition of nerve fiber layer (NFL) can be observed in the peripapillary retina. Sommer et al. (1977) reported that consistent abnormalities of NFL begins as early as five years before they developed glaucomatous field defect by Goldmann perimetry. Quigley et al. (1980) emphasized the NFL examination is as sensitive in detecting eyes with field loss as the optic disc configuration. On the other hand Pederson and Anderson (1980) reported that by their retrospective study of ocular hypertension, generalized expansion of disc cup was the first change, preceding field loss by several years. I attempted hereupon to reveal the first appearing finding and the mode of progression of POAG.

## Demonstration of Example

This is 36 year old patient with Behçet's disease, whose fundus shows optic disc vasculitis and the corresponding localized various

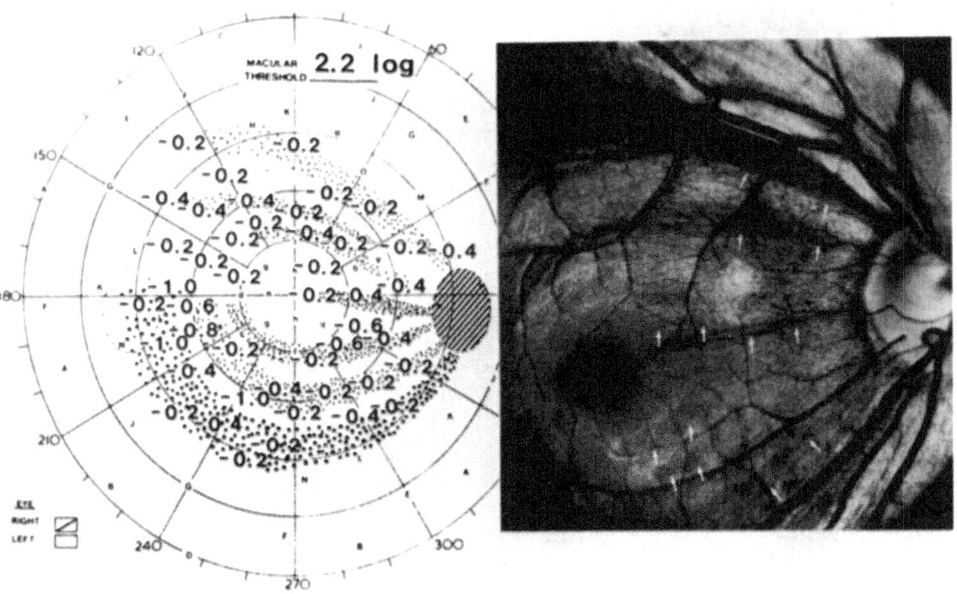


**Fig. 1.** Various grades of NFL abnormalities and their corresponding visual sensitivity reduction measured by Friedmann visual field analysed Mark II. in Behcet's disease

NFL defects from deep wedge-shaped defect to fine slit defect and fine thinning. Goldmann perimeter could demonstrate only the corresponding arcuate scotoma of the dark wedge-shaped NFL defect, and the other slight NFL abnormalities could not be detected. Goldmann perimetry, therefore, is not suitable for the early detection of slight NFL damage. Friedmann visual field analyser Mark II (FVFMII) could detect the corresponding sensitivity reduction not only as small scotomata but also as reduced area (Fig. 1). Figure 1 is showing the reduced sensitivity area overlapped with the NFL defects. It is noticeable that the finest NFL thinning area induces only 0.2log.u. reduction, which level is generally scarcely accepted as abnormal. Only when 0.2–0.4log.u. reduction is areal, then the reduction can be estimated as significant pathological (Iwata et al. 1981). Disc cup expansion corresponding fine NFL thinning could not be detected, except for thick wedge defect. These results indicate that NFL thinning precedes by far cup expansion and visual field abnormality measured by Goldmann perimeter.

**Posner-Schlossman' Syndrome as POAG Model**

Posner-Schlossman's syndrome repeats the crisis of IOP elevation to 45 mmHg or more of 3–10 days duration, and during its long course often develops glaucomatous nerve damage. The IOP level during the crisis resembles POAG but a little high. From the retrospective analysis of such 5 cases the mode of progression of NF damage, disc cupping, field defect and the correlation among them were disclosed (Iwata et al. 1982). Figure 2 shows the results. The earliest appearing sign is a slit-like NFL defect and the corresponding sensitivity reduction is smaller than 0.4log.u.. Cup expansion and Goldmann isopter depression in this stage are not recognized. With progression of the nerve damage the number and the width of NFL defect increase and finally grow wedge-shaped dark defect, which induce localized rim notch in optic disc and sure depression of Goldmann isopter. Besides the wedge defect diffuse general-thinning of NFL is combined around optic disc and forms generalized expansion of optic cup.

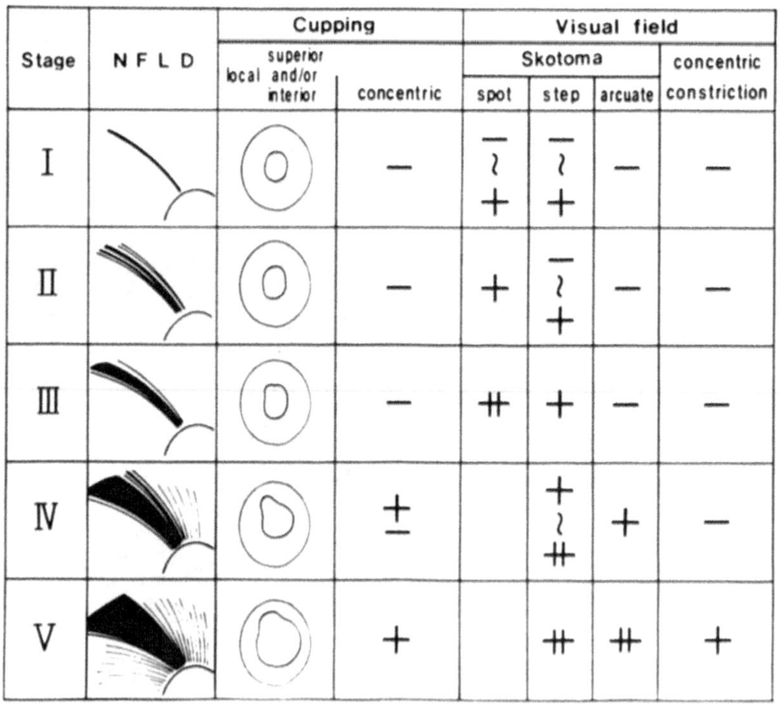


**Fig. 2.** The mode of progression of damage in optic nerve and visual field in earliest to early stage in Posner-Schlossman's syndrome

**Pair Eyes with Asymmetrical Early POAG**

In early stage of POAG the IOP usually relatively low and fluctuate between 20–30 mmHg, often under 27 mmHg. Therefore, the mode of appearance of NFL attrition may be much milder than Posner-Schlossman's syndrome, and it is very interresting to clarify whether the first appearing sign is the slit-like NFL defect or not. The natural history of early POAG may be reproduced by arranging the obtained findings from the slightest to the advanced, and by comparing a little advanced eye to scarcely advanced eye between pair eyes in early stage. I attempted to arrange the findings of 10 cases with asymmetrical early POAG. Figure 3 shows one of such cases. The IOP fluctuated between 20–30 mmHg in both eyes. The left eye shows a little advanced finding than the right eye, and the optic cup elongates to inferior pole, from which extends wege-shaped NFL defect. A slight round extension of the cup to superior pole is observed and the corresponding NFL thinning is recognized (arrows) by precise stereophotography. This thinning is so slight that it is easily overlooked without stereophotography. This thinning looks like raugh combed hair. The corresponding reduction of visual sensitivity is 0.4–0.6log.u. by FVFMII. The right eye shows no abnormal cupping and no local notch. However, under sharp focus on NFL in upper Bjerrum area, a slight but sure NFL thinning is exposed. The appearance looks like partially raugh combed hair (RCH) and partially fine combed hair (FCH). These thinnings do not cause any cup expansion. The corresponding reduction of visual sensitivity is 0.6log.u. for RCH, 0.4–0.2log.u. for FCH respectively. It should be noticed that the inferior Bjerrum area of the right eye FCH is also recognized, however, the corresponding visual field showed only two points reduction of 0.4 and 0.2log.u., and they developed within half a year into areal reduction. This is an evidence to indicate that FCH thinning begins at least a half-year before it develops minimum glaucomatous field abnormality by FVFMII. Goldmann perimetry could not detect any abnormality on the right eye. The findings of this case and other 9 cases are summarized as follows.

1. Where there is cup expansion, there is always NFL abnormality, which is recognized only by precise stereophotography.

2. Even on the occasion of no cup expansion, slight abnormality of NFL in Bjerrum area exists in the earliest stage.

3. Therefore, NFL abnormality in

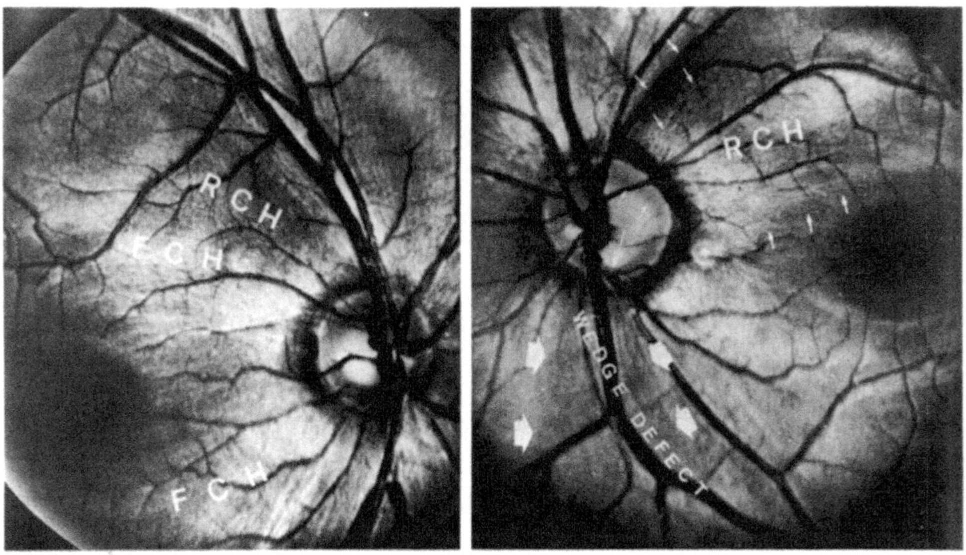


**Fig. 3.** Pair eyes in a case with asymmetrical early POAG. The left eye is a little advanced and the right eye is scarcely advanced. The earliest and a little advanced NFL abnormalities with cup expansion were demonstrated

Bjerrum area may precede the observable cup expansion.

4. The NFL abnormality may begin with the thinning of FCH, and it begins at least a half-year before it develops minimum glaucomatous field abnormality by FVFMII. FCH thinning develops into RCH thinning, then into darker NFL defect.

5. The corresponding sensitivity reduction is smaller than 0.4log.u. for RCH.

6. Abnormality by Goldmann perimetry occurs much later when NFL damage becomes wedge-shaped defect.

Figure 4 is showing the comparison between asymmetrical pair eyes in each ten cases of early POAG. Vertical shows the grade of NFL abnormality from the fine thinning of FCH to the advanced wedge-shaped NFL defect. Horizontal shows the grade of visual sensitivity reduction measured by FVFMII. In each eye superior and inferior Bjerrum area were observed.

In pair eyes open mark indicates scarcely advanced eye and closed mark indicates a little advanced eye. C and P mark mean disc cup expansion and pallor corresponding NFL abnormality respectively. It is remarkable that the scracely advanced eyes are distributed mainly in the area of FCH, RCH narrow than 30° and of smaller than 0.4log.u. reduction. In this group only one Bjerrum area showed local cup expansion and pallor. On the other hand a little advanced eyes are distributed mainly in the area of wide RCH and NFL defect. This group is mainly accompanied by local cup expansion and pallor. Goldmann perimetry does not detect the earliest abnormalities of NFL, and it is detected later when NFL attrition reaches a certain volume. The observed history of progression itself may display the true natural history of the earliest POAG.

**Summary.** The natural history of POAG in the early stage, when the IOP fluctuates within middle 20s of mmHg, was exposed by precise observation applying fundus color stereophotograph of 6 x 6 cm large size with 8 magnifications in pair eyes with asymmetrical early POAG. The first appearing clinical sign is slight thinning of NFL like fine combed hair (FCH) in Bjerrum area, then develops into raugh combed hair (RCH) thinning, and finally into NFL defect, which is observed as dark slit or wedge. In FCH thinning visual field shows a minimum glaucomatous abnormality of 0.2–0.4 log.u. reduction of areal sensitivity, which range is usually estimated as physiological in screening test.

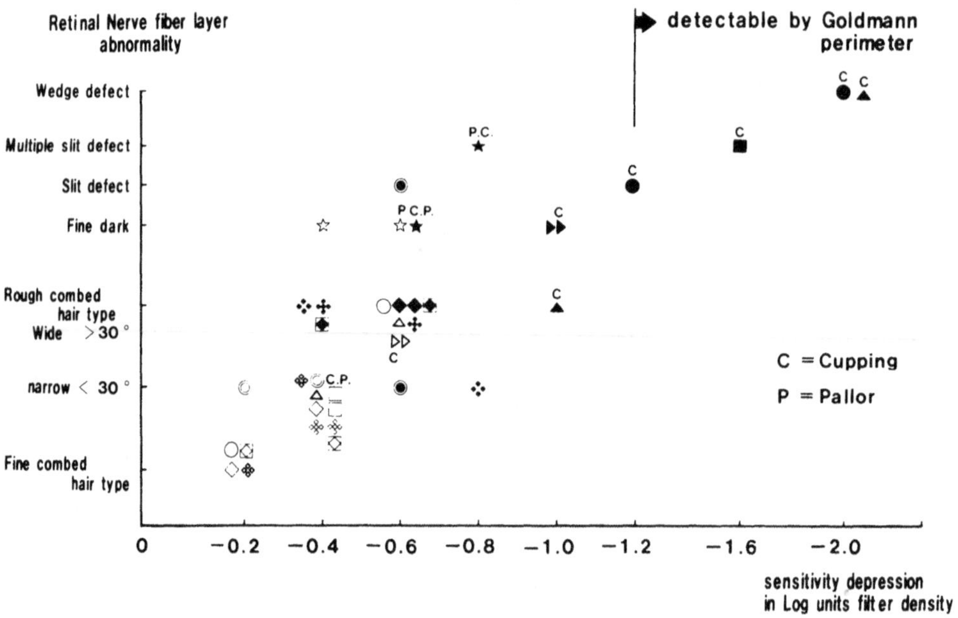


**Fig. 4.** Historical display of the mode of progression of glaucomatous damage observed in pair eyes of 10 cases with asymmetrical early POAG. *Open mark* shows scarcely advanced eyes and *closed mark* shows a little advanced eye

The FCH thinning may begin at least a half-year before the development of such field abnormality.

When the IOP level reaches to 35–45 mmHg, like Posner-Schlossman's syndrome, then the appearing first sign may be slit-like defect of NFL and not the FCH thinning. The visual field abnormality in FCH stage can not be detected by Goldmann perimetry.

Enlargement of disc cup and disc pallor is recognized later, when the NFL thinning becomes larger and deeper. NFL assessment is the most sensitive, objective means to find true glaucoma in the earliest stage and differentiate from ocular hypertension.

## References


Aulhorn E (1979) Pros and Cons of Quick-Tests in Glaucoma Perimetry. In: Krieglstein GK, Leydhecker W (eds) Glaucoma Update. Springer-Verlag, Berlin Heidelberg New York, p 79–88

Bengtsson BO, Krakau CET (1979) Automatic Perimetry in Secondary Prevention of Glaucoma. In: Krieglstein GK, Leydhecker W (eds) Glaucoma Update. Springer-Verlag Berlin Heidelberg New York, pp 71–78

Hoyt WF, Frisén L, Newman NM (1973) Fundoscopy of nerve fiber layer defects in Glaucoma. Invest Ophthalmol 12:814–829

Iwata K, Nanba K, Abe H (1981) Typical Slit-like Retinal Nerve Fiber Layer Defect and Corresponding Scotoma. Acta Soc Ophthalmol Jpn 85:1761–1803

Iwata K, Nanba K, Abe H (1982) Die beginnende Fundusveränderung infolge rezidivierender kleiner Krisen beim Posner-Schlossman-Syndrom. Klin Monatsbl Augenheilkd 180:20–24

Pederson JE, Anderson DR (1980) The Mode of Progressive Disc Cupping in Ocular Hypertension and Glaucoma. Arch Ophthalmol 98:490–495

Quigley HA, Miller NR, George T (1980) Clinical Evaluation of Nerve Fiber Layer Atrophy as an Indicator of Glaucomatous Optic Nerve Damage. Arch Ophthalmol 98:1564–1571

Sommer A, Pollack I, Maumenee E (1977) The Nerve Fiber Layer in the Diagnosis of Glaucoma. Arch Ophthalmol 95:2149–2156

Krieglstein G.K./Leydhecker W. (eds)
Glaucoma Update II


# The Computer-Perimetric Differentiation of Chronic Glaucoma, Low Tension Glaucoma, and Ischemic Neuropathy

G.K. Krieglstein and E. Gramer, Würzburg

Update computerized perimetry offers a variety of principle advantages in detecting [1] and assessing [2] localized changes of the central visual field. Within the different technical approaches, adaptive test strategies appear more promising than suprathreshold techniques with respect to sensitivity [3] and specificity [4, 5]. Utilizing these modern computer perimeters it was a great temptation to reevaluate the topography of the early visual field defect in different types of glaucoma. Since the role of ischemia in the individual glaucomatous eye as an etiological parameter of the disease is still obscure, it was a justified hope of this study to gain some more information on the question whether ischemia or IOP is the major villain in the individual glaucoma problem. If one concentrates on early visual field defects which could be identified with more reliability by computerized perimetry, one should expect a perimetric equivalent corresponding to the primary pathophysiology of the disease.

## Methods

Over a period of 4 years the computer perimeter Octopus was used at the Univ. Eye Hospital Würzburg to examine a total of 10 000 eyes with glaucoma or sustained elevated IOP. 1000 eyes of those exhibited glaucomatous field changes. Out of these 1000 eyes 301 (215 patients) were selected with early glaucomatous defects up to stage II according to the definition of Aulhorn [6]. The central visual fields (30° excentricity) of these eyes were examined with the Octopus usig program 31 (6° grid; adaptive strategy) and had a visual acuity of 0.5 or better. Pathological threshold determinations in the 73 test points were chosen for the evaluation of the topography of the early glaucomatous defect within the central visual field (Fig. 1). Sensitivity loss of at least 10 dB was defined as a relative defect, and nonrecognition at maximum luminosity as an absolute defect. A second series of 71 glaucomatous field defects (69 patients examined with the computer perimeter Competer (instrument according to the design of Heijl/Krakau; using the threshold program with an adaptive test strategy) served as a control group for the evaluation of the frequency distribution of defects. The sensitivity of this technique is equivalent to the Octopus in a conjoint test area [7]. However, it uses a denser grid of stimuli within 15° excentricity. This renders a high degree of detectability of scotomas close to the fixation point.

The results of the open angle glaucomas were compared to a group of early defects in anterior ischemic neuropathy of 12 eyes and of 21 eyes with low tension glaucoma. To avoid wrong projection of small defects a group of inflammatory optic nerve lesions (50 eyes with retrobulbar neuritis, 17 eyes with papillitis) were evaluated as control series to provide adequacy of the perimetric technique for studying the topography of field changes in the early disease. The latter three groups of ischemic neuropathy, low tension glaucoma, and neuritis have been investigated like the open angle glaucomas with program 31 of the Octopus. To include the aspect of IOP as further differentiation the diurnal IOP fluctuations of the above optic nerve diseases were compared as well.

## Results

The frequency distribution of early glaucomatous defects in the central visual field in 301 eyes in comparison to low tension glaucoma and ischemic neuropathy is presented in Fig. 2. In chronic open angle glaucoma the early defects dominate in the upper nasal

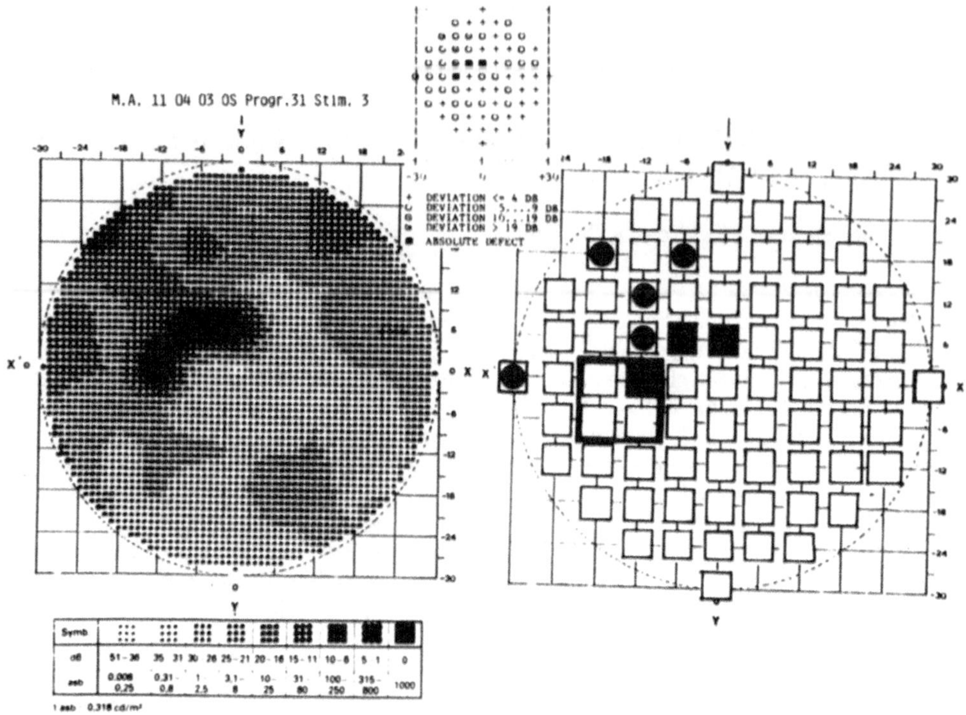


**Fig. 1.** Scheme for evaluation of frequency distribution of early visual field defects in different optic nerve diseases utilizing the computer perimeter Octopus. The *left side* shows a grey scale print of a glaucomatous defect of a left eye. The *right side* shows the locations of pathological retinal threshold determinations (*full circle* means relative sensitivity loss, *full square* absolute sensitivity loss). The four stimuli locations marking blind spot are labelled by an *open square*

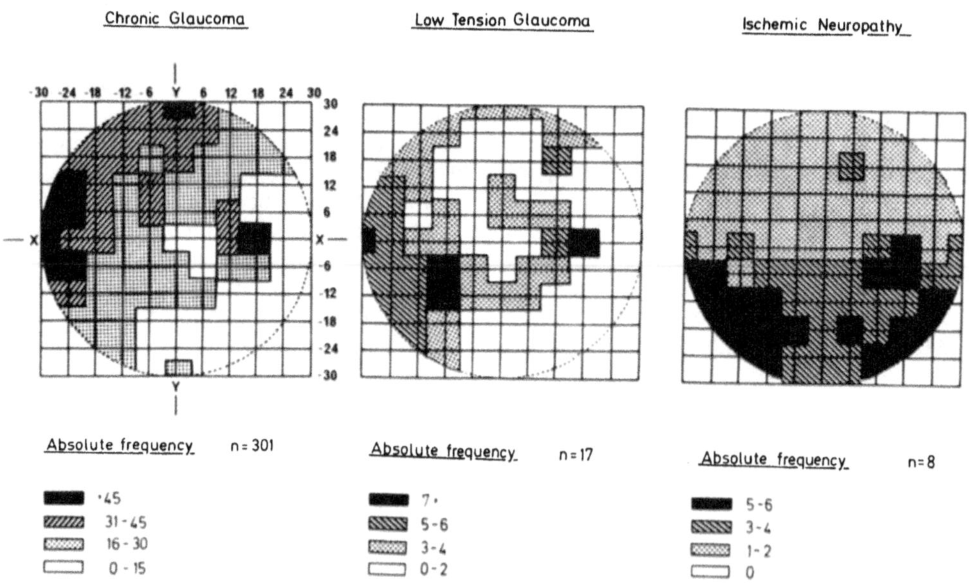


**Fig. 2.** Frequency distribution of absolute visual field defects in different optic nerve diseases verified by computerized perimetry

quadrant. Especially between 10° and 30° excentricity there is an increasing frequency of absolute scotomas. Defects in the upper half of the central field are closer to fixation point than in the lower half.

In low tension glaucoma the lower nasal quadrant represents the area of highest risk for developing an early defect (Fig. 2, *middle*). The visual field changes are similar to chronic glaucoma with respect to excentricity. In ischemic neuropathy both lower quadrants are equally affected (Fig. 2, *right side*). Early defects rarely occur in the upper quadrants. Scotomas due to ischemia in the central visual field within 30° are usually more peripherally located than scotomas of a comparable size in the glaucomas.

The frequency distribution of early absolute and relative defects in chronic glaucoma verified with the threshold program of the Competer is given in Fig. 3. These results confirm the topography obtained from the Octopus series both with respect to location and excentricity. As to absolute scotomas, there was an increasing frequency of defects beyond 5–10° excentricity. The evaluation of the early defects due to inflammatory optic nerve affections gave a clearcut predominance of the very centre of the field.

A typical greyscale print of central visual field changes in the four optic nerve diseases studied is presented in Fig. 4.

The relation between diurnal IOP fluctuations and the topography of central visual field changes in different optic nerve problems is illustrated in Fig. 5. The mean fluctuations in the inflammatory processes were 5.35 and 4.16 mmHg and not essentially different from normals. The mean diurnal fluctuation in the ischemic nerve lesions was somewhat higher with 6.62 mmHg, but not significantly different. The low tension glaucomas had a significant higher diurnal fluctuation with 8.09 mmHg on the average, indicating that some pathophysiology of IOP is involved. As was to be expected, the mean IOP diurnal change in the chronic glaucomas was the highest with 11.72 mmHg.

## Comment

If one concentrates on the early visual field damage, the perimetric differentiation between chronic glaucoma, low tension glaucoma, and ischemic neuropathy appears feasible.

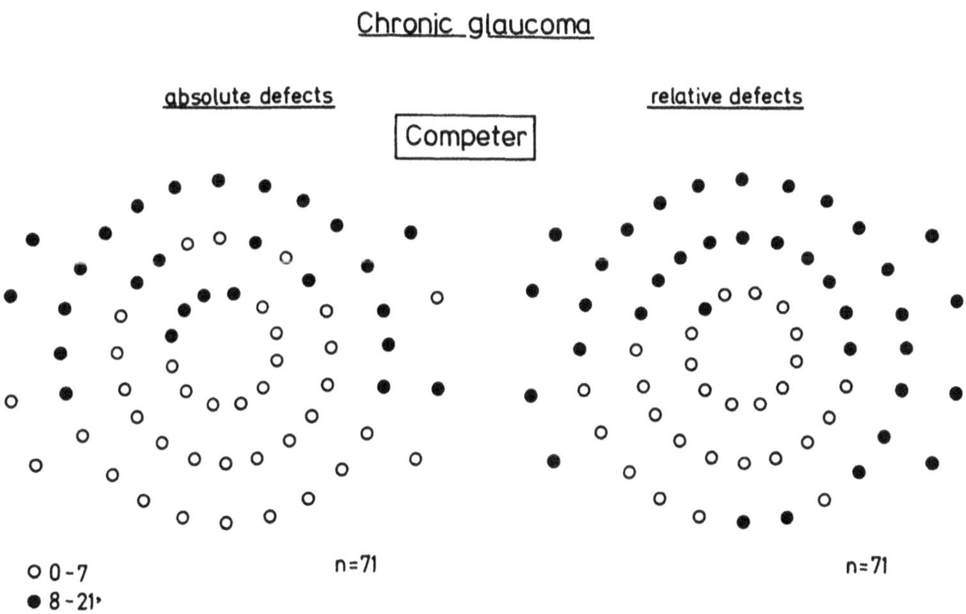


**Fig. 3.** The frequency distribution of relative and absolute glaucomatous visual field defects examined with the computer perimeter Competer according to Heijl and Krakau

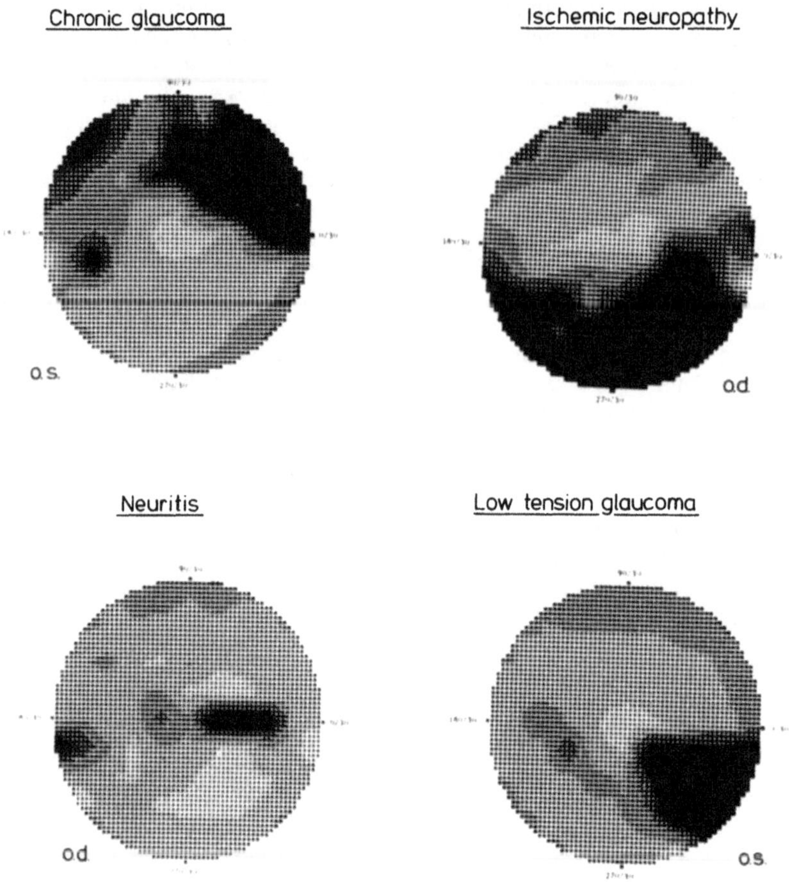


**Fig. 4.** Examples of typical locations of early defects in the central visual field in four optic nerve lesions

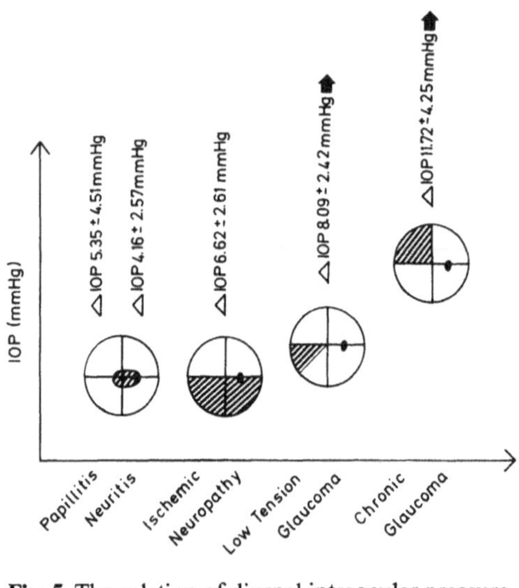


**Fig. 5.** The relation of diurnal intraocular pressure variations and topography of visual field defects in four optic nerve diseases

In chronic glaucoma the high risk area undoubtedly is the upper nasal quadrant. In this respect the results from computerized perimetry are not in full agreement with manual perimetry, in which the defects are also most frequently located in the upper nasal quadrant but closer to fixation point [8]. Of course, taking into account that isolated glaucomatous scotomas are the smaller, the closer they are to fixation point it can be argued that this study may have missed a good part of those within 10° because of the 6° test grid of program 31 of the Octopus. However, with the denser test grid of the Competer the location of the defects in terms of excentricity could be reproduced. An other indication for the correctness of the computer perimetric topography of field defects is derived from the neuritis results which gave exact central scotomas in agreement with the etiology of the disease [9].

In ischemic neuropathy the field changes were primarily in the lower quadrants as established with Tübinger manual static perimetry before [10].

In low tension glaucoma the topography of the early field defects corresponded to a middle position between chronic glaucoma and ischemic neuropathy. Again, the majority of the defects were in the nasal half of the field like in chronic glaucoma, but in the lower quadrant like in ischemic neuropathy.

The diurnal fluctuations of IOP that had been significantly higher than in normals, ischemic or inflammatory optic nerve diseases disclosed the pathophysiology of IOP. This means that considerable IOP elevations can occur within statistically normal limits and probably exert disadvantageous effects on nerve function.

Depending on the etiological mechanism in the foreground, the location of the first field defect may be in the upper nasal quadrant (primarily pressure) or in the lower nasal quadrant (mixed, pressure and ischemia) or in both lower quadrants (primarily ischemia). Since one can only influence IOP and very little or not arterial perfusion pressure, this bears some information on tension tolerance of the optic nerve and the necessity of lowering IOP. If the perimetric examination points out that ischemia is involved the IOP should be therapeutically lowered as much as possible [11].

The knowledge about specific topography of the early defect in the different types of glaucoma implies not only advantages in terms of classification and therapeutic concepts but opens a new horizon in early diagnosis itself. As we know, optic disc changes are of low specificity in dissolving the grey zone between physiologically elevated IOP and early glaucoma. Gloor [12] found that there are considerable disc changes without reproducible perimetric equivalent in terms of scotoma. Airaksinen [13] found a false negative rate of more than 60% when using the disc for the follow-up of ocular hypertension. On the other hand, there can be definite loss of retinal axons prior to field defects [14]. Does this phenomenon account for any visual dysfunctions, or do these axons represent just spare mechanisms without the imminent potential of field loss? Gloor [12] described increasing fluctuations of threshold determinations with computerized perimetry in locations of future field defects, and he suggested that localized threshold instability may be a preocursor of field loss and probably the effect of diffuse axonal loss.

Here computerized perimetry comes in with its capability of looking into the visual pathophysiology before the field defect shows up. The development of statistical programs for evaluation of perimetric data on a more objective basis [14] and the development of programs enabling the observer to entrust the computer with specific tasks (as for instance the Octopus computer language Sargon [15]) are helpful in that direction. Perhaps, with the most endangered area of the field in mind we can lay some stress on threshold instability there and compare it to a low risk area in an intra-individual comparison, thus providing better prognostication of field loss than the inspection of the disc will ever do.

## References


1. Krieglstein GK, Schrems W, Gramer E, Leydhecker W (1981) Detectability of early glaucomatous field defects. A controlled comparison of Goldmann versus Octopus perimetry. Doc Ophthalmol Proc Series, Junk Publishers/The Hague-Boston-London 26:19–24
2. Gramer E, Krieglstein GK (1981) Zur Verlaufskontrolle der retrobulbären Neuritis mit Hilfe des Computerperimeters Octopus. Klin Monatsbl Augenheilkd 179:418–423
3. Krieglstein GK, Glaab E, Gramer E (1981) Das Computer-Perimeter Fieldmaster-200. Eine vergleichende, kontrollierte klinische Studie zur Sensitivität und Spezifität in der Glaukomperimetrie. Klin Monatsbl Augenheilkd 179:340–345
4. Gramer E, Steinhauser B, Krieglstein GK (1982) The Specificity of the Automated Suprathreshold Perimeter Fieldmaster 200. Albrecht Von Graefes Arch Klin Exp Ophthalmol 218: 253–255
5. Neuhann T, Greite HJ (1981) Reliability of visual field examination in clinical routine. Doc Ophthalmol Proc Series, Junk Publishers/ The Hague-Boston-London 26:57–61
6. Aulhorn, E (1969) Glaukom-Gesichtsfeld. Ophthalmologica 158:469–487
7. Gramer E, Gerlach R, Krieglstein GK (1982) Zur Sensitivität des Computerperimeters Competer bei frühen glaukomatösen Gesichtsfeldausfällen. Eine kontrollierte Studie. Klin Monatsbl Augenheilkd 180:203–209

8. Aulhorn E (1976) Einfache perimetrische Methoden für die Erfassung der glaukomatösen Frühausfälle. Glaukom-Symposion Würzburg 1974 Enke Verlag, Stuttgart
9. Trobe JD, Glaser JS (1978) Quantitative perimetry in compressive optic neuropathy and optic neuritis. Arch Ophthalmol 96:1210–1216
10. Aulhorn E, Tanzil M, Litricin V (1979) Vergleich der Gesichtsfeldausfälle bei der Apoplexia papillae und beim Glaukom. Ber Dtsch Zusammenkunft Ophthalmol Ges 76: 633–640
11. Abedin S, Simmons RJ, Grant NM (1982) Progressive low-tension glaucoma. Ophthalmology 89:1–6
12. Gloor, B (1983) Die Computerperimetrie in der langfristigen Beurteilung des Glaukoms. In: Krieglstein GK, Leydhecker W (Hrsg) Medikamentöse Glaukomtherapie. J.F. Bergmann Verlag, München, S 59–72
13. Airaksinen, PJ (1983) Beziehung zwischen den Cup-Disc-Quotienten und der retinalen Nervenfaserschichtläsion bei Frühglaukom. In: Krieglstein GK, Leydhecker W (Hrsg) J.F. Bergmann Verlag, München, S 101–103
14. Quigley HA, Addicks EM, Green WR (1982) Optic nerve damage in human glaucoma. Arch Ophthalmol 100:135–146
15. Bebie H, Fankhauser F (1981) Statistical program for the analysis of perimetric data. Doc Ophthalmol Proc Series 26:9–10
16. Fankhauser F, Jenni A (1981) Programs Sargon and Delta. Albrecht Von Graefes Arch Klin Exp Ophthalmol 216:41–48

## Discussion

**Greve to Krieglstein:** The problem with the analysis of so-called low tension glaucoma is that we deal with a very heterogeneous group. The distribution of visual field defects in the sub-groups may be quite different. The example in the frequency of centrocecal and temporal defects in myopic low tension glaucoma as opposed to emmetropic low tension glaucoma. A second example is a group that has been called ischemic glaucoma. If one takes this sub-group of low tension glaucoma one finds that the layer defect is five times more frequent in the upper half than in the lower half.

These findings are not in agreement with the findings reported by Krieglstein. It *seems very attractive* to be able to distinguish certain high *risk areas* in the visual field of sub-groups of glaucoma. As the selection of the groups may determine the outcome of a study of such high rish areas. It *seems* not justified at present to state that the lower half of the visual field has an increased risk of developing visual field defects in low tension glaucoma.

**Drance to Krieglstein:** We have reported a large number of low tension glaucoma fields compared with a large number of chronic open angle glaucoma fields and found no difference in position, extent, closeness to fixation proving the discs have matched for the same stage of tissue involvement. The LTG cases are likely otherwise to be more advanced because they are selected by symptoms, which may mean major defects or by the obvious disc change seen on routine examination, whereas, glaucoma patients are followed because of elevated IOP so that early field defects are spotted. The high prevalence of major haemodynamic crises in a series is due to selection because people know of an interest in these cases. However, not even the shock like cases showed the difference in field defects from COAG which some observers suggested we would find.

In answer to Greve I agree completely in trying to identify various mechanisms of LTG which he proposes such as sclerotic LTG, focal infarctions etc. particularly if these can be reliably done. I would however, suggest that the same groups should be identified in glaucoma patients with elevated IOP . . . unless one assumes that anything over any given pressure is automatically pressure induced which is epidemiologically untenable. I do agree that these groups may help us in understanding the entire disease.

Krieglstein G.K./Leydhecker W. (eds)
Glaucoma Update II


# Use of Multivariate Analysis in the Prognostication of Ocular Hypertension

Y. Kitazawa, F. Go, S. Shirato and Y. Akiba, Tokyo

It is well recognized that only a small percentage of subjects with ocular hypertension develop primary open-angle glaucoma [1-3]. The identification of the patients at high risk of developing glaucoma is of utmost, clinical importance for the rational treatment of the patients with elevated intraocular pressure (IOP) alone. The quantitative determination of the risk has been attempted by previous investigators and multivariate analytic techniques have been advocated by some groups of investigators [4-7]. Little attempts, however, have been made to validate the results from multivariate analyses using an independent second sample in a prospective study.

We carried out a prospective study of two independent groups of patients who had elevated IOPs but no demonstrable field loss. One group was utilized for the risk factor analysis to estimate the probability of visual field loss. The validity of the analytical results was tested using the other independent group.

## Methods

A total of 165 patients with ocular hypertension were observed without therapy. All the patients studied were divided into two groups according to the length of follow-up. The group 1 comprised 116 patients who were followed up for 10 years or more and the group 2 consisted of 49 patients who were observed for 3 years or more. All patients had ocular hypertension at the initiation of the observation period, i.e. IOP was 22 mmHg or greater in the presence of normal open angles by gonioscopy and no visual field changes were demonstrated. All risk factors were recorded at the beginning of the observation period. IOP was measured with a Goldmann applanation tonometer and tonography was taken with an electronic tonometer coupled with a recorder. Visual field examination was done by means of quantitative kinetic perimetry with a Goldmann perimeter. The cup/disc ratio was determined by comparing the horizontal diameter of the cup estimated by contour to that of the disc on ophthalmoscopic examination. Glaucomatous visual field loss was defined as a paracentral scotoma over 5 degrees or a nasal step over 10 degrees that was confirmed by static perimetry with a Friedmann visual field analyzer and/or a Goldmann perimeter. The recorded values from one eye were used for each patient; in the group that developed visual field loss, the values for the first eye to demonstrate a field defect, and in the group that failed to develop a field loss one eye was chosen at random. The risk factors analysed in the study are summarized in Table 1.

### *Statistical Methods*

Using a multiple regression and a linear discriminant analysis the relative importance of risk factors was calculated. The contribution of the factors to the probability of developing a field defect was calculated using a multiple logistic function that is expressed as follows [8];

**Table 1.** Parameters for follow up

| | |
|---|---|
| 1 | Age (year) at the beginning of observation |
| 2 | Sex (6, male; 9, female) |
| 3 | IOP (mmHg) |
| 4 | Tonographic outflow facility (µl/min/mmHg) |
| 5 | Po/C |
| 6 | Horizontal Cup/disc ratio estimated by contour |
| 7 | Difference in horizontal Cup/disc ratio among a pair of eyes |
| 8 | Family history of glaucoma (0, negative; 1, positive) |

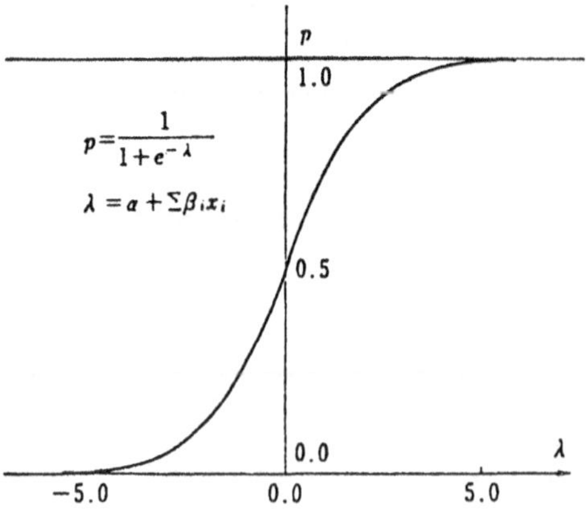


**Fig. 1.** Relationship between *P* (probability of risk) and λ in multiple logistic function

$$P = \frac{1}{1 + e^{-\lambda}}$$

In this function, P is the probability of risk, λ indicates the individual risk and is called the logit of risk. The exponent, λ, is expressed as follows;

$$\lambda = \alpha + \sum_{i=1}^{k} \beta i X i$$

were α is a constant, Xi are the values of the individual risk factors (eg, IOP): βi are the coefficients; and K is the total number of risk factors, Xi represent either discrete or continuous variables. As the exponent, λ, the logit of risk, attains a large negative value, P approaches 0, while as it attains a large positive value, P approaches 1 (Fig. 1). The relative significance of the various risk factors was tested by computing the estimate for each coefficient (βi) divided by the standard error of its estimate ($SE_{\beta i}$) yielding a value of t. The final solution of the logistic function was used to calculate the probability of risk in group 2 patients.

## Results

Of the 116 patients (group 1), glaucomatous field defects developed in one or both eyes of 13 patients (17 eyes) during the follow-up period, while 103 retained normal visual fields. The correlation of eight risk factors with the development of visual field defects was ranked using a stepwise multiple regression analysis. The order of correlation with the development of field loss was noted to be, age, IOP, family history, horizontal C/D-ratio, C-value, Po/C, difference in C/D-ratio and sex (Table 2). One factor, family history of glaucoma, was omitted because of very low prevalence and the uncertainty of information given by the patient. One other factor, Po/C, was excluded as this was strongly cross-correlated with IOP and C-value ($P < 0.001$). The remainder of six factors were used for the solution of multiple logistic function. The factor, the difference in C/D-ratio, was eliminated as this particular factor was noted not to significantly improve the ability of multiple logistic function to separate those who developed field defects from those who failed to. Consequently the remainder of five factors were used to compute the final multiple logistic function (Table 3).

The probability of risk computed using the final logistic function for group 1 patients was $0.181 \pm 0.100$ in 13 cases that developed field defects and was $0.103 \pm 0.091$ in 103 cases that failed to. The difference in the probability of risk was statistically highly significant between those who lost fields and those who failed to ($P < 0.01$). A cut off point that gives

**Table 2.** Risk factors ranked by stepwise multiple regression analysis

| Risk factor | $R^2$ |
|---|---|
| 1. Age | 0.06776 |
| 2. IOP | 0.07766 |
| 3. Family history | 0.08067 |
| 4. Horizontal C/D-ratio | 0.08362 |
| 5. Outflow facility | 0.08444 |
| 6. Po/C | 0.08457 |
| 7. Difference in C/D-ratio | 0.08466 |
| 8. Sex | 0.08467 |

**Table 3.** Coefficients of multiple logistic function

| Risk factor | βi | t-value |
|---|---|---|
| Age | 0.0552 | 2.43 |
| Horizontal Cup/disc-ratio | 0.1181 | 0.67 |
| IOP | 0.0394 | 0.63 |
| Outflow facility | -0.0111 | -0.22 |
| Sex | -0.0391 | -0.18 |
| Constant | -5.5141 | |

best separation of the visual field loss from the remainder was found to be P = 0.07, with this point there were 40 false positive cases and one false-negative cases.

Of the 49 patients in the group 2, four developed glaucomatous visual field defects in one or both eyes during the follow-up period of 3 years. The computed probability of risk was 0.178 ± 0.108 (n = 4) in the field loss group and 0.179 ± 0.098 (n = 45) in the remainder of cases that failed to develop field loss. The difference in the probability of risk was not of statistical significance between the field loss and the no-field loss groups. However, the probability of risk in the group 2 was 0.179 ± 0.098 (n = 49), that was significantly higher than that in the 103 cases in the group 1 which failed to develop field loss.

## Comment

Multivariate analytic techniques have been employed to evaluate the risk factors for the development of glaucomatous field defects in the ocular hypertensives [4–7]. Most analytic methods so far employed allow the simultaneous evaluation of multiple factors including the interrelationships of the factors and the combined effects of various factors on the development of a disease. However, not all the methods allow the estimation of the risk of developing field defects. It is one of the advantages of a multiple logistic function that this method of analysis can be used to compute the probability of risk for an individual to develop a disease [6, 8, 9]. Using a multiple logistic function Hart et al. calculated the probability of developing glaucoma in 82 ocular hypertensives. The computed logistic function could classify correctly 96.6% of eyes that developed glaucoma and 79.6% that did not [6]. The efficacy of their function was not, however, tested with an independent sample of patients with ocular hypertension. The ability of logistic function computed in the present study to separate the two groups of cases was apparently inferior to that of Hart et al. in that the function of our study yielded a considerably higher false positive rate. This seems to be due to a relatively small number of patients (13/116 = 11.2%) who developed glaucoma during 10 to 14-year period of observation. The incidence of a field defect becomes even smaller during the first 3-year

**Table 4.** Development of visual field defects and length of observation period

| Follow-up Period (years) | | |
|---|---|---|
| Follow-up period (years) | Cases with normal field | Cases that developed field loss |
| ⩽ 3 | 113 | 3 |
| ⩽ 6 | 111 | 2 |
| ⩽ 9 | 104 | 7 |
| ⩽ 12 | 99 | 0 |
| ⪵ 15 | 22 | 1 |
| total | | 13 |

period of observation, namely only 3 of 116 developed field loss (Table 4). This makes a striking contrast to the almost three times as high as the incidence of field defect in the second sample comprising 49 ocular hypertensives with 3-year follow-up who had a significantly, higher probability of risk estimated by using the function computed in the first 116 cases. The results appear to provide a further evidence that the present method of analysis may be useful in evaluating the risk of developing glaucoma in ocular hypertensives.

## References

1. Armaly MF (1969) Ocular pressure and visual fields. A ten-year follow-up study. Arch Ophthalmol 81:25
2. Wilensky JT, Podos SM, Becker B (1974) Prognostic indicators in ocular hypertension. Arch Ophthalmol 91:200
3. Kitazawa Y, Horie T, Aoki S, Suzuki M, Nishioka K (1977) Untreated ocular hypertension. A long-term prospective study. Arch Ophthalmol 95:1180
4. Kitazawa Y (1978) Clinical features of the eye in the earliest stage of primary open-angle glaucoma. In: Rehak S, Krasnov MM, Paterson GD (eds) Recent Advances in Glaucoma, Proceedings of the International Glaucoma Symposium, Prague (1976). Prague, Avicenum Czechoslovak Medical Press, p 159
5. Armaly MF, Krueger D, Maunder C (1979) Summary report of "Biostatistical Analysis of the Collaborative Glaucoma Study" In: Krieglstein GD, Leydhecker W (eds) Glaucoma Update, International Glaucoma Symposium,

Nara, Japan (1978) Springer-Verlag, Berlin Heidelberg New York, p 131

6. Hart WM, Yablonski M, Kass M, Becker B (1979) Multivariate analysis of the risk of glaucomatous visual field loss. Arch Ophthalmol 97:1455
7. Drance SM, Schulzer M, Thomas B, Douglas GR (1981) Multivariate analysis in glaucoma. Use of discriminant analysis in predicting glaucomatous visual field damage. Arch Ophthalmol 99:1019
8. Truett J, Cornfield J, Kannel W (1967) A multivariate analysis of the risk of coronary heart disease in Framingham. J Chronic Dis 20:511
9. Kass M, Hart WM, Gordon M, Miller JP (1980) Risk factors for the development of glaucomatous visual field loss in ocular hypertension. Surv Ophthalmol 25:155

## Discussion

**Perkins to Kitazawa:** We have been discussing the factors which increase the risk of a patient with ocular hypertension developing a field defect. It also important to define factors which reduce the risk of a field defect, so we can be less stringent in our follow up of people who have a low risk. As Dr. Kitazawa has shown and previous studies have shown, age and tension are the most reliable risk factors and for the patients under the age of 60 years and with tensions less than 25 mmHg the risk is less than 0.1%. Such patients do not need as frequent follow up as elder patients or patients with tensions above 25 mmHg.

Another important factor is the refraction. In a follow up of with patients with ocular hypertension Dr. Phelps and I found that only 1 in 46 hypermetropes and 3 in 56 emmetropes developed field defects in a mean follow up of 7 years, whereas 6 out of 19 myopes developed field defects. Refraction therefore is an important factor in the prognosis of ocular hypertension.

**Kass to Kitazawa:** Dr. Kitazawa should be commended for undertaking such an arduous project. Attempts to make predictions must be validated in prospective studies and repeated in second populations.

Other risk factos could have been included, e.g. vascular disease (diabetes, hypertension, hemodynamic crises, coronary artery disease), refractive error, race.

It is interesting that Dr. Kitazawa finds a sensitivity of 92% and a specificity of 71% in Group I. This is very similar to our findings in a retrospective study done a few years ago in St. Louis. It is reasuring that studies done on two such different populations yield similar results.

Table 4 of Dr. Kitazawa's paper demonstrates that the risk of developing glaucoma remains relatively constant over a 15-year period. Some ophthalmologists have worried that the rate of development of glaucoma would increase rapidly after a certain period of time. These data are reassuring.

The fact that Dr. Kitazawa's model does not predict the development of glaucoma in Group II as well may not be a shortcoming of the model. Group II appears to be different with respect to age, mean cup/disc ratio and the rate of development of glaucoma. The conversion rate in Group II, 4% per year, is much higher than Group I or that generally reported in the literature. It seems that some bias in selection or testing affected the composition of Group II. The model for predicting the development of glaucoma derived from Group I may be useful for assessing risk in a more representative group of patients with ocular hypertension. The model predicts a very high rate of conversion for Group II which may be true as times passes.

**Kitazawa to Perkins:** The cut-off point of IOP of 25 mmHg or more in the individuals above age 40 is not inconsistent with the results of our study. However, let me point out the age in the field loss patients was 49.0 ± 11.6 years old (n = 13) in group 1 and 49.0 ± 8.4 years old (n = 6) in group 2 and IOP of the patients was 25.7 ± 3.8 mmHg in group 1 and 24.8 ± 1.9 mmHg in group 2 respectively. The mean value of the two factors agrees well with your point, however, the large standard deviation limits the prognostic value of a single factor. With regards to the inclusion of refractive condition into the risk factors we will certainly repeat our analysis to see if to include refractive condition will improve prognostication.

**Kitazawa to Kass:** The reason for a higher probability of risk in the group 2 patients seems to be due to the age, i.e. it was higher by about 10 years in the group 2 which was 48.7 years in the group 2 (n = 49) and was 38.0 years (n = 116) in the group 1 on the average at the initiation of the study.

The point I feel most important is that the results of our study have provided a further evidence of the practical usefulness and significance of applying multivariate analysis for the prognostication of ocular hypertensives. The significantly higher incidence of field loss in the group 2 patients supports this conclusion which had significantly higher probability of risk at the time of enrollment into the study.

Krieglstein G.K./Leydhecker W. (eds)
Glaucoma Update II


# "Follow-up" Perimetric Study on Primary Open Angle Glaucoma and Ocular Hypertension

I. Azuma, Takatsuki/Osaka

## Introduction

Detailed perimetric examinations and simplified perimetric examinations for screening, play a very important role in the diagnosis of chronic glaucoma. When ocular hypertension (OH) or primary open angle glaucoma (POAG) is diagnosed, the patient should be monitored during the process of therapy with particular attension to regulation of intraocular pressure (IOP). However, all during this period, it is often difficult to conduct detailed and frequent perimetric examinations.

Intraocular pressure of an glaucomatous eye may sometimes exeed the normal upper limit during medical therapy, or there may be a need to change the drug therapy or to treat surgically if the IOP fluctuates markedly. However, no definite information is yet available about the indication for such changes in therapy. Today, we often change therapy when definite evidence of progress of visual field defects is obtained. However, at this point, we often find that it is too late to conduct the surgical operation. From the above described point of view, I thought it might be of help if I could use a very simplified perimeter and measure visual fields on a routine basis in practice in an attempt to follow any changes in IOP and to monitor the progress of the disease.

For this purpose, I developed a perimeter, which I named "follow-up perimeter", and today, I would like to report on its use and some results of my experience.

## Apparatus (Fig. 1)

The central fixation target is first lighted in a perimeter with background luminance of 0.1 abs. and thus, fixation of the eye to be examined is confirmed. Next, the starting button is pushed, and then, the visual target luminance is increased at a constant rate of 26.3 digital value/sec. at five points, that is, the central fixation point (CFP) and the paracentral points (5°), temporal superior (TS), temporal inferior (TI), nasal superior (NS) and nasal inferior (NI). It is convenient for us to measure the time to recognize the target of each point in digical values. Normal recognition time (visual sensation time) is about 5 seconds at each point.

## Patients and Methods

Thirty-three normal volunteers (65 eyes), 14 patients (28 eyes) with OH and 27 patients (51 eyes) with POAG were studied. Measured

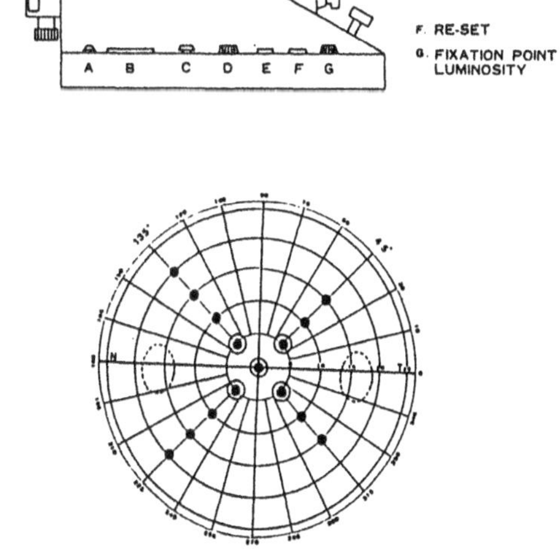


**Fig. 1.** Outline of "follow-up perimeter"

values at each point were compared by sex, age and degree of visual field defects. In the normal eyes, mydriasis was induced by tropicamide, and miosis by pilocarpine, and the results were compared between these two conditions.

Some patients were observed over a long period. The results of the "follow-up perimetry" as well as changes in IOP and the Goldmann perimetric findings are investigated.

**Table 1.** Visual sensation time

| Point \ Group | Normal | OH | POAG |
|---|---|---|---|
| C.F.P. | 141 ± 15 | 146 ± 17 | 159 ± 22 |
| T.S. | 129 ± 15 | 138 ± 15 | 153 ± 31 |
| T.I. | 132 ± 19 | 143 ± 16 | 159 ± 32 |
| N.I. | 134 ± 16 | 141 ± 15 | 157 ± 25 |
| N.S. | 128 ± 13 | 135 ± 15 | 159 ± 34 |

Digital number × 0.037 sec; (mean ± S.D.)

## Results

The visual recognition time in normal subjects and the patients with OH or POAG is shown in Table 1.

1) In the normal eyes, the visual recognition time was longer in women than in men ($p < 0.01$). It was significantly prolonged with increased age, in order of young, middle aged, elderly ($p < 0.05$ to 0.01). The results did not differ significantly whether in mydriasis or in miosis.

2) In the patients with POAG, the results did not differ significantly between sexes. However, the results differed between the young group and the elderly group ($p < 0.05$). At some points of measurement, the degree of the visual field defects was significantly related ($p < 0.05$) to visual recognition time.

3) The normal volunteers were compared with the patients with POAG. The results were high significantly different between the two groups at all points ($p < 0.01$). The normal volunteers were also very significantly different from the patients with OH at four points ($p < 0.01$) except the point NS ($p < 0.05$). The patients with OH differed significantly ($p < 0.01$) from those with POAG at 3 points (TS, NI and NS) (Fig. 2).

To clarify the practical value of the "follow-up perimeter", a few examples are given.

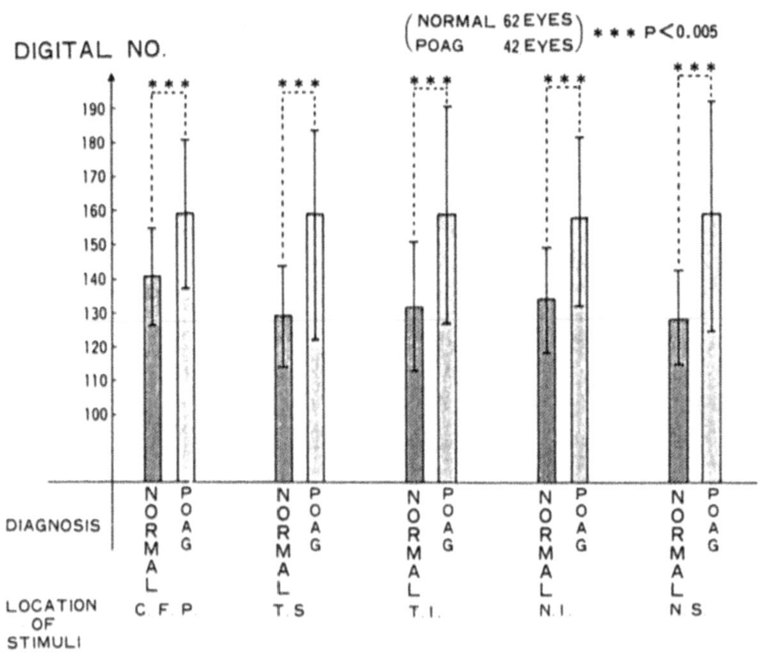


**Fig. 2.** Visual sensation time (normal vs POAG)

*Case (1) 73 y.-o. male, POAG (Fig. 3, 4)*

Since Feb. 1978 he was treated on the left eye with miotics and the IOP was good controlled. Goldmann's visual field showed no progressive change during the two years. Since 1980 the rising IOP was observed and difficult to control with potent medical treatment. As a matter of course, progressive field change was found, and finally, trabeculectomy was done successfully in July '80. Follow-up perimetry was occasionally performed and a prolongation of the visual recognition time was confirmed all that while in 1980.

*Case (2) 51 y.-o. male, POAG*

Since Dec. 1977 he was treated with Pilo-Ocusert 20. The IOP showed sometimes slight increase, but usually remained in normal range. Both physician and patient were satisfactory to the drug therapy. However, in the past several years, the visual field of this case was showing a progressive change, and also the data obtained from "follow-up perimeter" had certainly shown an aggravation. There is a great possibility that the occasional visual field examinations may be taken to be unchanged.

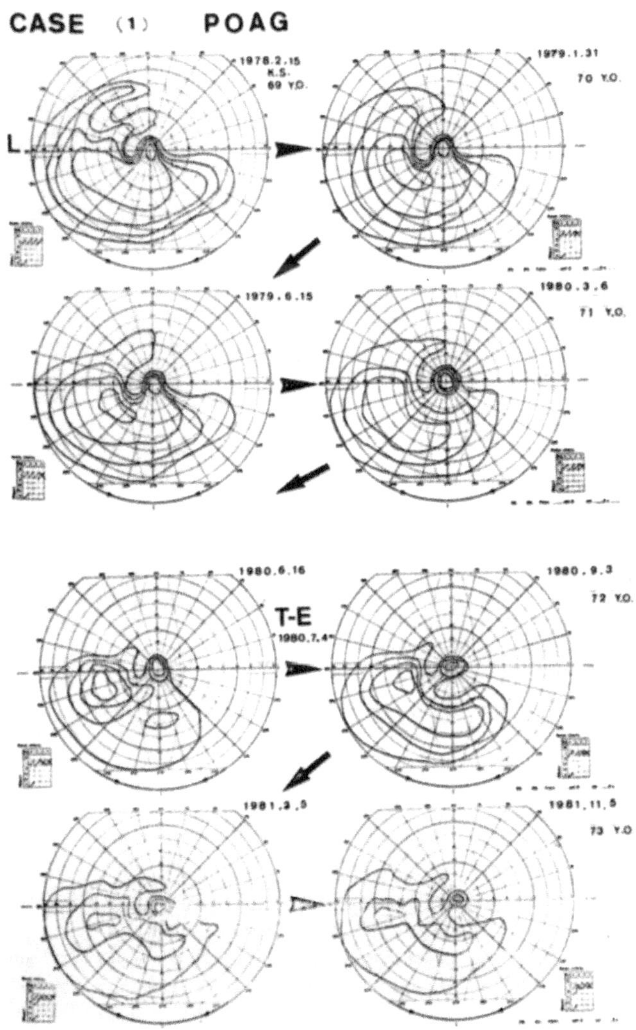


**Fig. 3.** (See text)

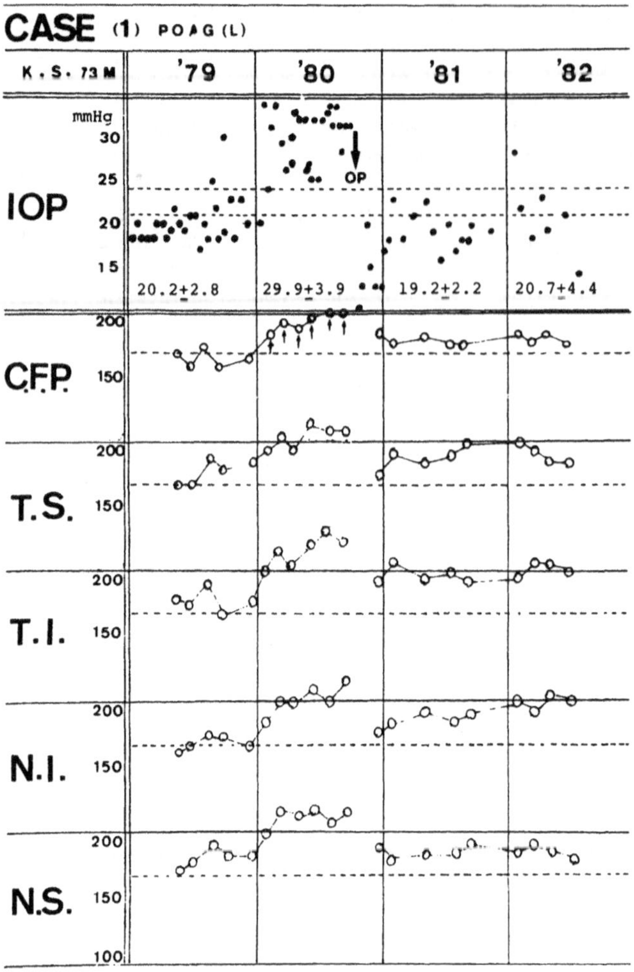


**Fig. 4.** (See text)

*Case (3) 47 y.-o. male, POAG*

This is a rare case with POAG. Over a long period of time, he did not wish to treat medically. Since he was diagnosed POAG in 1970, the periodical examinations of IOP, visual field and optic disk were made. In the last two years he agreed to treat with a beta-blocker. The visual recognition time obtained by "follow-up perimeter" shows an evident tendency of aggravation.

Many efforts to improve the apparatus and the accumulation of data on a lot of condition examples are needed hereafter.

## Conclusion

"Follow-up perimetry" can be performed easily and frequently in the field of clinical practice. It will be useful in judging validity of the treatment for individual case of chronic glaucoma.

## References

1. Armaly MF (1969) Ocular pressure and visual fields. A ten-year follow-up study. Arch Ophthalmol 81:25–40
2. Azuma I et al. (1974) On the Correlation between IOP and Visual Field in Glaucoma. Acta Soc Ophthalmol Jpn 78:1171–1178
3. Azuma I et al. (1975) A Study for the Visual Function of the Primary Open-Angle Glaucoma. Acta Soc Ophthalmol Jpn 79:1119–1130
4. Azuma I (1975) Problems on Diagnosis for Glaucoma. Acta Soc Ophthalmol Jpn 79:1687–1714

5. Azuma I, Yamaji S (1976) Critical Pressure in Glaucoma. Acta Soc Ophthalmol Jpn 80:803–820
6. Yamaji S (1978) Studies on Critical Pressure in Glaucoma-Estimation during Diurnal Variation of IOP and Visual Field at Selected Points. Acta Soc Ophthalmol Jpn 82:592–609
7. Azuma I et al. (1981) Design of a Follow-Up Campimeter for Glaucoma. Rinsho Ganka 35:1210–1217
8. Azuma I et al. (1981) Clinical Application of "Follow-Up Perimeter" to the Chronic Glaucoma. Acta Soc Ophthalmol Jpn 85:1622–1634
9. Goldmann H (1972) Open-Angle Glaucoma. Br J Ophthalmol 56:242–248
10. Goldmann H (1975) An analysis of some concepts concerning chronic simple glaucoma. Am J Ophthalmol 80:409–413

## Discussion

**Azuma to Krakau:** Illumination of the visual target is increasing continuously at a constant velocity from zero setting.

We estimated the visual field function at a given point as the visual recognition time.

Krieglstein G.K./Leydhecker W. (eds)
Glaucoma Update II


# Diurnal Pressure Curve in Surgically Treated Congenital Glaucoma in Comparison to Normal Patients of the Same Age Group

N. Calixto, S. Cronemberger Sobrinho, and F.J. Moreno, Belo Horizonte

It is a widely known fact that the intraocular pressure (Po) changes during the course of the day. The importance of the diurnal pressure curve (DCPo) in the diagnosis and in the control of the treatment in patients with primary glaucoma is recognized by many authors. Nevertheless, we do not know of a systematic study of the DCPo in patients with congenital glaucoma (CG) treated by surgery. We have found only two references in the literature available to us. (1) Thiel (1930) described the oscillations of the Po in an 8-year-old child with "hydrophthalmus with glaucomatous cup," who showed a good therapeutic response to pilocarpine and eserine. The behavior of the Po (four measurements/-day) was similar to that found in primary glaucoma [2]. Pau (1952) studied the DCPo in ten patients (20 eyes examined) with advanced CG. Of the 20 eyes, three were atrophic and 17 were buphthalmic (three with total cataracts). The age-range was 7–46 years. Only five patients (25%) were surgically treated (Elliot's trephination). Nine of the eyes were blind (no light perception), one was able to perceive light, six with projection of light, and only four (20%) had vision between 0.02 and 0.3. Pau confirmed the findings of Thiel in relation to the similar behavior of the Po of the primary glaucoma and CG patients.

The purpose of this paper is to present our findings for the DCPo, systematically obtained in 29 patients (48 eyes) with CG treated by surgery in comparison with 35 normal patients of the same age-group.

## Material and Methods

### *Normal Subjects*

Thirty-five eyes (35 subjects) were randomly chosen using a table of aleatory numbers; the age of the subjects ranged from 6 to 15 years. The subjects had emmetropic eyes, which were normal under ophthalmologic examination, and their family histories were negative for eye diseases (20 males and 15 females).

### *Congenital Glaucoma*

We examined 29 patients (48 eyes) with CG, which was gonioscopically characterized prior to surgery (see Table 1 for the congenital anomalies in the camerular sinus). The age-range was the same as in the normal group, that is, 6–15 years. Seventeen eyes (35%) required additional eyedrops (epinephrine or a combination of epinephrine plus pilocarpine). Thirty-one eyes (65%) did not require any additional medication (14 males and 15 females). The mean time interval between the surgery and the DCPo was 7 years. The mean age in both groups was 11.0 and 10.8 years, respectively. Initially, we studied 43 patients with CG but we excluded 14 patients because they were older than 15 years of age and, therefore, older than the normal group, which did not permit a suitable comparison.

We used the Goldmann applanation tonometer and the Haag Streit slit lamp model 900 for the daily measurements and the Perkins portable tonometer for the measurements at 6 a.m. when the subjects were in bed.

The following surgery was performed – (1)

**Table 1.** Types of anomalies in the camerulan sinus

| | |
|---|---|
| 1. Remnants of the pectinate ligament (in 11 eyes also with Barkan's membrane) | 33 eyes (69%) |
| 2. Metaplasia of the pectinate ligament | 8 eyes (17%) |
| 3. Aplasia of the pectinate ligament | 4 eyes (08%) |
| 4. Barkan's membrane only | 3 eyes (06%) |

basal iridencleisis (Evans' technique); (2) goniotomy; (3) trabeculotomy; (4) trabeculectomy. In rare cases, we combined trabeculotomy with trabeculectomy.

We followed the Sampaolesi method for the evaluation of the DCPo, that is, seven measurements of Po/day calculating the arithmetic mean of the measurements (Pm) and the standard deviation of the seven measurements (V).

## Results and Discussion

Tables 2 (normal patients) and 3 (CG) show that measurements were taken in each eye every 3 h (we did not measure the Po at 3 a.m.). As previously mentioned, in the CG group eyedrops were used in those eyes requiring additional medication.

In a plane of coordinates (Fig. 1), the value of Po the ordinate was marked as and the hour

**Table 2.** Diurnal curve of pressure in normal subjects

| Subject | Sex | Age | Time 0600 | | 0900 | | 1200 | | 1500 | | 1800 | | 2100 | | 2400 | | Pm | V |
|---|---|---|---|---|---|---|---|---|---|---|---|---|---|---|---|---|---|---|
| | | | RE | LE[a] | RE | LE | RE | LE | RE | LE | RE | LE | RE | LE | RE | LE | | |
| 1. R.D.C. | M | 11 | 11 | - | 13 | - | 13 | - | 11 | - | 11 | - | 10 | - | 10 | - | 11.29 | 1.25 |
| 2. D.A.O. | F | 14 | - | 13 | - | 14 | - | 13 | - | 12 | - | 13 | - | 12 | - | 10 | 12.43 | 1.27 |
| 3. M.C.P.S. | F | 7 | 12 | - | 12 | - | 12 | - | 11 | - | 12 | - | 10 | - | 10 | - | 11.29 | 0.95 |
| 4. D.A.O. | F | 8 | - | 13 | - | 13 | - | 11 | - | 10 | - | 10 | - | 10 | - | 9 | 10.86 | 1.57 |
| 5. E.A.P. | M | 8 | - | 14 | - | 10 | - | 11 | - | 11 | - | 11 | - | 11 | - | 12 | 11.43 | 1.27 |
| 6. C.C.L. | M | 9 | - | 12 | - | 10 | - | 10 | - | 10 | - | 9 | - | 11 | - | 10 | 10.29 | 0.95 |
| 7. T.A.O. | M | 12 | 13 | - | 12 | - | 12 | - | 10 | - | 11 | - | 11 | - | 12 | - | 11.57 | 0.98 |
| 8. R.F. | F | 10 | 13 | - | 11 | - | 11 | - | 11 | - | 10 | - | 10 | - | 10 | - | 10.86 | 1.07 |
| 9. A.F.N. | M | 15 | 10 | - | 13 | - | 11 | - | 11 | - | 10 | - | 10 | - | 10 | - | 10.71 | 1.11 |
| 10. C.C.R.F. | F | 15 | 13 | - | 10 | - | 10 | - | 9 | - | 8 | - | 10 | - | 10 | - | 10.00 | 1.53 |
| 11. A.S.L. | F | 11 | 12 | - | 10 | - | 10 | - | 10 | - | 12 | - | 10 | - | 10 | - | 10.57 | 0.98 |
| 12. J.A.G.R. | F | 11 | - | 13 | - | 13 | - | 12 | - | 11 | - | 11 | - | 12 | - | 10 | 11.71 | 1.11 |
| 13. E.F.S. | M | 9 | - | 11 | - | 10 | - | 10 | - | 10 | - | 10 | - | 10 | - | 9 | 10.00 | 0.58 |
| 14. F.A.P.R. | M | 10 | 15 | - | 12 | - | 13 | - | 12 | - | 13 | - | 11 | - | 11 | - | 12.43 | 1.40 |
| 15. R.R.M. | F | 14 | - | 13 | - | 12 | - | 10 | - | 10 | - | 11 | - | 11 | - | 9 | 10.86 | 1.35 |
| 16. J.C.A. | F | 12 | - | 12 | - | 12 | - | 11 | - | 12 | - | 12 | - | 10 | - | 12 | 11.57 | 0.79 |
| 17. R.A.S.A. | M | 13 | - | 14 | - | 10 | - | 10 | - | 10 | - | 11 | - | 9 | - | 10 | 10.57 | 1.52 |
| 18. A.L.C. | M | 9 | - | 13 | - | 11 | - | 10 | - | 11 | - | 10 | - | 10 | - | 10 | 10.71 | 1.11 |
| 19. A.R.F. | M | 12 | - | 14 | - | 10 | - | 11 | - | 12 | - | 12 | - | 10 | - | 14 | 11.86 | 1.68 |
| 20. M.C.P.S. | F | 15 | 11 | - | 14 | - | 10 | - | 11 | - | 10 | - | 10 | - | 10 | - | 10.86 | 1.46 |
| 21. R.P. | M | 11 | 15 | - | 14 | - | 12 | - | 12 | - | 10 | - | 12 | - | 11 | - | 12.29 | 1.70 |
| 22. R.S.C. | F | 10 | 12 | - | 10 | - | 11 | - | 11 | - | 13 | - | 14 | - | 13 | - | 12.00 | 1.41 |
| 23. J.R.S. | M | 9 | - | 12 | - | 10 | - | 10 | - | 9 | - | 9 | - | 10 | - | 9 | 9.86 | 1.07 |
| 24. E.M.D.C. | F | 9 | 13 | - | 9 | - | 10 | - | 10 | - | 10 | - | 11 | - | 11 | - | 10.57 | 1.27 |
| 25. L.M.M. | F | 10 | 15 | - | 10 | - | 9 | - | 11 | - | 12 | - | 9 | - | 10 | - | 10.86 | 2.12 |
| 26. P.S.P. | M | 12 | - | 15 | - | 11 | - | 10 | - | 9 | - | 10 | - | 10 | - | 10 | 10.71 | 1.98 |
| 27. E.C.O. | M | 6 | 14 | - | 10 | - | 9 | - | 10 | - | 9 | - | 9 | - | 8 | - | 9.86 | 1.95 |
| 28. R.A.P. | M | 10 | 14 | - | 14 | - | 12 | - | 14 | - | 13 | - | 12 | - | 11 | - | 12.86 | 1.21 |
| 29. J.C.D. | F | 7 | 13 | - | 12 | - | 10 | - | 10 | - | 11 | - | 11 | - | 9 | - | 10.86 | 1.35 |
| 30. A.R. | M | 11 | 13 | - | 11 | - | 12 | - | 10 | - | 12 | - | 12 | - | 10 | - | 11.43 | 1.13 |
| 31. R.S.P.A. | M | 12 | - | 14 | - | 14 | - | 13 | - | 13 | - | 14 | - | 12 | - | 13 | 13.29 | 0.76 |
| 32. J.G.F.R. | M | 13 | - | 10 | - | 10 | - | 9 | - | 8 | - | 8 | - | 8 | - | 8 | 8.14 | 2.04 |
| 33. N.V.S. | M | 11 | 14 | - | 12 | - | 13 | - | 12 | - | 12 | - | 14 | - | 10 | - | 12.43 | 1.40 |
| 34. J.R.A. | M | 14 | 15 | - | 12 | - | 11 | - | 13 | - | 13 | - | 11 | - | 13 | - | 12.57 | 1.40 |
| 35. M.R.A. | F | 15 | - | 15 | - | 13 | - | 13 | - | 13 | - | 13 | - | 14 | - | 12 | 13.29 | 0.95 |
| $\bar{x}$ | | 11.00 | 13.03 | | 11.54 | | 11.00 | | 10.86 | | 11.03 | | 10.77 | | 10.46 | | | |
| $\delta$ | | 2.45 | 1.40 | | 1.52 | | 1.26 | | 1.31 | | 1.52 | | 1.40 | | 1.42 | | | |

[a] RE, right eye; LE, left eye; Pm, arithmetic mean; V, standard deviation

**Table 3.** Diurnal curve of pressure (DCPo) in 29 patients (48 eyes) with congenital glaucoma treated by surgery

| Patient | Sex | Age | Time 0600 | | 0900 | | 1200 | | 1500 | | 1800 | | 2100 | | 2400 | | Pm | | V | | Medication |
|---|---|---|---|---|---|---|---|---|---|---|---|---|---|---|---|---|---|---|---|---|---|
| | | | RE | LE[a] | RE | LE | RE | LE | RE | LE | RE | LE | RE | LE | RE | LE | RE | LE | RE | LE | |
| 1. A.M.F. | F | 8 | 11 | 11 | 14 | 15 | 17 | 12 | 15 | 12 | 14 | 13 | 13 | 12 | 12 | 13 | 13.71 | 12.57 | 1.98 | 1.27 | epilo 4% |
| 2. A.D.M. | M | 9 | 18 | 20 | 18 | 18 | 18 | 18 | 18 | 20 | 18 | 19 | 19 | 19 | 17 | 17 | 18.00 | 18.71 | 0.58 | 1.11 | epilo 4% |
| 3. B.J.F. | F | 13 | - | 19 | - | 24 | - | 28 | - | 34 | - | 32 | - | 37 | - | 32 | - | 29.43 | - | 6.21 | epinephrine 1% |
| 4. C.F.C. | F | 10 | 12 | 16 | 14 | 20 | 14 | 22 | 14 | 23 | 12 | 18 | 12 | 18 | 12 | 18 | 12.86 | 19.29 | 1.07 | 2.50 | - |
| 5. C.H.S. | M | 8 | 12 | 11 | 10 | 15 | 12 | 15 | 12 | 13 | 12 | 14 | 9 | 12 | 11 | 11 | 11.14 | 13.00 | 1.21 | 1.73 | - |
| 6. C.S.C. | M | 10 | 12 | 12 | 13 | 12 | 11 | 11 | 11 | 10 | 10 | 10 | 8 | 8 | 8 | 9 | 10.43 | 10.29 | 1.90 | 1.50 | - |
| 7. D.F.G. | F | 14 | 10 | 15 | 12 | 11 | 16 | 22 | 10 | 14 | 14 | 20 | 14 | 13 | 12 | 12 | 12.57 | 15.29 | 2.23 | 4.15 | epilo 2% |
| 8. E.G.K. | M | 6 | 14 | 13 | 12 | 15 | 12 | 15 | 11 | 13 | 12 | 22 | 12 | 23 | 10 | 16 | 11.86 | 16.71 | 1.21 | 4.11 | - |
| 9. E.G.P. | M | 13 | - | 11 | - | 21 | - | 29 | - | 26 | - | 23 | - | 28 | - | 14 | - | 21.71 | - | 6.92 | epilo 4% |
| 10. G.L.N.C. | M | 15 | 12 | - | 15 | - | 17 | - | 13 | - | 12 | - | 18 | - | 18 | - | 15.00 | - | 2.71 | - | epinephrine 1% |
| 11. G.O.L. | M | 15 | 10 | 10 | 14 | 14 | 16 | 16 | 14 | 16 | 14 | 15 | 16 | 16 | 12 | 13 | 13.57 | 14.29 | 1.99 | 2.21 | - |
| 12. H.G.B. | F | 10 | - | 13 | - | 17 | - | 17 | - | 16 | - | 13 | - | 15 | - | 14 | - | 15.00 | - | 1.73 | - |
| 13. H.L.O. | M | 10 | - | 11 | - | 11 | - | 13 | - | 12 | - | 10 | - | 11 | - | 12 | - | 11.86 | - | 1.35 | - |
| 14. J.Q.R. | M | 10 | - | 20 | - | 20 | - | 26 | - | 16 | - | 14 | - | 13 | - | 14 | - | 17.57 | - | 4.69 | - |
| 15. J.R.M. | M | 10 | - | 13 | - | 15 | - | 15 | - | 14 | - | 14 | - | 14 | - | 16 | - | 14.43 | - | 0.98 | - |
| 16. J.C.O. | F | 12 | 15 | 15 | 20 | 20 | 18 | 18 | 17 | 17 | 17 | 17 | 14 | 14 | 14 | 14 | 16.43 | 16.43 | 2.23 | 2.23 | - |
| 17. K.S.V. | F | 11 | 11 | - | 11 | - | 12 | - | 12 | - | 12 | - | 13 | - | 12 | - | 11.86 | - | 0.69 | - | - |
| 18. L.C.G. | M | 8 | 10 | 11 | 16 | 16 | 17 | 16 | 12 | 12 | 14 | 14 | 12 | 12 | 14 | 14 | 13.57 | 13.57 | 2.44 | 1.99 | - |
| 19. L.M.F.G. | F | 8 | 11 | 16 | 16 | 16 | 14 | 14 | 8 | 10 | 12 | 12 | 10 | 12 | 10 | 11 | 11.57 | 13.00 | 2.70 | 2.38 | - |
| 20. M.A.R. | F | 12 | 12 | 14 | 13 | 14 | 12 | 16 | 14 | 18 | 12 | 14 | 10 | 16 | 12 | 16 | 12.14 | 15.43 | 1.21 | 1.51 | epilo 2% |
| 21. M.C.G. | F | 14 | 17 | 11 | 16 | 9 | 15 | 18 | 16 | 18 | 15 | 19 | 14 | 18 | 16 | 12 | 15.57 | 16.43 | 0.98 | 3.41 | epilo 2% |
| 22. M.C.S.B. | F | 11 | 8 | 17 | 8 | 12 | 7 | 14 | 6 | 12 | 5 | 15 | 5 | 13 | 6 | 14 | 6.43 | 13.86 | 1.27 | 1.77 | - |
| 23. M.D.S. | F | 14 | 12 | 16 | 12 | 18 | 18 | 17 | 18 | 17 | 16 | 16 | 15 | 16 | 16 | 14 | 15.29 | 16.29 | 2.50 | 1.25 | epinephrine 1% |
| 24. O.A.M. | F | 8 | 8 | 10 | 22 | 18 | 26 | 16 | 20 | 12 | 24 | 16 | 20 | 12 | 12 | 8 | 18.86 | 13.14 | 6.52 | 3.63 | - |
| 25. R.V. | F | 14 | 15 | 15 | 18 | 16 | 14 | 12 | 16 | 10 | 16 | 12 | 14 | 14 | 20 | 12 | 16.14 | 13.00 | 2.19 | 2.08 | RE- epilo 2% – LE- |
| 26. S.R. | M | 11 | - | 9 | - | 12 | - | 15 | - | 15 | - | 16 | - | 16 | - | 15 | - | 14.00 | - | 2.58 | - |
| 27. S.E.S. | M | 11 | - | 12 | - | 14 | - | 14 | - | 14 | - | 15 | - | 10 | - | 8 | - | 12.43 | - | 2.57 | - |
| 28. V.R.L. | F | 8 | 16 | 16 | 15 | 16 | 12 | 16 | 16 | 16 | 14 | 15 | 10 | 14 | 12 | 14 | 13.57 | 15.29 | 2.30 | 0.95 | - |
| 29. W.R.A. | M | 9 | 18 | 10 | 16 | 11 | 14 | 8 | 12 | 8 | 16 | 8 | 14 | 8 | 12 | 8 | 14.57 | 8.71 | 2.23 | 1.25 | RE- epinephrine 1% LE |
| $\bar{x}$ | | 10.76 | 13.15 | | 15.31 | | 15.94 | | 14.65 | | 14.94 | | 14.29 | | 13.31 | | | | | | |
| δ | | 2.46 | 3.08 | | 3.39 | | 4.53 | | 4.74 | | 4.36 | | 5.22 | | 4.01 | | | | | | |

[a] RE, right eye; LE, left eye; Pm, arithmetic mean; V, standard deviation

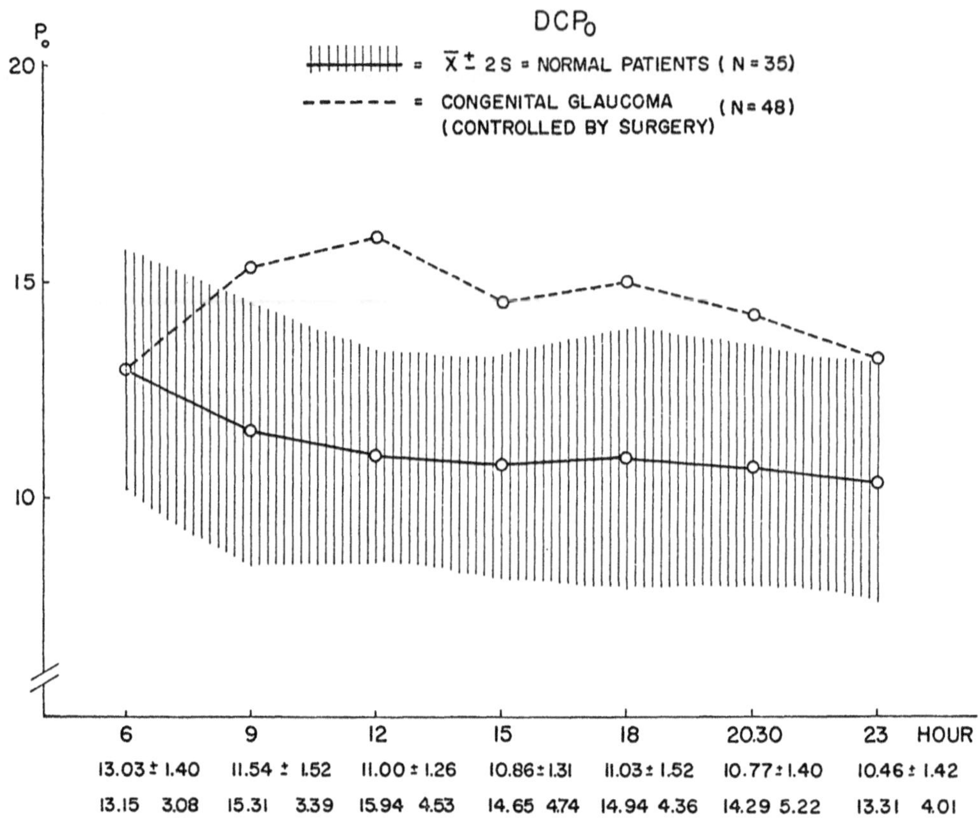


**Fig. 1.** (See text)

of the measurement as the abscissa. The mean value of Po in both groups was plotted in this graph (in the normal group we plotted also the normal range of variation as $\bar{x} \pm 2s$). Under each hour when a measurement was taken, we have given the corresponding values (mean ± standard deviation) of both groups for that hour.

We obtained astonishing results: whereas in the normal group (as indeed in patients with primary glaucoma) the most common highest value of Po was at 6 a.m. in bed, in the CG group the highest value was at 12 (noon). There was also a big difference in lowest values: In the normal group it occurred at midnight but in the CG group it was at 6 a.m. for the great majority of the eyes. Figures 2 and 3 emphasize the differences between the two samples, but here instead of the value of Po at the ordinate we have entered the frequency percentage of the incidence of maximal and minimal values of Po in each hour of measurement.

At 6 a.m., the patterns showed by the two groups were reversed, that is, in the normal group the highest value of Po, statistically obtained, occurred at 6 a.m., while in the CG group the lowest value of Po, likewise statistically obtained, also occurred at 6 a.m. In the normal group, the highest values of Po were clustered around 6 a.m.; in the CG group, the highest values of Po were much more distributed around the clock.

We believe these findings to be significant, but at same time we admit that we do not have any explanation for them. More data need to be obtained not only from our clinic but also from other glaucoma clinics in different countries.

Our findings are obviously quite different from those of Thiel (1930) and Pau (1952).

## Conclusions

1. The DCP$_0$ of eyes with CG treated by surgery is different from the DCPo of normal

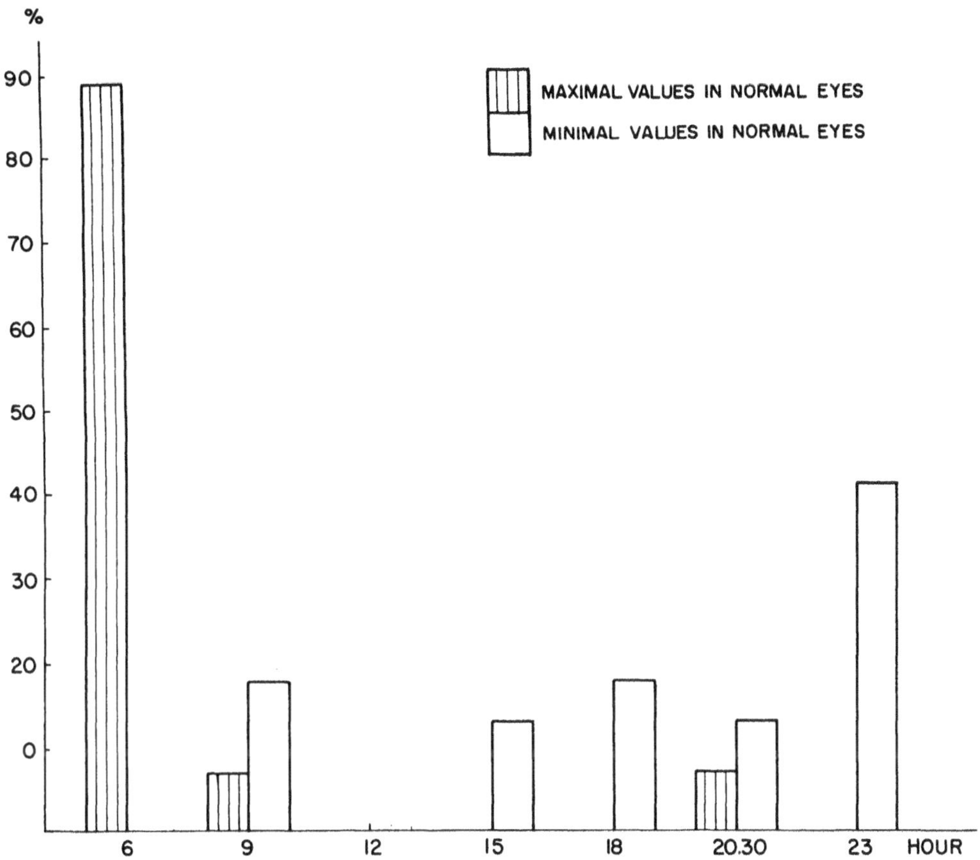


**Fig. 2.** (See text)

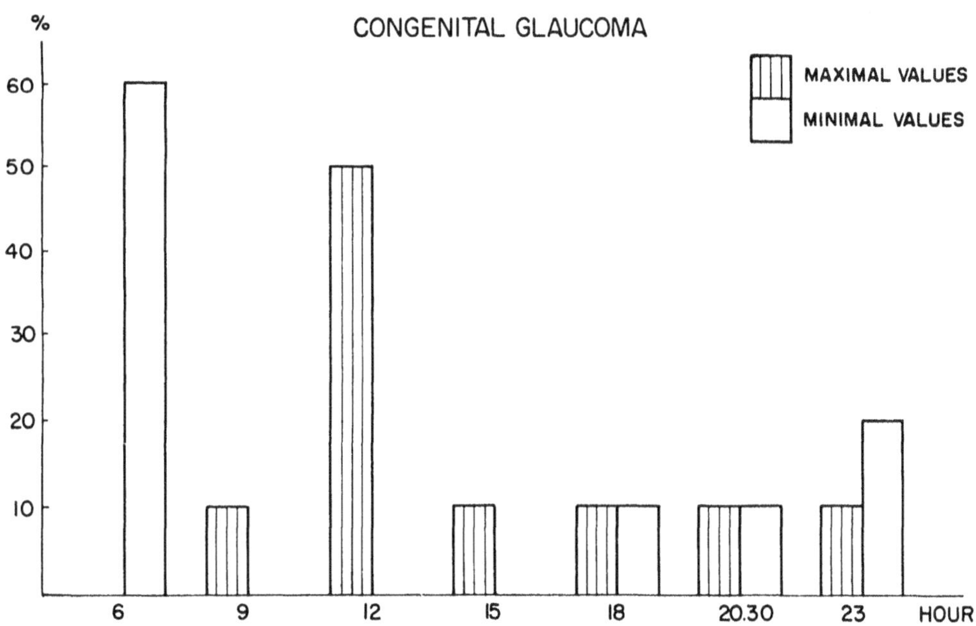


**Fig. 3.** (See text)

eyes in the same age-group, according to our findings.

2. At 6 a.m., we measured the highest value of Po in the normal group and the lowest value of Po in the CG group.

3. The highest value of the Po in the CG group was at about noon and the range of the maximal values was more diverse than in the normal group.

4. We do not have an explanation for the different patterns of the two groups.

## References


1. Calixto N, e Cronemberger S° S (1981) Curva Diária de Pressão Intraocular no Glaucoma Congênito. Rev Bras Oftalmol 40:284–290
2. Pau H (1952) Augendruckschwankungen beim kindlichen Glaukom. Klin Monatsbl Augenheilkd 118:468–471
3. Sampaolesi R (1961) Semiologia del glaucoma: tonometria, curvas tensionales diarias. Congresso Argentino de Oftalmologia, Rosario, Relato Oficial Vol I 289–294
4. Thiel R (1930) Der Hydrophthalmus, Buphthalmus. In: Schiek und Brückner (Hrsg) Kurzes Handbuch der Ophthalmologie. Band IV. Springer, Berlin Heidelberg, S 828–842

Krieglstein G.K./Leydhecker W. (eds)
Glaucoma Update II
© Springer-Verlag 1983

# Visual Sensitivity to Intraocular Pressure

M.E. Langham, Baltimore

A central problem of glaucoma that remains unresolved is the nature of the relations between intraocular pressure (IOP), the ocular vascular perfusion pressure, and the development of irreversible loss of vision. The complexity of this problem is reflected in the wide disparity in the susceptibility of the visual system to increased IOP. The difficulty in deciding whether a patient with ocular hypertension is in danger of visual loss is matched by the paradox of the low tension glaucoma patient who continues to lose vision in spite of an apparent well controlled IOP. In this paper I will describe new approaches to define the visual response of human subjects to sustained change in the ocular perfusion pressure including measurement of the visual response to transient experimentally induced increments of intraocular pressure.

The methodology used in these studies comprised objective hemodynamic and visual measurements. First, the ocular perfusion pressure was measured using a modification of the procedure described by Langham and To'mey [1] and Langham, Preziosi and To'mey [2]. This procedure uses the Langham pneumatic tonometer to measure the relationship between pulse amplitude and intraocular pressure (PA/IOP relation). In order to simplify recording and analysis of the pulsatile component of the intraocular pressure, a new instrument was developed in collaboration with Digilab Laboratories (Cambridge, Mass. U.S.A.) which included a 2 channel recorder for separating the intraocular pressure pulse recordings from the steady state intraocular pressure printed digitally (Fig. 1); this OCVM system is now available commercially. The OCVM includes a modified scleral suction cup system controlled by a motor driven syringe for increasing stepwise the intraocular pressure. The visual response was measured using the Heijl-Krakau automatic perimeter [3-5].

The intraocular pressure pulses and the PA/IOP relations are identical in pairs of eyes of normal subjects of all ages (Fig. 1). In young subjects, the PA/IOP relation is sigmoid in form, whereas in older patients the form of the relationship is sometimes hyperbolic [1]; this latter form is characteristic of eyes with relative ischemia, such as in patients with moderate stenosis of the internal carotid artery [2].

The PA/IOP curve is bounded at its lower limit by the intraocular pressure and at its upper limit by the ciliary arterial systolic pressure. The difference between these two pressures is the ocular perfusion pressure. It is to be noted that the intraocular pulse is generated by the ciliary arterial circulation and that the measurement of the ophthalmic arterial pressure by this procedure differs from that of traditional retinal arterial ophthaldynamometry. When the IOP is increased sufficiently to extinguish the pulse, vision fades sequentially inwards from the periphery and blood flow to both the retinal and ciliary arteries ceases.

Major changes in the form of the PA/IOP relation are present in patients with unilateral and bilateral stenoses of the internal carotid arteries [2]. A representative example of the PA/IOP relations in pairs of eyes of a patient with a unilateral occlusion of the internal carotid artery is shown in Fig. 2. In this representative patient, the ophthalmic arterial pressures were 78 mmHg and 27 mmHg in the eyes contralateral and ipsilateral to the stenotic artery, respectively. The corresponding ocular perfusion pressure were 57 and 11 mmHg.

Patients with severe stenosis of one internal carotid artery provided an excellent opportunity to determine the visual response to a sustained large unilateral decrease of the ocular perfusion pressure. This was studied in

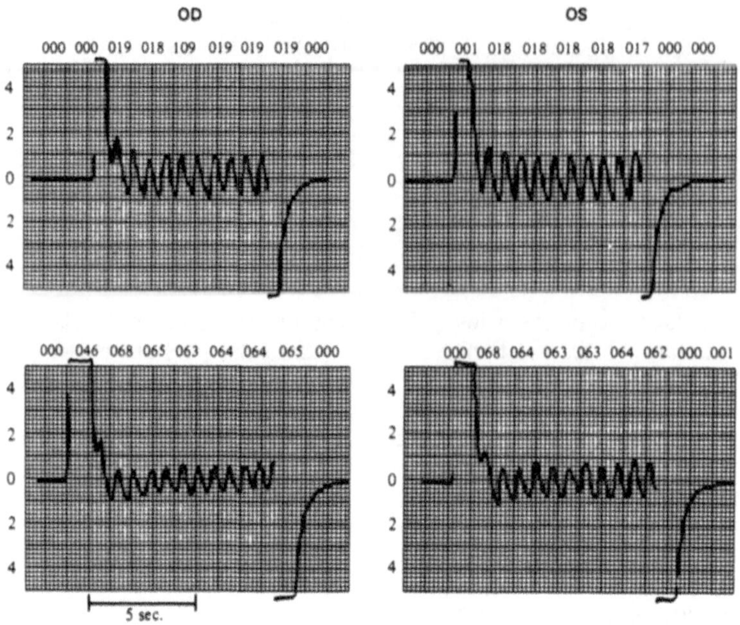


**Fig. 1.** Representative recordings of the intraocular pressure pulses and the digital print-out of the mean intraocular pressure in pairs of eyes of a normal subject using the Langham OCVM instrument. The *ordinate* gives the *amplitude* of the intraocular pressure pulse; *absence* of pulse is shown by the *zero line*. The intraocular pressure is averaged over successive 2 sec intervals and printed at the corresponding time interval. **(a)** and **(b)** are recordings on the left and right eyes prior to and after the intraocular pressure had been increased using a scleral suction cup

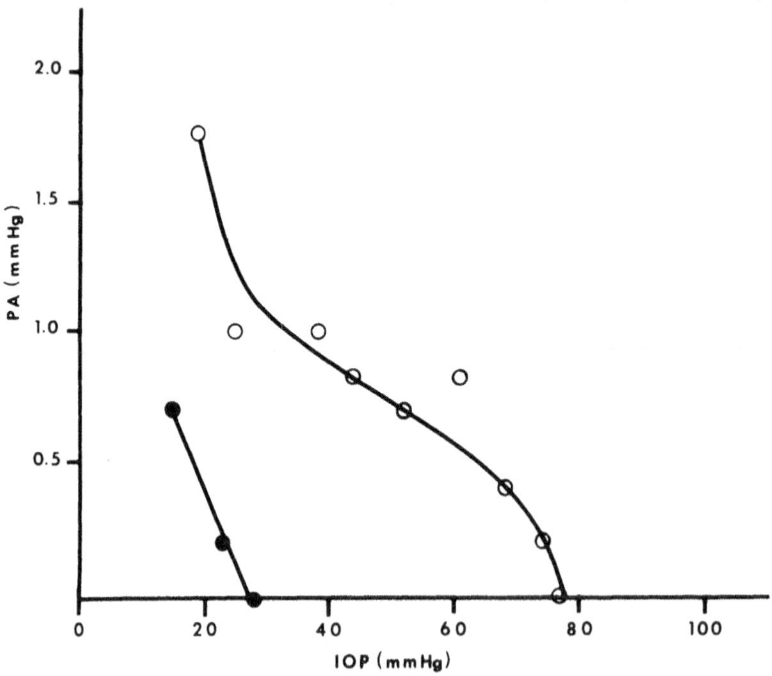


**Fig. 2.** The PA/IOP relations in the eyes of a patient with severe unilateral stenosis of the right internal carotid artery. ○--○ and ●--● are the PA/IOP relations in the non affected and affected eyes, respectively

**Table 1.** Comparsion of the visual performance index (VPI) in pairs of eyes of patients with severe unilateral or bilateral stenoses of the internal carotid arteries. Intraocular pressure (IOP), brachial arterial pressure (BrAP), Ophthalmic arterial pressure (OAP), and ocular perfusion pressure (OPP) are recorded in mmHg. % Stenosis are values for the right and left internal carotid arteries based on arteriographic studies

| IOP | | BrAP | OAP | | OPP | | VPI | | % Stenosis | |
|---|---|---|---|---|---|---|---|---|---|---|
| O.D. | O.S. | | O.D. | O.S. | O.D. | O.S. | O.D. | O.S. | Rt. | Lt. |
| 17 | 14 | 148/74 | 75 | 46 | 58 | 32 | 399 | 422 | 0 | 50 |
| 14 | 10 | 160/90 | 90 | 42 | 76 | 32 | 467 | 522 | 0 | 100 |
| 13 | 14 | 110/60 | 70 | 40 | 57 | 26 | 366 | 374 | 30 | 95 |
| 18 | 11 | 184/82 | 80 | 28 | 62 | 17 | 455 | 410 | 15 | 95 |
| 15 | 13 | 120/80 | 35 | 45 | 20 | 32 | 415 | 410 | 75 | 90 |
| 11 | 12 | 125/68 | 45 | 55 | 34 | 43 | 410 | 400 | 75 | 75 |

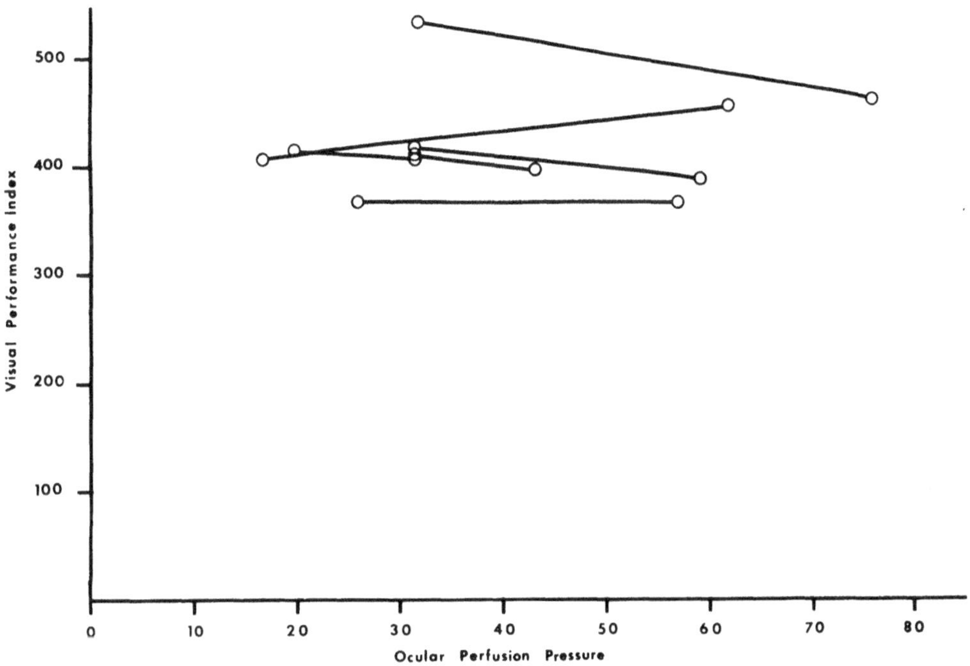


**Fig. 3.** The visual performance indices in pairs or eyes of patients with either unilateral or bilateral severe stenoses of the internal carotid arteries. The results on pairs of eyes are represented by the 2 *circles* joined by the connecting *straight line.* The visual performance (central field) was measured using Heijl-Krakau automatic perimeter (screening program)

six patients and the results are summarized in Table 1 and Fig. 3. The vision and ocular hemodynamic studies were completed prior to the radiological studies, which confirmed the presence of a severe stenosis in one or both internal carotid arteries. In all patients the visual performances in the central field were similar to those found in patients of similar age without cervical arterial occlusive disease. Furthermore, the visual performances in pairs of eyes were similar in spite of the very large difference in the ocular perfusion pressures. In 2 patients with severe bilateral stenoses of the internal carotid ar-

**Table 2.** The visual response to a transient increase of intraocular pressure in normal and glaucoma patients. VPI (I) and VPI (II) are the visual performance indices in the undisturbed eye (I) and in the same eyes with the IOP increased to 50 mmHg

| Parameter | Normals | Glaucoma |
|---|---|---|
| IOP | 14.9 ± 0.74 (7) | 21.3 ± 1.34 (10) |
| OAP | 78 ± 2.5 (7) | 92 ± 3.6 (10) |
| BrAP (systolic) | 122 ± 3.2 (7) | 144 ± 6.3 (10) |
| BrAP (diastolic) | 77 ± 1.8 (7) | 86 ± 3.1 (10) |
| VPI (I) | 473 ± 10.7 (7) | 374 ± 38.6 (10) |
| VPI (II) | 477 ± 10.1 (7) | 264 ± 43.8 (10) |
| I - II | -4 ± 7.5 (7) | 110 ± 26.6 (10) |

teries and corresponding very large decreases of the ocular perfusion pressures, the visual performances were normal.

No abnormalities in the form of the PA/IOP relation and no abnormalities of the ocular perfusion pressures were found in 10 patients with open angle glaucoma (Table 2). In individual patients the form of the PA/IOP relations in pairs of eyes were closely similar even when there was a marked difference in visual loss between pairs of eyes.

Establishment of the PA/IOP relation and the ocular perfusion pressure provided the basis to the analysis of the visual sensitivity to intraocular pressure (Fig. 4). The quantitative automatic central visual field perimeter developed by Krakau and his colleagues [3–5] was used to measure the visual response to transient experimentally induced increased intraocular pressure in normal and glaucoma subjects. The protocol of this study was to measure the visual response of the central field in the undisturbed eye and then to repeat the study with the intraocular pressure increased to approximately 50 mmHg using the scleral suction cup system. Finally, the test was repeated after removal of the cup from the eye to determine the time course of the recovery of vision. No major technical problem was found in the application of this procedure to normal and glaucoma patients.

In normal subjects the visual performance was unaffected when the intraocular pressure was increased from its normal average value of 15 mmHg to a mean value of 50 to 60

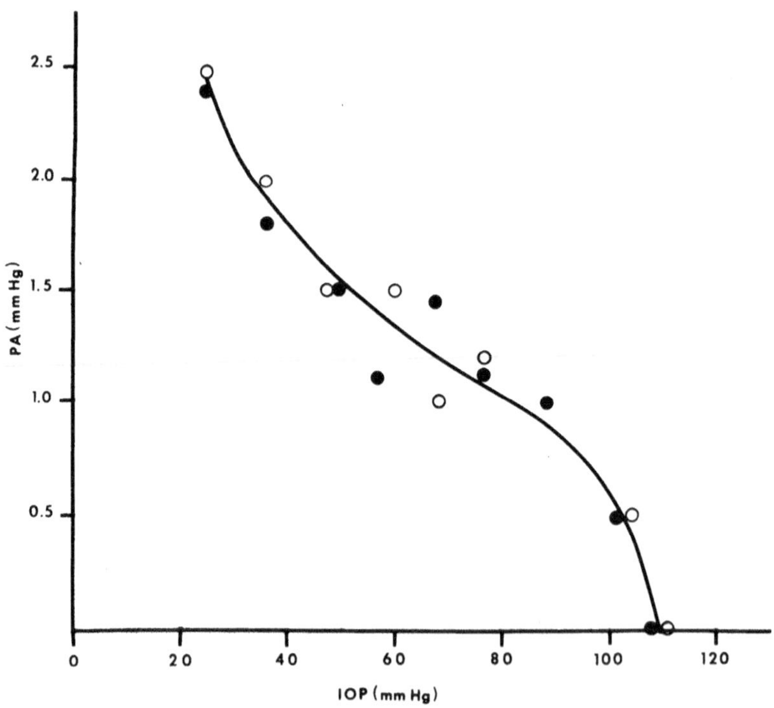


**Fig. 4.** The PA/IOP relation in left (○--○) and right (●--●) eyes of a glaucomatous patient

mmHg. This increased intraocular pressure corresponded to a decrease of 50 to 60% of the ocular perfusion pressure.

The stability of the visual performance to increased intraocular pressure in normal subjects was not found in patients with either open angle glaucoma or low tension glaucoma. The results of visual performance in 10 randomly chosen glaucoma patients are summarized in Table 2. All patients were either under medical therapy or treatment had been discontinued 2 weeks prior to this study. None of the patients were under treatment with a miotic drug. The visual performances in the undisturbed eyes of the glaucoma eyes was less than in nonglaucoma patients. In 7 of the 10 patients the visual performance decreased significantly when the intraocular pressure was increased to an average of 50 mmHg; in the remaining three patients the visual performance remained unchanged at the increased IOP. These findings are consitent with the studies of Gaffner and Goldmann [6], Harington [7], and Drance [8] that the retinal sensitivity of some glaucomatous eyes decreased with transient increase of intraocular pressure.

The loss of retinal sensitivity with increased intraocular pressure in the glaucomatous eyes was unrelated to the level of the ocular perfusion pressure. In individual patients with unequal glaucomatous damage in pairs of eyes and asymmetry of visual loss, the visual response to increased intraocular pressure was greatest in the more affected eye. However, in the same patients the PA/IOP relations and the ocular perfusion pressures were identical in pairs of eyes.

The conclusion from these observations that the ocular perfusion pressure is not the critical parameter determining the visual loss to increased intraocular pressure in the glaucomatous patient was supported by comparison of the results in normal and glaucoma patients. In the group of 10 glaucoma patients the average ophthalmic arterial systolic pressure and the ocular perfusion pressure exceeded those in normal eyes (Table 2). Nevertheless, when the intraocular pressure in normal and glaucomatous eyes were increased to similar levels, the loss of retinal sensitivity occurred only in the glaucoma group.

More drammatic evidence that the ocular perfusion pressure was not the critical parameter determining the visual loss to increased intraocular pressure was documented in individual patients with low tension glaucoma. In one such patient the intraocular pressure was 16.5 mmHg in both eyes. The PA/IOP curves were identical in the two eyes, and the ophthalmic arterial pressure was 100 mmHg in both eyes (Fig. 5). The glaucomatous damage and field loss were more severe in the right eye; the visual performance indices in the undisturbed eyes were

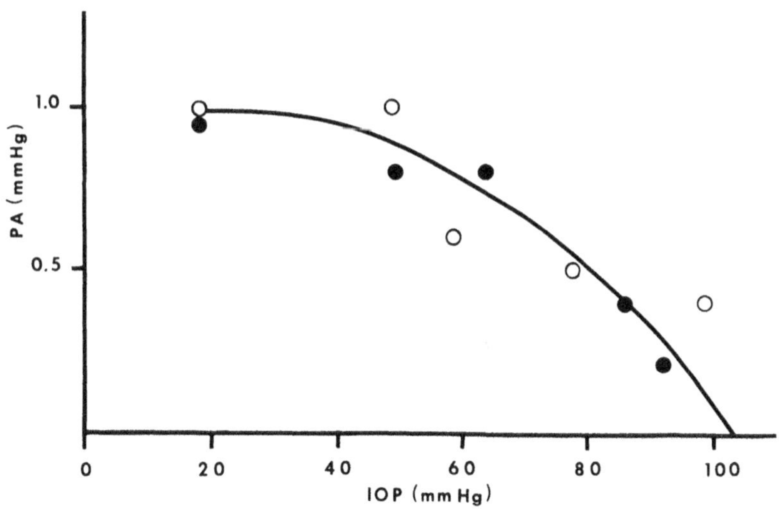


**Fig. 5.** The PA/IOP relation in the right (O--O) and left (●--●) eyes of a patient with low tension glaucoma (see text). The visual loss was more severe in the right eye (Fig. 6)

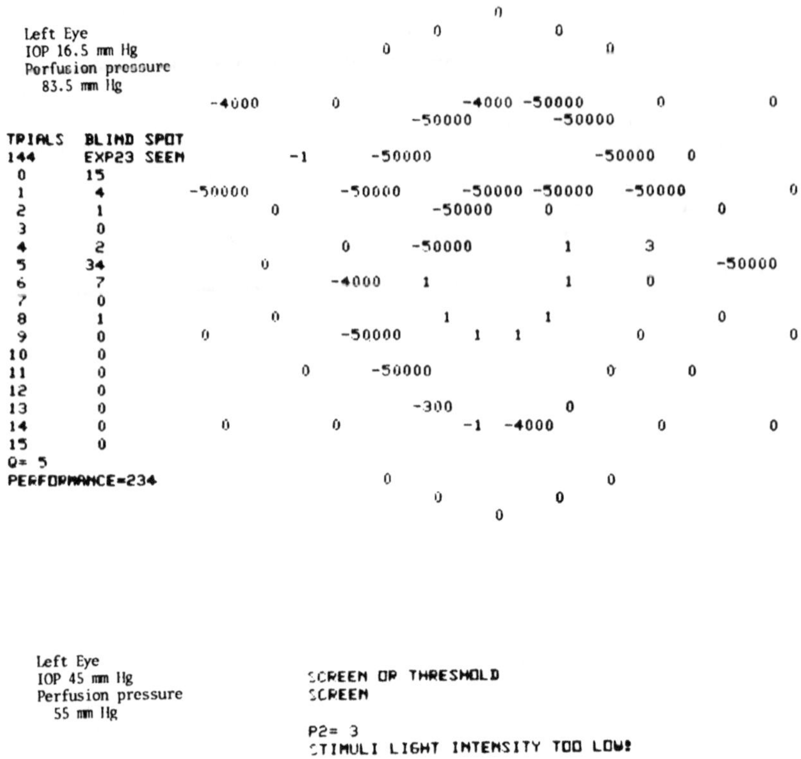


**Fig. 6.** The central visual field and the visual performance index on the right eye of a patient with low tension glaucoma recorded at an intraocular pressure of 16.5 mmHg. At an experimentally induced intraocular pressure of 45 mmHg the visual performance index became zero within 2 min. In the contralateral eye, the visual performance index was 423 at 16.5 mmHg and 167 at an intraocular pressure of 45 mmHg

234 (O.D.) and 423 (O.S.). In the right eye the visual performance decreased to zero within 1 to 2 min when the intraocular pressure was 45 mmHg (Fig. 6); in the left eye the visual performance decreased to 167 at the same intraocular pressure. After removal of the scleral suction cup the visual performances recovered to 230 (O.D.) and 435 (O.S.).

The rapid onset and reversibility of the visual loss to increased intraocular pressure in glaucomatous eyes makes it highly probable that the mechanism is due to a localized ischemia. In this respect there are two principal physiologic functions of the ocular vascular circulation [9]. The first is to provide blood flow to the tissues within the eye. The finding that the PA/IOP relation, the ophthalmic arterial pressure, and the ocular perfusion pressure in glaucomatous eyes were not impaired indicates that changes in blood flow within the eye were not the cause of the visual sensitivity to increased IOP. The second function of the ocular circulation is to provide blood flow to the scleral envelope and to the neurons passing through the scleral foramen. The collagenous septae bridging the scleral foramen provide the framework and support for the microcirculatory vessels. These septae and the attached vessels are under the influence of the compression force exerted by the intraocular pressure and are also influenced by the stretching forces induced by the circumferential tension within the scleral shell. The present findings point strongly to this specific cribosal region as the site for ischemia to develop and that this ischemia causes the visual loss at increased pressure. It is pertinent to note that a similar pressure sensitivity of intrascleral vessels in the anterior segment to small compression forces in glaucomatous eyes was observed some years ago by Langham and Maumenee [10].

## References

1. Langham ME, To'mey KF (1978) A clinical procedure for the measurements of the ocular pulse/pressure relation and the ophthalmic arterial pressure. Exp Eye Res 27:17–25
2. Langham ME, To'mey KF, Preziosi TJ (1981) Carotid occlusive disease: effect of complete occlusion of internal carotid artery on intraocular pulse/pressure relation and on ophthalmic arterial pressure. Stroke 12:759–765
3. Heijl A, Krakau CET (1975) An automatic static perimeter, design and pilot study. Acta Ophthalmol (Copenh) 53:293–310
4. Heijl A, Krakau CET (1975) An automatic perimeter for glaucoma visual field screening and control. Construction and clinical cases. Albrecht Von Graefes Arch Klin Ophthalmol 197:13–23
5. Krakau CET (1978) Aspects on the design of an automatic perimeter. Acta Ophthalmol (Copenh) 56:389–405
6. Gaffner F, Goldmann H (1965) Experimentelle Untersuchungen über den Zusammenhang von Augendrucksteigerung und Gesichtsfeldschädigung. Ophthalmologica 130: 357–377
7. Harington DO (1960) Pathogenesis of the glaucomatous visual field defect. In: Newell FW (ed) Glaucoma, Transactions of the Fifth Conference. Josiah Macy Jr. Foundation, New York, pp 259–310
8. Drance SM (1962) Studies in the susceptibility of the eye to raised intraocular pressure. Arch Ophthalmol 68:478–485
9. Langham ME (1980) The temporal relation between intraocular pressure and loss of vision in chronic simple glaucoma. Glaucoma 2:427–435
10. Langham ME, Maumenee AE (1964) The diagnosis and treatment of glaucoma based on a new procedure for the measurement of intraocular dynamics. Trans Am Acad Ophthalmol Otolaryngol, pp 277–302

## Discussion

**Yablonski to Langham:** In 1979 I reported [1] that experiments in cats showed that the lamina cribrosa could easily be bowed back as a function of the hydrostatic pressure difference across the lamina cribrosa. The intracranial pressure which is transmitted down the optic nerve sheath to the area behind the lamina cribrosa and the intraocular pressure in front of the lamina cribrosa were independently altered. Increasing the difference between intraocular pressure and intracranial pressure by only 10 mmHg yielded definite distortion of the lamina cribrosa. Therefore it is apparent that the lamina cribrosa is quite flexible and its movement may account for the reversible cupping shown by Dr. Spaeth and for the pathophysiology of glaucomatous optic nerve head damage described by Dr. Quigley.

1. Yablonski ME, Ritch R, Pokorny KS (1979) Effect of decreased intracranial pressure on optic disc. ARVO [Abstr], p 165

Krieglstein G.K./Leydhecker W. (eds)
Glaucoma Update II


# Ultrasonographic Echometry in the Control of Congenital Glaucoma

C.A. de Carvalho and A.J. Betinjane, São Paulo

Ocular echometry is of greatest clinical significance in children, in whom the most significant changes in the dimensions of the different ocular structures occur. Ocular echometry, therefore, has particular value in the diagnosis and assessment of surgical therapy effectiveness in congenital glaucoma. In spite of the essential significance of tonometry by applanation in the clinical study of the disease, echometry allows for invaluable information as to the magnitude of the pathologic effects induced by an abnormal intraocular pressure in a given time interval. Echometry, therefore, can provide an assessment of the dynamics and magnitude of ocular changes caused by an anomalous intraocular pressure in eyes with congenital glaucoma.

A survey of the literature does not reveal many ultrasonographic echometric studies of congenital glaucoma. The authors of the present communication have found some biometric aspects in previous studies that are worthy of mention: (1) The echometric values of the anterior chamber, vitreous space, and total axial length of the eyeball are higher in eyes with congenital glaucoma than in normal eyes of any age-group; (2) both in normal eyes and in those with congenital glaucoma, the total axial length of the eyeball is an expression of the variations that take place in the axial length of the vitreous space.

The purpose of this paper is to study the variations in total axial length in eyes with congenital glaucoma in different age-groups, according to intraocular pressure levels observed postoperatively.

## Subjects and Method

This study considered 98 eyes with congenital glaucoma (group G) and 36 normal eyes (group N), which were used as a control group. The 98 eyes of group G comprised 74 patients of up to 15 years of age and including both sexes (41 males and 33 females). With regard to race, 68 were white, five black, and one oriental. The patients had definite congenital glaucoma diagnosed by means of applanation tonometry, biomicroscopy, gonioscopy, refraction, and in some cases ophthalmoscopic studies. All patients with congenital glaucoma were submitted to antiglaucomatous surgery (goniotomy, trabeculotomy, or trabeculotomy in association with concomitant trabeculectomy), or to more than one surgical procedure in some instances. The data in this report were collected in examinations that took place before or after such surgery.

Both the eyes with congenital glaucoma and the normal ones were divided into age-groups, as listed in Table 1. Eyes with congenital glaucoma (group G) were further subdivided into subgroups according to the levels of intraocular pressure after surgery. The congenital glaucoma was considered controlled (subgroup Gc) when intraocular pressure values were equal to a maximum of 15 mmHg; it was considered "suspect" of not being controlled (subgroup Gs) when intraocular pressure values ranged from 16 to 20 mmHg; and it was considered noncontrolled (subgroup Gnc) when intraocular pressure values were higher than 20 mmHg.

**Table 1.** Age-groups of subjects in the study

| Age-group | Number of eyes | |
|---|---|---|
| | Normal | Congenital glaucoma |
| I Up to 1 year | 10 | 16 |
| II 1-2 years | 8 | 10 |
| III 2-5 years | 7 | 23 |
| IV 6-10 years | 5 | 34 |
| V 11-15 years | 6 | 15 |

**Table 2.** Axial length in normal eyes and eyes with congenital glaucoma

| Age (years) | Normal (N) | | | Congenital glaucoma (G) | | | | | | | | |
|---|---|---|---|---|---|---|---|---|---|---|---|---|
| | | | | Controlled (Gc) | | | „Suspect“ (Gs) | | | Noncontrolled (Gnc) | | |
| | No. of eyes | Mean age | Axial length | No. of eyes | Mean age | Axial length | No. of eyes | Mean age | Axial length | No. of eyes | Mean age | Axial length |
| < 1 | 10 | 6 mo[a] | 19.64 ± 0.57 | 6 | 7 mo | 21.55 ± 0.63 | 4 | 5.7 mo | 23.40 ± 2.54 | 6 | 5.5 mo | 23.39 ± 1.20 |
| 1–2 | 8 | 1 y 3 mo | 20.79 ± 0.49 | 4 | 1 y 3 mo | 22.60 ± 0.54 | 3 | 1 y 2 mo | 24.77 ± 1.20 | 3 | 1 y 5 mo | 24.48 ± 0.79 |
| 2–5 | 7 | 3 y | 21.97 ± 0.55 | 15 | 3 y | 24.45 ± 1.55 | 5 | 3 y 2 mo | 25.04 ± 2.50 | 3 | 3 y 3 mo | 26.36 ± 1.34 |
| 6–10 | 5 | 7 y | 22.45 ± 1.12 | 18 | 7 y 3 mo | 24.75 ± 1.79 | 11 | 7 y 3 mo | 25.15 ± 2.86 | 5 | 6 y 8 mo | 26.84 ± 2.03 |
| 11–15 | 6 | 13 y | 23.40 ± 0.28 | 3 | 11 y 7 mo | 24.91 ± 0.60 | 9 | 12 y 2 mo | 25.90 ± 1.36 | 3 | 12 y | 26.43 ± 2.25 |

[a] mo, months; y, years

Method "A" ultrasonographic ocular biometry was performed in all eyes included in the study. A Kretz 7200 MA echograph model with an 8-MHz probe was employed used. A scleral shell was used (Ossoinig Scleral Shell, manufactured by Hansen Ophthalmic Development Laboratory, Iowa City, USA), filled with saline solution for immersion of the probe. Sound power ranged from 48 to 52 dB. We used a polaroid camera coupled to the echograph and always took two to three pictures of each eye. The initial values were obtained in microseconds and later converted into millimeters by taking into account the velocity of ultrasound in the various transparent media of the eye.

Echometry was performed under general anesthesia (methoxifluorane) in the younger children. The examination was done under local anesthesia of the external segment of the eyeball on those children who either were old enough or who showed the necessary willingness to undergo such an examination.

For the statistical evaluation, we used a variance analysis to a 5% level of significance to compare values of the total axial length in normal eyes (group N) to corresponding values in eyes with congenital glaucoma (controlled, "suspect", and noncontrolled subgroups). When there was statistical significance, the Scheffé test (at 5% level) was employed to check which values were statistically different from each other.

## Results

Table 2 shows the mean values and standard deviations of the axial length obtained in different age-groups, both in normal eyes and in those with congenital glaucoma (controlled, "suspect," and noncontrolled subgroups). Figure 1 illustrates our findings in normal eyes and in the three congenital glaucoma subgroups.

Table 3 shows the result of the Scheffé test to a 5% level of significance. It can be seen that in spite of normal postoperative intraocular pressure in the controlled congenital glaucoma eyes (Gc), the axial lengths of normal eyes were significantly different in age-groups I, II, and III, but were not significantly different in age-groups IV and V. The same was observed for the axial length of normal eyes, which were also significantly different from "suspect" congenital glaucoma eyes (Gs) in all age-groups, with the exception of age-group IV. On the other hand, normal eyes were significantly different from the noncontrolled congenital glaucoma subgroup (Gnc) in every one of the five age-groups. The test also showed non significantly different values for the axial length of the three congenital glaucoma subgroups (Gc, Gs, and Gnc) when each of them was testing against the other.

## Discussion

To characterize biometric values in eyes with congenital glaucoma, it is necessary to know the corresponding values in the normal eye as well as its physiologic changes. This has been done by the present authors and by others in the literature reviewed.

With regard to the axial length values in eyes with congenital glaucoma, one can

**Table 3.** Comparison between the axial lengths of normal eyes and eyes with congenital glaucoma

| | Age-group | | | | |
|---|---|---|---|---|---|
| Comparison | I | II | III | IV | V |
| N and Gc[a] | Significant | Significant | Significant | Nonsignificant | Nonsignificant |
| N and Gs | Significant | Significant | Significant | Nonsignificant | Significant |
| N and Gnc | Significant | Significant | Significant | Significant | Significant |
| Gc and Gs | Nonsignificant | Nonsignificant | Nonsignificant | Nonsignificant | Nonsignificant |
| Gc and Gnc | Nonsignificant | Nonsignificant | Nonsignificant | Nonsignificant | Nonsignificant |
| Gs and Gnc | Nonsignificant | Nonsignificant | Nonsignificant | Nonsignificant | Nonsignificant |

[a] N, normal; G, congenital glaucoma; Gc, controlled congenital claucoma; Gs, "suspect" congenital glaucoma; Gnc, noncontrolled congenital glaucoma
[b] $\Delta\alpha$, value found in the Scheffé test ($\alpha = 5\%$)

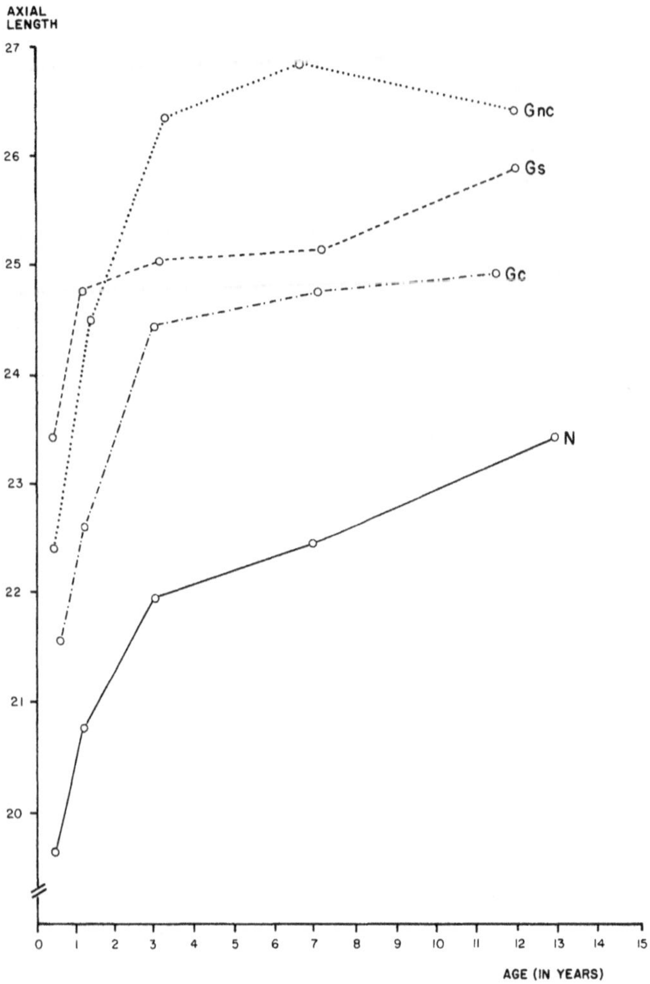


**Fig. 1.** Age of patients and axial length in normal eyes (*N*) and eyes with controlled (*Gc*), "suspect" (*Gs*), and noncontrolled (*Gnc*) congenital glaucoma

observe that those eyes classified in subgroups Gs ("suspect") and Gnc (noncontrolled) showed higher values than the corresponding values in subgroup Gc (controlled) in all age-groups (Table 2). Through the Scheffé test it was possible to observe that the axial length of eyes in subgroups Gc (controlled), Gs ("suspect"), and Gnc (noncontrolled) were statistically different from the corresponding normal values in age-groups I–III. After the age of 5 years (age-groups IV and V) the eyes of subgroup Gc (controlled) started to show axial length values similar to those of normal eyes. Conversely, the eyes of subgroup Gnc (noncontrolled) continued to show statistically higher values than the corresponding normal values, even for the older age-groups. Although "suspect" eyes (Gs) had shown values similar to normal eyes in age-group IV, axial length values were again statistically higher than those of normal eyes in age-group V (Table 3).

The undoubtedly interesting results cited above might be interpreted as a consequence of the very features of the pathology under study: The pathologic increase in the axial length, which takes place in the first years of life in congenital glaucoma, is of such a magnitude that the value reached remains abnormal even if the intraocular pressure returns to normal. However, after a given age (usually about 5 years), those eyes with surgically controlled intraocular pressure would tend to have an axial length similar to that in normal eyes. Eyes with persitent pathologic intraocular pressure will maintain an abnormal growth due to the continued presence of the pathologic growth factor (high intraocular pressure), a situation that could remain until the age of approximately 15 years.

On the other hand, by comparing axial length among subgroups Gc (controlled), Gs ("suspect"), and Gnc (noncontrolled), we can observe that there is no statistically significant difference in any of the age-groups studied (Table 3). This could also be interpreted as a consequence of the very features of the pathology responsible for the disease. Thus, the pathologic increase in the axial length varyies in patients of the same age-group with congenital glaucoma. The pathologic growth factor in children (high intraocular pressure) will bring about different effects on the axial length of the eye according to the time of onset, the length of time during which the eye remained untreated, and the level reached by the abnormal intraocular pressure. Thus, in congenital glaucoma the pathologic factor (high intraocular pressure) does not have a fixed standard behavior; the characteristics vary from eye to eye. It is, therefore, difficult, if not impossible, to standardize ocular biometrics for a population with the disease, even when eyes with the same level of intraocular pressure are considered.

It is important to stress that although there were no statistically significant differences between subgroups Gc (controlled), Gs ("suspect"), and Gnc (noncontrolled) in the different age-groups, it was possible to observe an unquestionable trend toward higher axial length values in the eyes of the "suspect" subgroup (Gs) and particularly in the noncontrolled subgroup (Gnc).

## Conclusions

1) Although the axial lengths of eyes with congenital glaucoma in the controlled (Gc), "suspect" (Gs), and noncontrolled (Gnc) subgroups were not statistically different in the several age-groups, a clear trend was observed for higher axial length values in those eyes that had higher intraocular pressure values (Gs and Gnc subgroups).
2) The eyes of patients with congenital glaucoma showed a higher axial length value when postoperative intraocular pressure was above 15 mmHg (subgroups "suspect" and noncontrolled). This fact was more significant at the age of approximately 3-5 years.
3) The axial length in patients with congenital glaucoma who had controlled intraocular pressure in the postoperative period (Gc) showed a tendency to have statistically similar values to the corresponding values of normal eyes in older age-groups.
4) By means of the biometric values obtained through ultrasonography (method "A" and standardized ecograph), it was possible to observe that those eyes with an intraocular pressure above 15 mmHg (applanation tonometry) did not show adequate control over the disease. Our results confirm that ultrasonographic biometry is a reliable clinical method for judging the efficiency of surgical treatment in congenital glaucoma.

## References


Baum G (1967) An evaluation of ultrasonic techniques used in measurements of the eye size. Am J Ophthalmol 64:926–936

Bechetoille A, Saraux H (1970) Biometric oculaire ultrasonique. Étude de 100 yeux appartenan à une population homogene. Ann Ocul 203:131–149

Betinjane AJ, Carvalho CA (1980) Biometria ocular ultrasonográfica. Procedimento para melhorar a precisão do método. Arq Bras Oftalmol 43:159–161

Blondhal S (1979) Ultrasonic measurements of the eye in the newborn infant. Acta Ophthalmol 57:1048–1056

Buschmann W, Bluth K (1974) Regelmäßige echographische Messung des Auges zur Kontrolle der Druckregulierung bei Hydrophthalmie. Klin Monatsbl Augenheilkd 165:878–884

Buschmann W, Bluth K (1974) Eine Echographische Methode zur Verlaufskontrolle angeborener Glaukome. Albrecht Von Graefes Arch Klin Exp Ophthalmol 192:313–329

Carvalho CA, Betinjane AJ (1980) Valores da biometria ultra-sonográfica obtidos em olhos normais de pacientes até 18 meses de idade. Rev Bras Oftalmol 39:479–482

François J, Goes F (1971) Ultrasonography in pediatric ophthalmology. J Pediatr Ophthalmol 8:221–233

François J, Goes F (1975) Oculometry of progressive myopie. Ultrasonography in ophthalmology. Bibl Ophthalmol 83:227–282

Gernet H (1963) Kompensatorisches Verhalten von Hornhautbrechkraft und Bulbusauge bei Buphtalmus. Klin Monatsbl Augenheilkd 143: 429–431

Gernet H (1967) Ultraschall-Briometrie des Auges. Klin Monatsbl Augenheilkd 151:853–871

Gernet H, Hollwich F (1969) Oculometrie des

Kindlichen Glaukoms. Ber Zusammenkunft Dtsch Ophthalmol Ges 69:341–348
Gernet H, Hollwich F (1969) Résultats oculmétriques à propos du glaucome infantile. Bull Mem Soc Fr Ophthalmol 82:41–47
Larsen JS (1971) The sagittal growth of the eye. I. Ultrasonic measurement of the depth of the anterior chamber from birth to puberty. Acta Ophthalmol 49:239–262
Larsen JS (1971) The sagittal growth of the eye. II. Ultrasonic measurement of the axial diameter of the lens and the anterior segment from birth to puberty. Acta Ophthalmol 49:427–440
Larsen JS (1971) The sagittal growth of the eye. III. Ultrasonic measurement of the posterior segment (axial length of the vitreous) from birth to puberty. Acta Ophthalmol 49:441–453
Larsen JS (1971) The sagittal growth of the eye. IV. Ultrasonic measurement of the axial length of the eye from birth to puberty. Acta Ophthalmol 49:873–886
Luyckx J (1966) Mesure des composantes optiques de l'oeil du nouveau-né pour echographie ultrasonique. Arch Ophthalmol 26:159–170
Luyckx J, Weekers JF (1967) Contribuition à l'étude des glaucomes par l'ultrasonographie. Ann Ocul 200:489–504
Pérez-Llorca Rodrigo J (1971) Biometrie echographic statique du segment anterieur et axe antero-posterieur de l'oeil humain vivant, du nouveau-né premature au vieillard chez les habitants de Cadix. Bull Soc Ophthalmol Fr 84:275–281
Sampaolesi R (1981) Ocular Echometry in the Diagnosis of Congenital Glaucoma. Doc Ophthalmol Proc Ser Vol. 29 Thijessen JM, Verbeek AM (eds) Dr. W. Junk Publishers, The Hague
Sampaolesi R, Caruso R (1982) Ocular Echometry in the Diagnosis of Congenital Glaucoma. Arch Ophthalmol 100:574–577
Saraux H, Bechetoille A (1972) Étude en temps de la croissance de 30 yeux adolescents ametropes. Ann Ocul 205:1103–1108

Krieglstein G.K./Leydhecker W. (eds)
Glaucoma Update II


# Ocular Echometry and the Diagnosis of Congenital Glaucoma and its Evolution

R. Sampaolesi, Buenos Aires

It is well known that the diagnosis of congenital glaucoma and the consequent indication of surgical treatment depend upon two factors: (1) the clinical symptoms, and (2) the intraocular pressure measured by applanation tonometry (Sampaolesi 1969; Sampaolesi et al. 1976; Sampaolesi et al. 1980; Sampaolesi and Viñas 1980. In 1971, we started performing echometry on eyes with congenital glaucoma and it became apparent that in those cases with borderline pressure levels which did not show any meaningful deviation from the normal, echometry seemed to furnish us with a new and helpful parameter. This led us to undertake a systematic study of ocular echometry in normal children in order to establish the mean values and their dispersion in relation to age. We further studied a group of patients suffering from congenital glaucoma by means of echometry, applanation tonometry, and the usual diagnostic procedures, and thus we were finally able to establish the comparative value of echometry and tonometry. In October 1974, at the Glaucoma Symposium in Wurzburg, I called attention to the value of echographic measurements, which has proved to be a supplement to the diagnosis and follow-up of congenital glaucoma; Buschmann and Bluth (1974) confirmed this.

In previous articles (Sampaolesi 1981; Sampaolesi and Caruso 1982), we described the method of echometry with the Kretz 7200 MA echograph and we showed the correlation between axial length and age in normal eyes (Fig. 1, small dots, 33 normal eyes). The

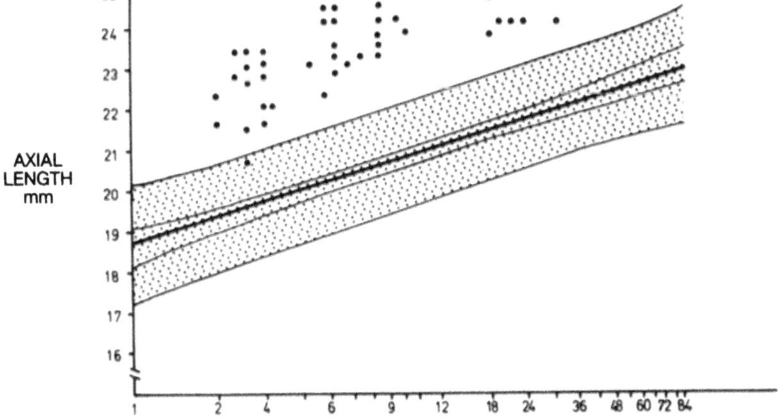


**Fig. 1.** Correlation between axial length and age. *Large dots* indicate congenital glaucoma (59 eyes), *small dots* signify normal range

**Table 1.** Correlation between axial length and age in subjects with normal eyes

| Age in months | Y Axial length | 95% Confidence Interval | |
|---|---|---|---|
| | | Line | Prediction |
| 1 | 18.7 | 18.2–19.1 | 17.3–20.1 |
| 2 | 19.4 | 19.0–19.7 | 18.0–20.7 |
| 3 | 19.8 | 19.4–20.1 | 18.4–21.1 |
| 4 | 20.0 | 19.8–20.3 | 18.7–21.4 |
| 5 | 20.3 | 20.0–20.5 | 19.9–21.6 |
| 6 | 20.4 | 20.2–20.7 | 19.1–21.8 |
| 7 | 20.5 | 20.3–20.8 | 19.3–21.9 |
| 8 | 20.7 | 20.5–20.9 | 19.4–22.0 |
| 9 | 20.8 | 20.6–21.1 | 19.5–22.2 |
| 10 | 20.9 | 20.7–21.2 | 19.6–22.3 |
| 11 | 21.0 | 20.8–21.3 | 19.7–22.4 |
| 12 | 21.1 | 20.9–21.3 | 19.8–22.4 |
| 18 | 21.5 | 21.3–21.8 | 20.2–22.8 |
| 24 | 21.8 | 21.5–22.1 | 20.5–23.1 |
| 30 | 22.0 | 21.7–22.3 | 20.7–23.3 |
| 36 | 22.2 | 21.9–22.5 | 20.8–23.5 |
| 42 | 22.3 | 22.0–22.7 | 21.0–23.7 |
| 48 | 22.5 | 22.1–22.8 | 21.1–23.8 |
| 54 | 22.6 | 22.2–22.9 | 21.2–23.9 |
| 60 | 22.7 | 22.3–23.1 | 21.3–24.0 |
| 66 | 22.8 | 22.4–23.2 | 21.4–24.1 |
| 72 | 22.9 | 22.5–23.3 | 21.5–24.2 |
| 78 | 22.9 | 22.5–23.3 | 21.6–24.3 |
| 84 | 23.0 | 22.6–23.4 | 21.6–24.4 |

axial length of normal eyes was found to increase with age according to the equation: axial length y = 18.7 + 2.245 (log x) (age in months).

The confidence interval of the normal growth curve allows the prediction of the maximum normal axial length for any given age (Table 1). In congenital glaucoma cases, in which the visual field and daily pressure curve cannot be evaluated, clinical echometry was proposed as a very valuable diagnostic and follow-up procedure. The correlative coefficient $r$ is 0.9044 ($P$0.01 significance), and the lineal confidence interval (related to each normal eye studied) and prediction confidence interval (related to the population of normal infants) were calculated.

The range of normal growth (normal area) of the axial length of the eye in children from birth up to the 7th year found by us is the same as the values determined by Gernet and Hollwich (1969), Grignolo and Rivara (1968), and Carvalho and Betinjane (1980). Prahs (1981) compared our findings with those of Buschmann and Bluth (1974) and those of Larsen (1971a–d) and Luyckx (1966).

In a second stage, the growth of normal eyes was compared with the correlation between axial length and age in 36 eyes with congenital glaucoma. Between 1979 and 1982, we examined 23 new cases of congenital glaucoma, 19 of which were diagnosed in children aged between 2 and 24 months and four in children aged between 30 and 72 months. Thus, with the first group, 36 eyes, and the second, 23 eyes, we have a total of 59 cases. Of all these cases, only one case was on the upper limit of the normal range (Fig. 1).

Table 2 shows the measurements of the anterior chamber depth, the length of the vitreous body, and the axial length, which are significantly higher among the group of glaucomatous eyes. This fact has been established by Gernet and Hollwich (1969) and Espiladora Couso et al. (1979) and reflects the effect of an increased intraocular pressure on a distensible eye.

The most interesting finding is that the lens thickness of glaucomatous eyes is notably reduced in these groups. This is an

**Table 2.** Echometry in normal and glaucomatous eyes

| Echometry | Normal eyes, mean ± SD | Glaucomatous eyes, mean ± SD | Independent Student's $t$ test[a] |
|---|---|---|---|
| No. of eyes | 33 | 22 | |
| Corneal thickness, mm | 0.54 | 0.64 ± 0.24 | |
| Anterior chamber depth, mm | 3.04 ± 0.51 | 3.57 ± 0.53 | −3.71 |
| Thickness of lens, mm | 3.85 ± 0.24 | 3.50 ± 0.25 | 5.30 |
| Length of vitreous body, mm | 13.25 ± 1.18 | 14.70 ± 0.93 | −4.82 |
| Axial length, mm | 20.97 ± 1.48 | 22.75 ± 1.05 | −4.84 |

[a] Significant difference ($P$0.001)

**Table 3.** Indices for evaluating normal and glaucomatous eyes

| | Normal eyes, mean ± SD | Glaucomatous eyes, mean ± SD | Independent Student's *t* test |
|---|---|---|---|
| 1. Anterior chamber depth divided by axial length, mm | 0.15 ± 0.02 | 0.15 ± 0.02 | −1.28[a] |
| 2. Length of anterior segment divided by length of vitreous body, mm | 0.57 ± 0.04 | 0.53 ± 0.05 | 3.51 |
| 3. Cornea thickness plus anterior chamber depth divided by length of vitreous body, mm | 0.27 ± 0.04 | 0.28 ± 0.03 | 1.27[a] |

[a] Nonsignificant difference

important contributing factor in the emmetropization of the glaucomatous eye, the axial length of which, when considered as an isolated factor, would warrant a higher myopia than that corresponding to the actual refractive state of the patients' eyes. (The other emmemtropia-inducing factors are the larger corneal radius and the deeper anterior chamber.)

The statistical study of the three indices listed in Table 3 shows that there is no significant difference between normal and glaucomatous eyes as far as the indices "anterior chamber depth divided by axial length" and "sum of the cornea thickness plus anterior chamber depth divided by length of the vitreous body" are concerned. However, the index length of anterior segment divided by length of the vitreous body discloses a highly significant difference; it is lower in glaucomatous children because it comprises the lens, the thickness of which decreases in eyes with congenital glaucoma.

On the basis of the results previously described, we propose that the echometric measurements of the axial length of the eyes of infants and children is a highly valuable variable in the diagnosis of congenital glaucoma. Our results confirmed the clinical value of echographic biometry for both the diagnosis of congenital glaucoma and the follow-up. Up until now, intraocular pressure (IOP) has been considered to be the fundamental variable in the diagnosis of congenital glaucoma. The essential difference between tonometry in adults and children resides in the practical impossibility of ascertaining the daily pressure curve of the latter. The second difference is the need to measure a child's IOP under general anesthesia, since even when using a reliable method such as that described in our previous articles (Sampaolesi et al. 1969), the IOP is never measured more than once daily. The daily IOP variability in hypertensive eyes is characteristic of the disease and occurs during a relatively short period (24 h), whereas increased axial length in congenital glaucoma reflects variations occurring over prolonged periods (days, months, or years) as a result of the increased mean IOP acting on a distensible eye. The IOP only reflects the situation at any given moment, whereas axial length furnishes information about what has happened in the course of the disease over a prolonged period. Furthermore, while IOP is a variable influenced by the anesthetic agents that are necessary for its measurement in children, echometric measurements are not altered by such agents.

Our experience has led us to consider axial length as the fundamental factor for the diagnosis of congenital glaucoma when occurring in conjunction with clinical symptoms, and it has the most direct bearing on whether surgery is indicated. Thus the fundamental basis for diagnosis in the presence of clinical symptoms is, first, axial length and, second, IOP.

In bilateral congenital glaucoma there is an echometrial asymmetry. Of 60 cases surveyed, 20 were unilateral and 40 were bilateral. In the latter, we found a manifest asymmetry in both the axial length and in each of the segments corresponding to the transparent media, and this is probably related to the fact that in glaucomatous children there is usually a difference between the IOP of the two affected eyes. This finding is in notable contrast to the values obtained for both normal infants and children (33 eyes) and bilateral megalocorneas (ten eyes) where symmetry was characteristic; Luyckx and Delmarcelle (1969) found the same in megalocornea cases.

The following cases show the importance of echometry both in the diagnosis and in the *follow-up* of congenital glaucoma. *Case 1* was a 3-month-old male infant brought in for examination in October 1978. Figure 2 and Table 4 indicate the signs of unilateral congenital glaucoma in the patient – a corneal diameter of 12 mm in the normal eye and a corneal diameter of 12.5 mm in the diseased one. The IOP under anesthesia with methoxyflurane was 10 mmHg in the healthy eye and 29 mmHg OS. Corneal thickness measurements were above normal because of edema, and vitreous and axial length were higher in the diseased eye than in the normal one. The infant under went a second exami-

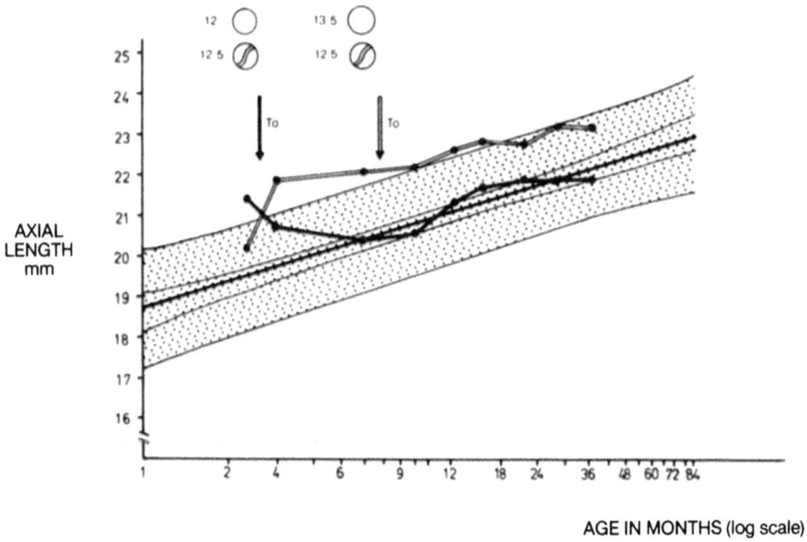


**Fig. 2.** Case 1. ═ right eye; — left eye. *Arrows* indicate surgery; *To*, trabeculotomy. *Small circles* indicate cornea with or without ruptures in Descement's membrane and endothelium. The *numbers* close to the *circles* are the corneal diameters in milimeters

**Table 4.** Echometric and IOP values in 3-month-old male infant (case 1- s.m.)

| Date | Corneal diameter | IOP | Echometry: Cornea | Anterior chamber | Cornea | Vitreous body | Axial length |
|---|---|---|---|---|---|---|---|
| October 1978 | 12 | 10 | .54 | 3.45 | 3.69 | 12.26 | 20.29 |
| | 12.5[a] | 29 | .78 | 3.06 | 3.94 | 13.02 | 21.15 |
| December 1978 | 12 | 8 | .54 | 3.45 | 3.69 | 13.41 | 21.44 |
| | 12.5 | 8 | .54 | 3.06 | 3.94 | 12.64 | 20.53 |
| February 1979 | 13.5[a] | 25 | .54 | 3.83 | 3.28 | 13.79 | 21.71 |
| | 12.5 | 12 | .54 | 3.06 | 3.69 | 12.64 | 20.29 |
| May 1979 | 13.5 | 10 | .54 | 3.83 | 3.69 | 13.79 | 22.20 |
| | 12.5 | 10 | .54 | 3.06 | 3.69 | 12.64 | 20.29 |

[a] Trabeculotomy

[b] The underlined figures indicate echometric values permitting the diagnosis of congenital glaucoma

nation in December 1978 after a trabeculotomy had been performed on the left eye. At this time, the IOP was completely normal. Another examination in February 1979 disclosed increased pressure in the previously normal eye, i.e., the IOP had risen to 25 mmHg OD, whereas it was found to be normal in the eye that had been operated up on. We performed surgery on the latter and in May 1979 the IOP was normal in both eyes. At that time, we had not yet analyzed the results of our first statistical survey, so we were still unaware of what factors determine the limits of normality.

During the first postoperative checkup in December 1978, *despite a normal IOP of 8 mmHg in both eyes, the length of the vitreous body was 13.41 mm in the eye that had been considered normal and 12.4 mm in the eye that had undergone surgery. The axial length was 21.44 mm in the "healthy" eye and 20.63 mm in the trabeculotomized eye.* The IOP was obviously normal in both eyes, yet the echometric values were already pointing towards glaucoma in the "healthy" eye, which, on further examination 2 months later, showed a distinctly pathologic IOP and corneal diameter. In the right eye, the vitreous length and the axial length increased after the IOP was lowered with surgery, but only with in the normal limits for that age. The left eye had a much higher preoperative IOP (29 mmHg) than the right eye. We often see that when a child has a high IOP, the axial length decreases after surgery. The progress was good but the surgery on the right eye was performed too late.

This case shows the importance of echometry in the diagnosis and follow-up.

**Echometry in the Follow-up of Congenital Glaucoma**

Echometry is undoubtedly a valuable method for controlling the progress of congenital glaucoma after surgery (Buschmann and Bluth 1974). There appear to be four different types of development (Fig. 3). (a) When the axial length does not increase and with time thus becomes within the normal range. Generally it is coincident with regulation of the IOP. The functional result depends on the axial length measured before surgery. An axial length of 23 or 24 mm in the eyes of children with congenital glaucoma signifies a good functional result (case 1 - Fig. 2, and case 2 - Fig. 3). When the axial length is greater than 25 mm, the functional result is poor (case 3). (b) When the axial length continues to increase in subsequent checkups and it deviates even further from the normal range. It is usually coincident with ocular hypertension. If this is not the case, it is neces-

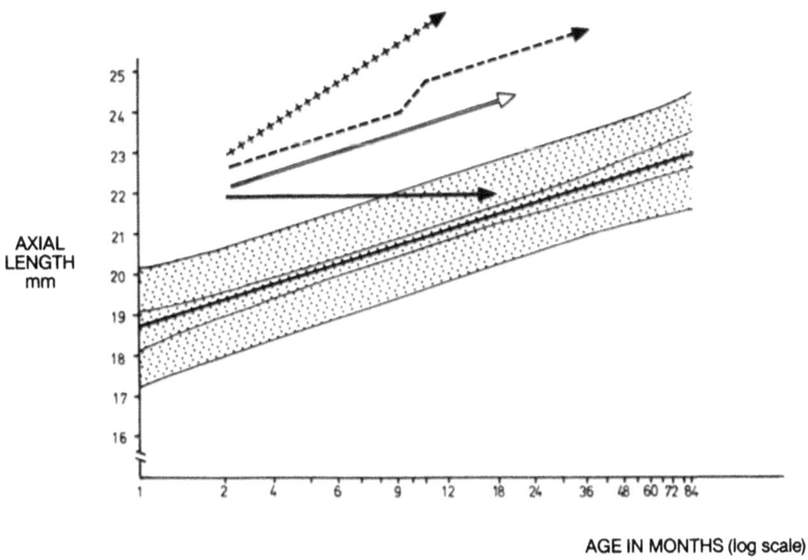


**Fig. 3.** The four different types of development of the axial length in congenital glaucoma

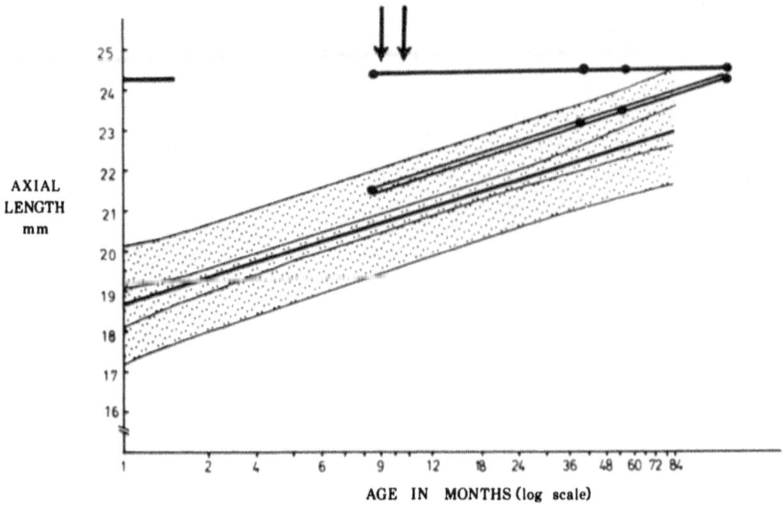


**Fig. 4.** Case 4. ══ right eye, — left eye. *Arrows* indicate surgery; *G*, goniotomy; *To*, trabeculotomy

sary to examine the child under anesthesia on different days and at different times in order to determine the hypertension (case 5 - Fig. 6c). (c) There are cases with regulated pressure after surgery in which the axial length does not increase initially but starts to do so between the ages of 2 and 4 years and later stops. This was also observed by Massim and Pellat (1982). We ignore the reason but a more frequent checkup of the ocular pressure is necessary (e.g., case 4 - Fig. 5). (d) In cases with good prognosis, the eye develops with a greater axial length but parallel to normal growth. Figure 3 summarizes the four different types of development.

If echometry is carried out 2 weeks after surgery, in most cases the axial length decreases to values lower than those before sur-

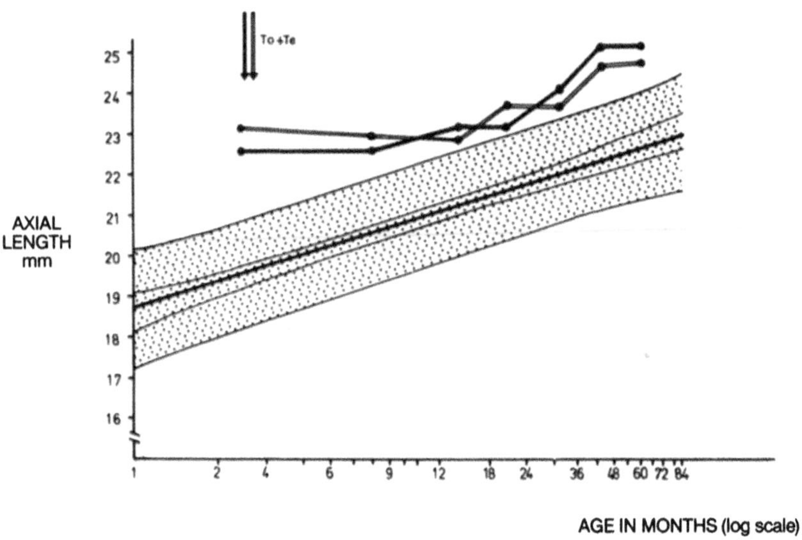


**Fig. 5.** Case 4. ══ right eye, — left eye. *Arrows* indicate surgery. *To + Te*, combined surgery - trabeculotomy and trabeculectomy. From the 3rd month until the 24th month, the axial length approached normal valves, but at the age of 36 months, both eyes started to grow again and then remained constant

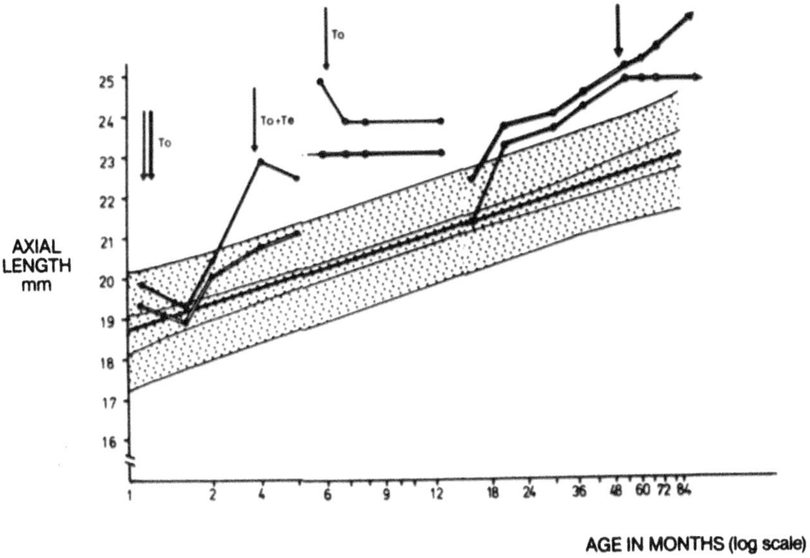


**Fig. 6.** ═ right eye; — left eye; *To,* trabeculotomy; *To + Te,* combined surgery. a) Case 2. Premature. b) Case 6. ═ right eye, myopic without congenital glaucoma; — left eye, myopic with congenital glaucoma. c) Case 5. Left eye, good progress, the growth of the axial length has stopped and the IOP is regulated. right eye, poor development

gery and after 2 months goes back to the original values. This phenomenon is more pronounced in myopic eyes (Fig. 6b).

The following cases show these kinds of development.

*Case 2* was a female, 9 months old and had unilateral congenital glaucoma. The patient had an IOP of 25 mmHg, a corneal diameter of 13.5 mm, and the axial length was 24.3 mm; there were no ruptures of the endothelium and Descemet's membrane. The normal eye had an IOP of 12 mmHg and a corneal diameter of 12 mm. The chamber angle of the glaucomatous eye showed persistent pathologic mesodermal tissue. A goniotomy was performed and since the IOP was not regulated, a trabeculotomy was performed after 1 month as a second operation. Progress was completely favorable and as can be seen in Fig. 4, the axial length remained constant until it fell within the normal area at the age of 7 years. After a follow-up of 11 years and 3 months the operated eye, with -0.25 spheric and -1.25 at 35° cylinder has a 0.7 vision and the non-operated eye a vision of 1.0. Stereoscopic vision is third grade. This case can be compared with case 3.

*Case 3* was a male, aged 7 months, with unilateral glaucoma. The patient had an IOP of 44 mmHg, a corneal diameter of 14.5 mm, and corneal edema in the OS. In the OD the patient had an IOP of 10 mmHg and a corneal diameter of 11.5 mm. This child was operated on at the age of 7 months, first by trabeculotomy, which proved to be insufficient, and then after 2 months by trabeculectomy. The axial length development was very good horizontal as in the preceding case, but at the time of the first examination, the glaucoma had already been developing for a long time and the corneal diameter was 14.5 mm, *the axial length 27 mm.* After 11 years and 7 months of follow-up, despite good evolution vision in the operated eye was only finger counting, whereas vision in the normal eye was 10/10. To obtain a good functional result it is, therefore, imperative to treat surgically as soon as possible. The closer the axial length is to the normal range, the better the prognosis of the retinal function.

*Case 4* was male, aged 3½ months and had bilateral congenital glaucoma with an IOP of 29 mmHg in the OD and 22 mmHg in the OS. The corneal diameter was 13.5 mm and there were ruptures of the endothelium and Descemet's membrane in both eyes. Trabeculotomy and trabeculectomy was performed immediately in both eyes. The IOP became completely normal - 10 mmHg in both eyes. A follow-up was carried out for 5 years. Refraction under cycloplegia was - OD, -2; OS, -3. From the age of 3 to 24 months, the axial length (Fig. 5) approached the normal range, but at the age of 3 years the axial length in both eyes started to increase again and then remained constant. We do not know the reason for this phenomenon but it has been observed in several cases in spite of normal intraocular pressure. We are unable to find an explanation for it. In a personal report recently received from Massim and Pellat (1982) these authors found the same phenomenon.

*Case 5* was male and aged 17 months. This was a rare case that came in late for examination. The patient had a bilateral flat anterior chamber and very high intraocular pressure - 25 mmHg OD and 27 mmHg OS. There were ruptures in the endothelium and Descemet's membrane.

In the right eye, in spite of two trabeculectomies, lensectomy, and vitrectomy performed by another ophthalmologist, the intraocular pressure remained very high - 50 mmHg. In the left eye, an iridectomy was performed using laser, and the intraocular pressure was regulated to within normal values. In Fig. 5c, the axial length of the OD continued to increase, while the OS reached the normal range. The right eye is an example of poor development (Fig. 5c).

*Case 6* was male and aged 6 months. This child had a unilateral congenital glaucoma; the intraocular pressure was 20 mmHg in the OD and 8 mmHg in the OS. The corneal diameter was 13.5 mm in the OD and 12 mm in the OS. The parents were myopic. Figure 5b shows that both eyes are myopic and do not fall within the normal range, but the eye with congenital glaucoma (the right eye) is larger than the eye with normal pressure.

*Case 7* was female and 12 days old. The patient had a bilateral glaucoma and was a premature born in the 6th month of pregnancy. There was an IOP of 30 mmHg in the OD and 40 mmHg in the OS. We performed a bilateral trabeculotomy. The IOP in the OD became regulated but a second intervention (trabeculectomy) was necessary in the OS at the age of 4 months because the IOP had again reached 33 mmHg. After surgery, the IOP was regulated and the axial length started to approach the normal range.

The development of the axial length in both eyes can be seen in Fig. 5a to be completely in accordance with IOP development. The axial length in both eyes at the time of the diagnosis was within the normal range, this being due to the fact that the child was born in the 6th months of pregnancy. The values appearing in the figure do not actually correspond to the real age. It is important to note that when the IOP was not regulated by the first operation, the OD immediately went beyond the normal range.

Grignolo and Rivara (1968) found the following ocular axial length values for premature babies: 6 months, 12.08 mm; 7 months, 14.41; and 8 months, 16.83 mm. The above case, with an IOP of 30 and 40 mmHg, had an axial length of 19.3 mm in the OD and 19.9 mm in the OS, that is, 3 mm more than the value considered normal for this age.

There are cases of high IOP in which the axial length of the eye does not increase. This happens generally after the age of 5 years, probably because by that time the sclera has lost its elasticity. Leydhecker (1973), Ytterborg (1960), and Dannheim (1969) have called attention to the variation in rigidity in children of different ages.

## Conclusions

(1) Echometry is a valuable method in the diagnosis of congenital glaucoma. It is superior to measurements of intraocular pressure especially in children up to the age of 2 years. The enlargement of the eye is a consequence of the increased IOP. The intraocular pressure is subject to daily variations and can be affected by anesthetics. Axial length is not affected by any of these factors, especially by the latter. Echometry is of great help in cases of critical ocular pressure, successive checkups show that the eye continues to grow and development is abnormal. Echometry is, in our experience, the most important parameter in the diagnosis of congenital glaucoma, followed by ocular pressure measurements of means of applanation, gonioscopy, and examination of the optic nerve.

(2) In cases of megalocornea and in normal children, echometry shows symmetry in the values of axial length in both eyes in

contrast to congenital glaucoma in which asymmetry is characteristic.

(3) Echometry is also a very useful parameter to control the evolution of cases of operated congenital glaucoma. The development of IOP and the axial length generally coincide: If the axial length stops increasing, the IOP is regulated; if the axial length continues to grow and derivates from normal values, the IOP increases. Whenever both parameters do not coincide, i.e., the axial length increases whereas the IOP is normal, it is necessary to keep a very close control of the IOP to detect hypertension, and in these cases further surgery will be necessary.

## References


Buschmann W, Bluth K (1974) Regelmäßige echographische Messung der Achsenlänge des Auges zur Kontrolle der Druckregulierung bei Hydrophthalmie. Klin Monatsbl Augenheilkd 165:878–886

Buschmann W, Bluth K (1974) Eine echographische Methode zur Verlaufskontrolle angeborener Glaukome. Albrecht Von Graefes Arch Klin Exp Ophthalmol 192:313–329

Carvalho C, Bettinjane AJ (1980) Valores da biometria ultra-sonografica obtidos em olhos normais de pacientes até 18 meses de idade. Rev Bras Oftalmol 39:479–482

Dannheim R (1968) Bericht über die 69. Zusammenkunft der DOG, p 248

Espildora Couso J et al. (1979) Alteraciones Biométricas en el Control Tardío del Ojo con Glaucoma Congenito Operado, Glaucoma Symposium. The Panamerican Congress of Ophthalmology, Miami

Gernet H, Hollwich F (1969) Oculometrie des kindlichen Glaukoms. Ber Zusammenkunft Dtsch Ophthalmol Ges 69:341–348

Grignolo A, Rivara A (1968) Biometry of the human eye from the sixth month of pregnancy to the tenth year of life (measurements of the axial length, retinoscopy refraction, total refraction, corneal and lens refraction). Diagnostica ultrasonica in ophthalmologia, Brno: Univ. J.E. Purkyně, pp 251–257

Larsen JS (1971a) The sagittal growth of the eye. I. Ultrasonic measurement of the depth of the anterior chamber from birth to puberty. Acta Ophthalmol 49:239–262

Larsen JS (1971b) The sagittal growth of the eye. II. Ultrasonic measurement of the axial diameter of the lens and the anterior segment from birth to puberty. Acta Ophthalmol 49: 427–440

Larsen JS (1971c) The sagittal growth of the eye. III. Ultrasonic measurement of the posterior segment (axial length of the vitreous) from birth to puberty. Acta Ophthalmol 49:441–453

Larsen JS (1971d) The sagittal growth of the eye. IV. Ultrasonic measurement of the axial length of the eye from birth to puberty. Acta Ophthalmol 49:873–886

Leydhecker W (1973) Glaukom, Ein Handbuch. 2. Aufl. Springer Berlin Heidelberg New York, pp 58–75

Luyckx J (1966) Mesure des composantes optiques de l'oeil du nouveauné pour echographie ultrasonique. Arch Ophthalmol 26:159–170

Luyckx J, Delmarcelle Y (1969) Contribution of ultrasonography to the study of microcornea and megalocornea. In: Gitter KA, Keeney AH, Sarin LK et al. (eds) Ophthalmic Ultrasound. St. Louis, CV Mosby Co, pp 149–157

Massim M, Pellat B (1982) Ultrasonic Biometry in Congenital Glaucoma, a Clinical Study - Personal communication - Hópital National des Quinze-Vingts., 28 rue de Charenton 75571, Paris - Codex 12, France

Prahs B (1981) Des Mesures Biométriques dans les glaucomes congénitaux primaires. Bulletins et memoires de la Societé Francaise d'Ophthalmologie Congres 1981, pp 405–409

Sampaolesi R (1969) La pression oculaire et le sinus camerulaire chez l'infant normal et dans le glaucome congenital au-dessous de l'age de 5 ans. Doc Ophthalmol 26:497–515

Sampaolesi R, Reca R, Armando E (1976) Normaler intraocularer Druck bei Kindern bis zu 5 Jahren mit und ohne Allgemeinnarkose: Seine Wichtigkeit für die Frühdiagnose des angeborenen Glaukoms, Glaucoma Symposium, Würzburg, Germany, 1974

Sampaolesi R, Viñas R (1981) Resultados obtenidos con el tonómetro neumático. Segundo Simposio Sudamericano de Glaucoma - Iguazú, Brasil (1975). Panamericana - Buenos Aires, pp 42–47

Sampaolesi R, Reca R, Carro A, Armando E (1980) Estado actual del estudio continuado sobre el comportamiento de la presión intraocular de los niños desde el nacimiento hasta los 5 años. Segundo Simposio Sudamericano de Glaucoma - Iguazú, Brasil (1975) - Panamericana - Buenos Aires, pp 48–56

Sampaolesi R (1981) Ocular echometry in the diagnosis of congenital glaucoma. Docum Ophthal Proc Series Vol 29, JM Thijessen and AM Verbeek (eds) Dr. W. Junk Publishers, The Hague

Sampaolesi R, Caruso R (1982) Ocular Echometry in the Diagnosis of Congenital Glaucoma. Arch Ophthalmol 100:574–577

Ytterborg J (1960) On sclera rigidity. Oslo University Press

## Discussion

**Tarkkanen to Sampaolesi:** I congratulate the author on this excellent paper. Our experience is in agreement with the findings presented. The problem in borderline cases of infantile glaucoma is that the estimates of the intraocular pressure are inaccurate. The applanation tonometer has never been calibrated against infantile corneas in glaucomatous eyes. Our experience of echometry in 20 cases aged 4-48 months shows that the axial lengths in eyes with infantile glaucoma are greather than those of normal controls. Some of the borderline cases show an increase in axial length not attributable to normal growth. After surgery, an early decrease in the axial length down to 0.8 mm has also been noted. The anterior measurements, however, remained unchanged while only the postequatorial readings showed alterations.

**Spaeth to Sampaolesi:** We are impressed with the value of performing ultrasound examinations on children with congenital glaucoma. The test is a very important addition to the other test that are used in the diagnosis and treatment of children with, or suspected of having, congenital glaucoma. The author is to be congratulated for this important advance.

Krieglstein G.K./Leydhecker W. (eds)
Glaucoma Update II


# Prognosis of Goniotomy in Primary Infantile Glaucoma (Trabeculodysgenesis)

R.N. Shaffer, San Francisco

Frequently papers concerning congenital glaucoma are based on small numbers of cases and the specific type of congenital anomaly is not always clearly defined. Over the past 40 years over 400 cases of congenital glaucoma have been examined and treated in our offices.[1] Instead of the usual classification by syndrome, our patients are now being classified anatomically, based on the Hoskins' gonioscopic classification of the Developmental Glaucomas [1]. The anomalies are described in terms of the anatomic structures involved, namely, the iris, the trabecular meshwork and the cornea:

1. Iridocorneal Trabeculodysgenesis:
These developmental glaucomas include the spectrum of syndromes with abnormal iris attachments to the cornea, such as Rieger's, Axenfeld's and Peter's anomalies.

2. Iridotrabecular Dysgenesis:
The typical example of iridotrabecular dysgenesis is aniridia. Another example is familial hypoplasia of the iris.

Neither iridocorneal trabeculodysgenesis nor iridotrabecular dysgenesis respond well to goniotomy, nor to any other surgery. They should be controlled medically as long as possible.

3. Isolated Trabeculodysgenesis:
This is the typical primary congenital or infantile glaucoma. The onset of symptoms is usually in the first year of life. Gonioscopically the iris has a flat insertion into a thickened trabecular meshwork. Specimens which have been studied microscopically all show this flat insertion anterior to a poorly developed scleral spur as described by Maumenee [2, 3]. When symptoms develop between the first and twenty-first month of life, goniotomy is highly successful in controlling the glaucoma. The purpose of this paper is to point out the safety, the efficacy and the prognosis of goniotomy in the treatment of trabeculodysgenesis (primary congenital or infantile glaucoma).

## Surgical Complications

Over a 40-year period, 577 consecutive goniotomies were performed by Shaffer, Hetherington and Hoskins, using a slightly modified Barkan technique. Ocular complications were negligible as tabulated in Table 1. Most of the complications occurred some years ago when goniotomy was performed in eyes with marked hazing of the corneas. Such eyes are now treated by trabeculotomy. The one case of severe bleeding with blood-staining of the cornea occurred in a patient with Lowe's syndrome. The goniotomy was uneventful, but repeated hemorrhages occurred resulting in a blood-stained cornea. The second eye had an uneventful, successful goniotomy. The occasional shallow anterior chamber postoperatively has been largely eliminated by closure of the puncture wound with 9-0 Nylon suture.

The only alarming complication was six cases of cardiopulmonary arrest during anes-

**Table 1.** Complications in 577 consecutive goniotomies

| | |
|---|---|
| Hemorrhage | -- 2, severe, one lost vision |
| Iridodialysis | -- 4, small, without sequelae |
| Cyclodialysis | -- 2, small, without sequelae |
| Shallow Chamber | -- 5, lasting 1 to 2 days |
| Lens Injury, Infection | -- None |
| Cardio-pulmonary Arrests | -- 6, All recovered |

[1] Shaffer, Ridgway, van Herick, Hetherington, Hoskins

thesia. Fortunately all recovered. As a result of this experience, bilateral cases of trabeculodysgenesis are treated by bilateral goniotomies rather than subjecting the infant to two anesthetics. It is our opinion that the anesthetic risk markedly outweighs the risk of infection [4].

## Efficacy of Goniotomy Depending on Age of Onset of Symptoms

Table 2 documents the efficacy of 287 goniotomies which could be followed long enough to assess the success or failure of one or two goniotomies. Success seems to be dependent on the age of onset of symptoms and the presence or absence of iris hypoplasia or abnormal iris vascularity.

When signs and symptoms are present at birth, the anomaly is more severe. There is often considerable corneal edema both in the epithelium and the stroma. The anterior stroma of the iris is frequently hypoplastic with absence or irregularity of the collarette. Small blood vessels wander irregularly on the surface of the iris. These are not the prominent radial vessels frequently seen in blue-eyed babies. In general such patients with a combination of iris and trabecular anomalies are difficult to control. They fall into the classification of iridotrabecular dysgenesis.

There were 50 eyes with signs and symptoms identifiable at birth. As can be seen in Table 2, only 26% of these eyes were successfully treated by 1 or 2 goniotomies. The uncontrolled 74% required trabeculotomies, trabeculectomies and occasionally cryotherapy. Surprisingly, most of the 26% successes could be classified as isolated trabeculodysgenesis without iris anomalies.

**Table 2.** Efficacy of 287 goniotomies by age

| | Birth to 1 month | 1 to 24 months | Over 24 months |
|---|---|---|---|
| Number Cases | 50 | 205 | 32 |
| 1 Goniotomy | 8 (16%) | 129 (75%) | 11 (35%) |
| 2 Goniotomies | 5 (10%) | 66 (19%) | 1 ( 3%) |
| | 26% | 94% | 38% |
| Multiple operations | 37 (74%) | 10 ( 6%) | 20 (64%) |

## Signs and Symptoms Occurring from 1 to 24 Months of Age

In patients whose eyes showed isolated trabeculodysgenesis with signs and symptoms occurring between 1 and 24 months of age, goniotomy was almost 100% successful in controlling intraocular pressure. Of the 205 cases, 195 (94%) were controlled by 1 or 2 goniotomies.

## Signs and Symptoms Occurring After 24 Months

Few cases of late-developing isolated Trabeculodysgenesis are seen. There is a flat insertion of the iris into the trabecular meshwork. There are no iris abnormalities and sometimes there may be a beginning of an angle recess. It is well known that there is continuing development of the angle structures after birth. Alvarado has noted a continuing decrease in cellularity and increase in collagen in the trabecular meshwork through life [5]. Such changes are probably responsible for the poor response to goniotomy in children over 2 years of age. Of 32 such eyes, only 12 (38%) were cured by 1 or 2 goniotomies. Often multiple surgeries were needed to salvage some vision in these unfortunate children.

## Long-Term Prognosis of Successful Goniotomies

The mobility of young families makes the follow-up data of these cases very hard to obtain. It has been our observation that we tended to hear from referring doctors if pressures were uncontrolled, but did not hear if tensions were controlled. After a year or two, the frequent response was that the family had moved and left no forwarding address. A prospective study is currently under way which should provide more accurate follow-up information in the future.

Satisfactory information could be obtained in 82 successfully goniotomized eyes

**Table 3.** 52 successful goniotomies (tension 10–20) complications noted after 15 to 25 years

| | |
|---|---|
| Amblyopia (Vision 20/50 or less) | –20 (46%) |
| Tension 24 to 32 mmHg after 18 years | – 3 |
| Endothelial dystrophy after 17 years | – 2 |
| Retinal detachment after 20 years | – 2 |
| Visual loss from trauma after 20 years | – 2 |

whose pressure ranged between 10 and 20 mmHg without medication for a minimum of 5 years after the operation. 30 of these eyes had been followed 5 to 15 years, 52 eyes had been followed 15 to 25 years after successful goniotomy. Not until 15 years later did some complications other than amblyopia begin to appear. These are tabulated in Table 3.

As is well known, one of the major problems in these enlarged eyes is amblyopia. This is a deprivation amblyopia due to anisometropia, high degrees of astigmatism, breaks in Descemet's membrane lying in the visual axis, and perhaps from periods of corneal hazing before the glaucoma was cured. Patching was of limited value. Most of these eyes had full fields of vision with minimal or no damage to the optic nerves. A few cases with advanced glaucomatous cupping had field loss, but surgery stopped progression of damage. As shown in Table 3, 54% of the eyes had a vision between 20/20 and 20/40; 21%, between 20/50 and 20/100; and 25% had 20/200 or less.

## Late Complications

No new complications occurred in any of the 52 eyes until at least 15 years after successful goniotomies had been performed. Some new problems were noted after that time as is shown in Table 3. In 3 cases, an increase in intraocular pressure appeared, requiring medication. There were 2 cases of endothelial dystrophy with corneal edema; 2 retinal detachments occurred; and 2 eyes were lost due to trauma.

## Discussion

The Hoskins' anatomic classification of the Developmental Glaucomas is proving useful in predicting probable success or failure of goniotomy in any given case. In properly selected patients, namely those with isolated trabeculodysgenesis, goniotomy is amazingly successful. It can be quickly performed and produces a minimum of trauma to the eye. In skilled hands it has almost no complications at the time of surgery and fewer late complications than almost any other glaucoma operation. It is certainly less traumatic than trabeculotomy and should be used in preference whenever possible. Neither goniotomy nor trabeculotomy should be attempted by the occasional surgeon. These highly specialized operations are best performed at medical centers where there is a sufficient volume to ensure skillful anesthesia and surgery. Their best hope for vision lies in those first one or two operations. Parents and patients should be warned that complications can occur many years after a seemingly successful operation. Periodic examinations should continue to be performed throughout life.

**Summary.** The Hoskins' anatomic classification of the Developmental Glaucomas is proving to be a useful guide to therapy and to prognosis. In patients with isolated trabeculodysgenesis a cure can be expected in 95% of the cases after 1 or 2 goniotomies. In successful goniotomies, no complications appeared for 15 years. Then a few cases of increased pressure, endothelial dystrophy and retinal detachment have been noted. Periodic examinations should be performed throughout the patient's life.

## References

1. Hoskins H, Hetherington J, Shaffer R, Welling A (1981) Developmental glaucoma: diagnosis and classification. Symposium on Glaucoma. Trans Acad Ophthalmol, The CV Mosby Company, St. Louis, p 172
2. Maumenee AE (1958) The pathogenesis of congenital glaucoma: a new theory. Tranc Am Ophthalmol Soc 56:507
3. (1962) Further observations of the pathogenesis of congenital glaucoma. Tranc Am Ophthalmol Soc 60:140

4. Litinski S, Shaffer R, Hetherington J, Hoskins H (1977) Operative complications of goniotomy. Trans Am Acad Ophthalmol 83:78
5. Alvarado J, Murphy C, Polansky J, Juster R (1981) Age-related changes in trabecular meshwork cellularity. Invest Ophthalmol 21:5:714

## Discussion

**Kitazawa to Shaffer:** Could you tell us about your current thinking about how goniotomy works, that may be relevant to the actual operative procedure. Literally goniotomy means incision of the angle, when you do goniotomy, do you intend to cut the trabeculum superficially or to peel off so-called Barkans' membrane?

**Shaffer to Kitazawa:** In performing a goniotomy, the trabeculum is incised. The mechanism by which this effects a cure is still unknown.

Krieglstein G.K./Leydhecker W. (eds)
Glaucoma Update II


# Developmental Glaucoma

H.D. Hoskins Jr., R.N. Shaffer, I. Hetherington, San Francisco

*Terminology*

The terminology used to describe these rare diseases is confusing and inconsistent in the world's literature. It is necessary when discussing these syndromes to define terminology precisely. For the purposes of this discussion the following definitions will be used.

*Definitions*

1. Developmental Glaucoma: Glaucoma resulting from maldevelopment of some portion of the eye.
   a. Primary Developmental Glaucoma: Glaucoma resulting from maldevelopment of the aqueous outflow system.
   b. Secondary Developmental Glaucoma: Glaucoma resulting from damage to the aqueous outflow system due to maldevelopment of the some other portion of the eye (e.g. angle closure with PHPV or RLF).

2. Terminology relating to age of onset.
   a. Congenital: at or near birth
   b. Infantile: during the first three years of life
   c. Juvenile: in childhood after the first three years of life.

3. Terminology relating to structural maldevelopment.
Goniodysgenesis: maldevelopment of the iridocorneal angle.
   a. Trabeculodysgenesis: maldevelopment of the trabecular meshwork.
   b. Iridodysgenesis: maldevelopment of the iris.
   c. Corneodysgenesis: maldevelopment of the cornea.

4. General Terms
   a. Buphthalmos: "Ox Eye" implying a large eye due to the effects of elevated intraocular pressure. It does not imply etiology or appropriate therapy.
   b. Primary Congenital Glaucoma (Primary Infantile Glaucoma): A specific syndrome consisting of glaucoma in infancy associated with an isolated trabeculodysgenesis which responds well to goniotomy and may be inherited in a recessive mode.

## Structural Changes in the Anterior Segment in Developmental Glaucoma

*Primary Developmental Glaucoma*

Primary developmental glaucoma has as its hallmark some maldevelopment of the iridocorneal angle (goniodysgenesis). The angle is comprised of the peripheral cornea and iris, and the trabeculum. Thus, goniodysgenesis is comprised of trabeculodysgenesis, iridodysgenesis or corneodysgenesis either singly or in some combination.

Trabeculodysgenesis

Trabeculodysgenesis is the hallmark of primary developmental glaucoma. Barkan [1] suggested that in primary congenital glaucoma there was an impermeable membrane overlying the surface of the trabeculum and it was this membrane which was divided by goniotomy allowing aqueous to escape from the eye.

Scanning electron microscopic studies of specimens [2] taken from infants with this disease have not often demonstrated a membrane covering the surface of the trabeculum. These specimens show an anterior insertion of the iris with thickened and heavy uveal tissues with some evidence of compression of the intertrabecular spaces.

This does not exclude persistence of a membrane as a possible cause of developmental glaucoma. Many more specimens will need evaluation before all forms of trabeculodysgenesis will be known. Clinically, trabe-

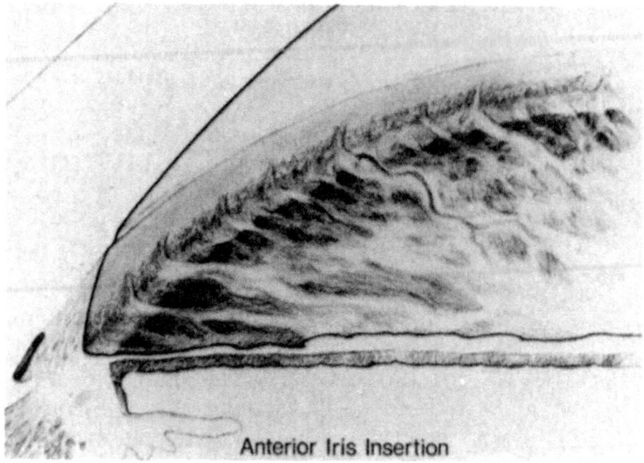


**Fig. 1.** The iris inserts anteriorly into a thickened trabecular meshwork. In blue eyes the peripheral anterior stroma is quite thin allowing a good view of the pigmented arcades. The actual junction of the surfaces of the iris and trabeculum may be difficult to see due to the transparency of the tissue. In the brown eye the junction is easily seen

culodysgenesis can be divided into three major groups.

*a. Anterior plane of iris insertion.* In this condition, the plane of the iris is flat and abuts directly into the trabecular surface at or anterior to the level of the scleral spur. The trabeculum appears thickened and translucent. If one raises his angle of observation, it is possible to see the ciliary body through this thickened, translucent trabeculum. In our experience, this form of isolated trabeculodysgenesis without other developmental anomalies in the eye is the most common type of developmental glaucoma (Fig. 1).

*b. Posterior plane of iris insertion.* In this situation, the iris inserts posterior to the scleral spur and the ciliary body can be seen anterior to the level of iris insertion. The angle recess, however, is not completely formed. The iris abuts into a continuation of the trabecular surface as it courses posteriorly internal to the scleral spur. The trabeculum is thickened and does not provide a clear crisp view of the ciliary body. This may represent a slightly more mature angle than the one described above (Fig. 2).

*c. Anterior insertion of iris stroma (wrap-around insertion).* In these cases, the iris stroma appears to wrap around the angle wall to insert anterior to the scleral spur sometimes as far forward as the Schwalbe line. This iris stroma may be either sheet-like with no obvious perforations, or it may be a dense meshwork on the surface of the trabeculum. This so-called "wrap-around" angle configuration is the least common form of isolated trabeculodysgenesis in our experience (Fig. 3).

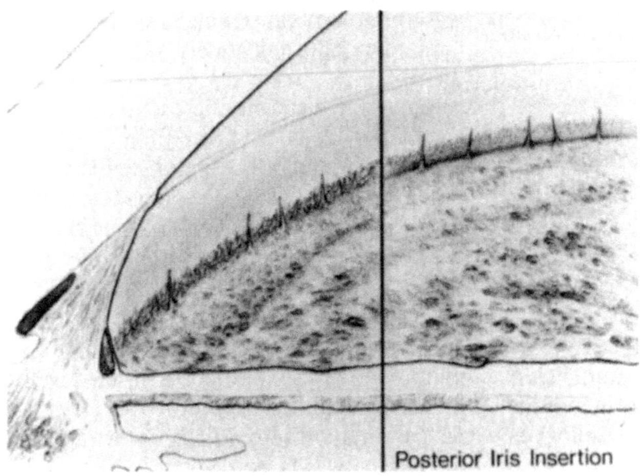


**Fig. 2.** Posterior insertion of the iris into the trabecular band allows one to see the ciliary body rather indistinctly through the thickened trabecular meshwork. *(Right side* of picture). If the peripheral iris stroma turns upward onto the trabeculum, it may obscure the view of the ciliary body. (*left side* of picture)

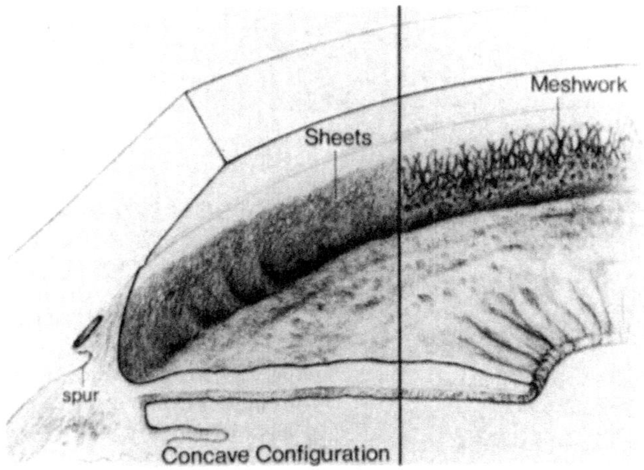


**Fig. 3.** Concave or "Wrap around" iris insertion into the trabecular *meshwork* may take the form of a solid *sheet* of iris stroma covering the angle recess and posterior trabeculum, or it may be a dense *meshwork* of iris tissue

All of the above forms of trabeculodysgenesis which occur in the absence of other ocular anomalies respond to goniotomy when it occurs in the infant.

## Iridotrabeculodysgenesis

When malformation of the trabecular meshwork is accompanied by maldevelopment of the iris, iridotrabeculodysgenesis is present. Although some authors consider hypoplasia of a portion of the anterior stroma of the iris a usual finding in developmental glaucoma, our studies indicate that this is not true. In the infant eye, the anterior stroma of the iris is poorly developed normally.

When one looks at the central iris, the anterior stroma is usually present with a normal collarette in infants both with and without glaucoma. As the eye stretches under the influence of elevated intraocular pressure, there may be no associated increase of iris stroma and, therefore, that which is present may appear thinner. We have found true hypoplasia of the anterior iris stroma to be uncommon in glaucoma presenting in infancy.

*a. Hypoplasia of anterior stroma.* Cases of marked hypoplasia of the iris stroma associated with glaucoma show absence or irregularity of the collarette with varying remnants of anterior stroma. These cases usually demonstrate a dominant mode of inheritance with high penetrance. Onset of the glaucoma varies from infancy to late adulthood. The correlation of the appearance of the iris with glaucoma is very high so that those patients with hypoplasia of the iris are destined to develop glaucoma at some time [3, 4, 5].

*b. Vascular anomalies.* In some cases of developmental glaucoma occurring in infancy there are irregularly wandering vessels present on the surface of the iris. These differ from simple prominence of iris vessels which is often seen in blue eyes of infants. Occasionally these vessels cross the pupillary margin to migrate over the surface of the lens. The pupil is often distorted and irregular. Such appearance carries a grave prognosis and all patients we have seen with this particular finding have required multiple surgeries and often continue to require medical treatment.

*c. Structural defects.* Loss of integrity of the iris structure may be manifest as holes, colobomas, or nearly complete absence of the iris such as aniridia.

In general, patients with a combination of iris and trabecular anomalies respond less well to therapy, may have onset of their disease at a later date, and may have dominant modes of inheritance as opposed to patients with isolated trabeculodysgenesis.

## Iridocorneotrabeculodysgenesis

Macrocornea and microcornea are associated with developmental glaucoma as well as isolated corneal opacities and structural defects. Most commonly there are iridocorneal adhesions, hypoplasia of the anterior iris stroma and some form of corneal opacity or struc-

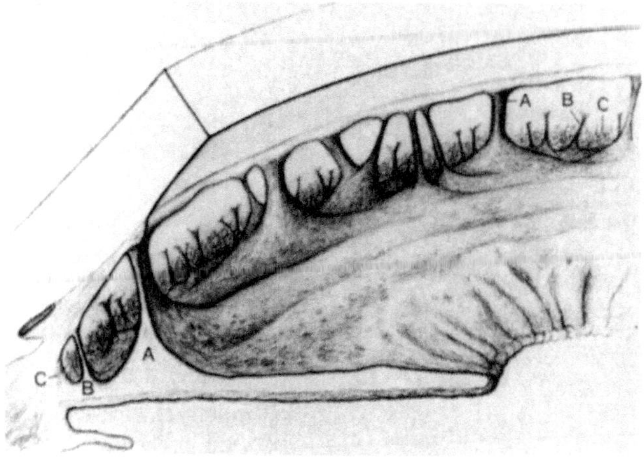


**Fig. 4.** Bridging iridocorneal "filaments" *(A)* are to be differentiated from "iris processes" *(B)*. These are both different from the wispy junctional tissue that joins the iris to the trabeculum *(C)*. Since all three structures which form the angle are involved, this represents a type of Iridocorneal-trabeculodysgenesis

tural change. Iridocorneotrabeculodysgenesis can be divided into the following.

*a. Peripheral.* Iridocorneal adhesions are limited to the periphery of the anterior chamber and are attached to a prominent cordlike Schwalbe line which is known as posterior embryotoxon. Axenfeld anomaly is typical of this subgroup (Fig. 4).

*b. Midperipheral.* Iridocorneal attachments extend out toward the center of the cornea with broad areas of iridocorneal apposition. Microcornea or macrocornea may exist. The iris has hypoplasia of the stroma, hole formation and pupillary anomalies. Rieger anomaly is typical of this group.

*c. Central.* Central iridocorneal adhesions occur between the collarette and the central cornea. The peripheral cornea may be clear. Glaucoma is not constantly seen in this group. Peter anomaly is typical of this group.

Occasionally, maldevelopment of the central portion of the cornea may result in adhesions between lens, iris and cornea with no anterior chamber formation (anterior chamber cleavage syndrome, anterior staphyloma). This is an extreme form of central iridocorneodysgenesis.

## Therapy

The choice of therapy in the developmental glaucomas is dependent upon a variety of factors. Most important of these is the structural defect present. Also, age, corneal clarity and associated systemic syndromes can influence the choice of therapy.

*General Considerations*

Isolated trabeculodysgenesis, as occurs in primary congenital glaucoma, is highly responsive to goniotomy or trabeculotomy. Although long-term data is not available for trabeculotomy, the long-term follow up data for goniotomy indicates excellent results approaching 90% control of the glaucoma. In these cases, medical therapy has a generally poor result.

When other defects are associated with trabeculodysgenesis, the success rate of goniotomy and trabeculotomy falls. In iridotrabeculodysgenesis, in which only the iris defect is hypoplasia of the anterior stroma, good response to goniotomy has been noted. However, when the iris defect is one of abnormal vessels which appear to wander somewhat irregularly across the surface of the iris, then the prognosis is extremely grave. In such cases, multiple surgeries are usually needed. If the angle can be easily visualized, then goniotomy is a reasonable first attempt. If not, the trabeculotomy would be the initial procedure of choice.

We have frequently noted an anterior insertion of iris stroma in patients with aniridia. This is not an acquired process but rather is present at birth. The stroma of the stump of the iris seems to sweep up across the angle. Although synechial formation may cause some glaucoma in patients with aniridia, many of them have glaucoma without synechial formation. In the presence of this developmental anomaly, we prefer trabeculotomy for the initial operation when medical therapy fails.

In patients with Axenfeld or Rieger anomaly (iridocorneal trabeculodysgenesis), surgical therapy does not have a good prognosis and medical therapy is used initially. Often this is unsuccessful and surgical intervention becomes necessary. In such cases, the surgery should be tailored to the specific case. Patients with peripheral iridocorneal adhesions such as Axenfeld syndrome may respond to goniotomy if the angle is not completely covered and the patient is under three years of age. The bridging iris bands can be bypassed or, if they are quite delicate, be incised with a goniotomy knife. In general, however, we prefer trabeculotomy as the initial operative procedure in these cases. Often they subsequently require trabeculectomy or even standard filtering operations to control the pressure.

In those patients with midperipheral iridocorneal adhesions such as might occur in Rieger anomaly, there is often little available angle open. If sufficient trabeculum is available, then trabeculotomy can be attempted if medical therapy has not succeeded. Otherwise, trabeculectomy should be the initial procedure. It should be performed away from the areas of iridocorneal attachment.

**References**


1. Barkan O (1955) Pathogenesis of Congenital Glaucoma. Gonioscopic and Anatomic Observations of the Anterior Chamber in the Normal Eye and in Congenital Glaucoma. Am J Ophthalmol 40:1
2. Maglio M, McMahon C, Hoskins HD Jr, Alvarado J (1983) Scanning Electron Microscopy of the Trabecular Meshwork in Primary Open Angle Glaucoma. I. Potential Artifacts. (submitted for publication)
3. Jerndal T (1972) Dominant Goniodysgenesis with Late Congenital Glaucoma. Am J Ophthalmol 74(1):28-33
4. Martin JP, Zorab EC (1974) Familial Glaucoma. Br J Ophthalmol 58:536–542
5. Weatherill JR, Hart CT (1969) Familial Hypoplasia of the Iris Stroma Associated with Glaucoma. Br J Ophthalmol 53:433–438


## Discussion

**Leydhecker to Hoskins:** I have always objected the term juvenile glaucoma. Primary open angle glaucoma can start at an age as early as five or six years. I have published these observations (Simple glaucoma before the age of 30 years, Ophthalmologica Basel (1979) 178:32-36). Glaucoma in young persons can, furthermore, be an abortive self-arresting congenital glaucoma or secondary glaucoma.

Krieglstein G.K./Leydhecker W. (eds)
Glaucoma Update II


# Bubble-free Gonioscopy

R. Smith, London

The communication is in the form of a film which illustrates the behaviour of the air bubble under a conventional single-mirror Goldmann goniolens and a specially modified version.

The standard Zeiss 4-mirror goniolens has a small corneal segment (9 mm) and a flattish corneal curvature (7.72). This lens is extremely bubble-free and can be placed against a moist cornea without the addition of saline or methocell. In contrast, the normal Goldmann single mirror lens has a corneal contact diameter of 11 mm and a corneal radius of curvature of 7.4 mm. There appears also to be a flatter "scleral" section, giving a total diameter of 14 mm. This lens frequently traps air and can very rarely be used without the addition of saline or methocell. Sometimes air bubbles can be a considerable nuisance and waste a good deal of time in the clinic. However, the steep corneal clearance and the relatively large size of the mirror give exceptional optical clarity when free of bubbles.

The lens shown in the film is a standard Goldmann single mirror lens which has been subjected to a simple modification.

The contact surface has been flattened in the contact lens department of Moorfields to give a radius of curvature of 8.4 mm. The original lens which was modified by a commercial firm also had a part of the rim removed and was given a back curve of 8.5 mm.

This lens was unfortunately lost soon after it was delivered but performed very well.

In practice, the modified lens saves time in the clinic as it is not necessary to add saline or methocell to it, provided that the cornea is anaesthetised and moist.

The lens is simply picked up and placed on the eye with the patient sitting normally at the slit lamp.

As will be seen in the film, there may be an air bubble but it will be peripheral and will not interfere with the gonioscopic view. Frequently there is no bubble.

Another use of the lens is during or prior to surgery. The lens can be placed on the eye and viewed vertically down the operating microscope.

A simple fundus lens on the low-curve principle and a goniotomy lens have also been made. The goniotomy lens has proved particularly useful. Again, it is simply held on the cornea with one finger during goniotomy. No fluid is needed and no bubbles interfere with the view.

The diameter of contact is 12 mm, radius 8.4 and slope of inclined face 45°. It is very simply made in any contact lens department out of a piece of perspex rod.

## Discussion

**Leydhecker to Smith:** I have published a similar goniotomy lens in 1969 (Klin Monatsbl Augenheilkd 154:111-112), which has the advantage to have a built - in glass-fibre optic, so that the chamber angle is illuminated. This lens is completely bubble-free and needs no contact-fluid. In addition, I have published in the same paper a new goniotomy knife, or needle, which is perforated so that the anterior chamber is never lost during goniotomy, the chamber angle is widened by constant infusion of sterile BSS and haemorrhages are avoided by working with increased pressure and inflating air into the anterior chamber immediately after the operation through the same perforated needle. These instruments are in use in several hospitals and can be ordered from the firm Klein in Heidelberg.

# Subject Index

J. Lang

# Clinical Anatomy of the Head

**Neurocranium - Orbit - Craniocervical Regions**

Translated from the German by R. R. Wilson, D. P. Winstanley
1983. 388 color photographs and 189 diagrams. XIV, 489 pages
ISBN 3-540-11014-3

**Contents:** Synopsis of the Skull. - Diploic Veins, Meninges and Scalp. - Orbit and Contents. - Anterior Cranial Fossa, the Approach to the Orbit and the Ethmoid Bone. - The Floor of the Orbit. - Pituitary Region and Anterior Cranial Fossa: Approaches via the Cranium. - Transnasal Approach to the Pituitary Region. - Cisternae and Vessels of the Pituitary and Diencephalon. - Cavernous Sinus and Trigeminal Ganglion. - Cerebral Ventricles of the Anterior and Middle Cranial Fossae. - Floor and Contents of the Middle Cranial Fossa. - Midbrain and Adjacent Structures. - Posterior Cranial Fossa and Contents. - Craniocervical Junction. - Skull: Data for Computed Tomography. - References. - Subject Index.

*Clinical Anatomy of the Head* is an unusually instructive, full-color atlas emphasizing the neurocranium, the orbita and craniocervical transitional regions. The result of cooperative efforts involving leading clinicians, it provides neurosurgeons, neuroradiologists, neuropathologists, ophthalmologists and otorhinolaryngologists with a practice-oriented anatomical foundation for their work.
The presentation is based on investigations undertaken with the aim of clarifying problems of immediate interest to clinicians today. The carefully selected full-color photographs are supplemented by drawings and tables showing mean and limit values as well as structural variants.

# Computer Reformations of the Brain and Skull Base

**Anatomy and Clinical Application**

By R. Unsöld, C. B. Ostertag, J. DeGroot, T. H. Newton
1982. 237 figures including 76 plates in color. VI, 234 pages
ISBN 3-540- 11544-7

**Contents:** General Considerations. - Orbit and Paranasal Sinuses. - Anterior Cranial Fossa. - Temporal Lobe and Insula. - Sella, Pituitary Gland, Suprasellar Cistern, and Parasellar Area. - Supratentorial Periventricular Structures. - Quadrigeminal Cistern. - Occipital Lobe. - Prepontine and Cerebellopontine Cisterns. - Cerebellum and Fourth Ventricle. - Lower Brain Stem, Cisterna Magna, Posterior Skull Base. - Index. I. - Index. II.

The first guide to the optimal use of computer reformation in almost every conceivable plane of the brain and skull base regions is provided in this book. It contains detailed descriptions of normal anatomy in the clinically most important section and reformation planes and compares them with normal CT anatomy. Diagnostic techniques and approaches are then described and illustrated on the basis of case histories.
Functional and pathologic anatomy of the cranial compartments is covered with a view toward localizing the symptoms most often encountered in clinical practice. The optimal choice of section and reformation plane prior to radiologic examination itself is facilitated by an index of clinical signs indicating the location of the suspected lesion or papathologic process. A brief description of common surgical approaches is also provided to allow radiologists to correctly interpret lesions resulting from earlier operations.
With its wealth of information, concise presentation and handy format, this book will prove an indispensable manual for work at the light box and at the CT console.

Springer-Verlag
Berlin
Heidelberg
New York
Tokyo

GPSR Compliance

*The European Union's (EU) General Product Safety Regulation (GPSR) is a set of rules that requires consumer products to be safe and our obligations to ensure this.*

*If you have any concerns about our products, you can contact us on ProductSafety@springernature.com*

In case Publisher is established outside the EU, the EU authorized representative is:

Springer Nature Customer Service Center GmbH
Europaplatz 3
69115 Heidelberg, Germany

**Batch number: 10704763**

Printed by Printforce, the Netherlands